THE COMPLETE
Clean Eating
COOKBOOK

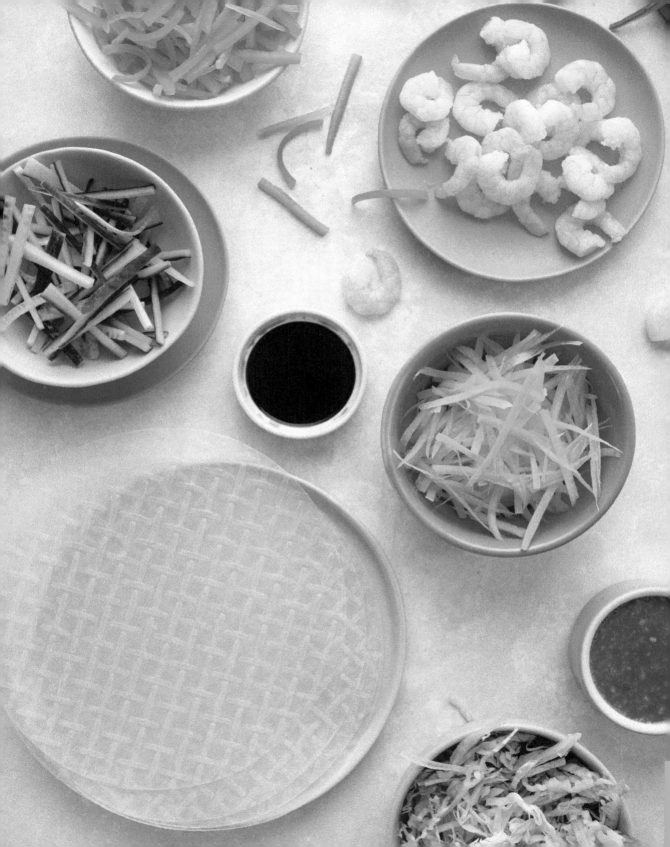

THE COMPLETE

Clean Eating

Eating

COOKBOOK

200 | Fresh Recipes and 3 Easy
Meal Plans for a Healthy Diet

LAURA LIGOS, MBA, RDN, CSSD

ROCKRIDGE
PRESS

Interior and Cover Designer: Lisa Forde
Photo Art Director/Art Manager: Sue Bischofberger
Editor: Bridget Fitzgerald
Production Editor: Kurt Shulenberger

Photography: © 2019 Darren Muir, all except pp. 72, 188, and 286; © Nadine Greeff, pp. 72, 188, and 286.

Author photo © Rachel Holt, Owner at Reach Creative

ISBN: Print 978-1-64152-606-7 | eBook 978-1-64152-607-4

R0

To my husband for always believing in me and supporting my dreams, no matter how big. To my friends for the endless laughs and kitchen messes.

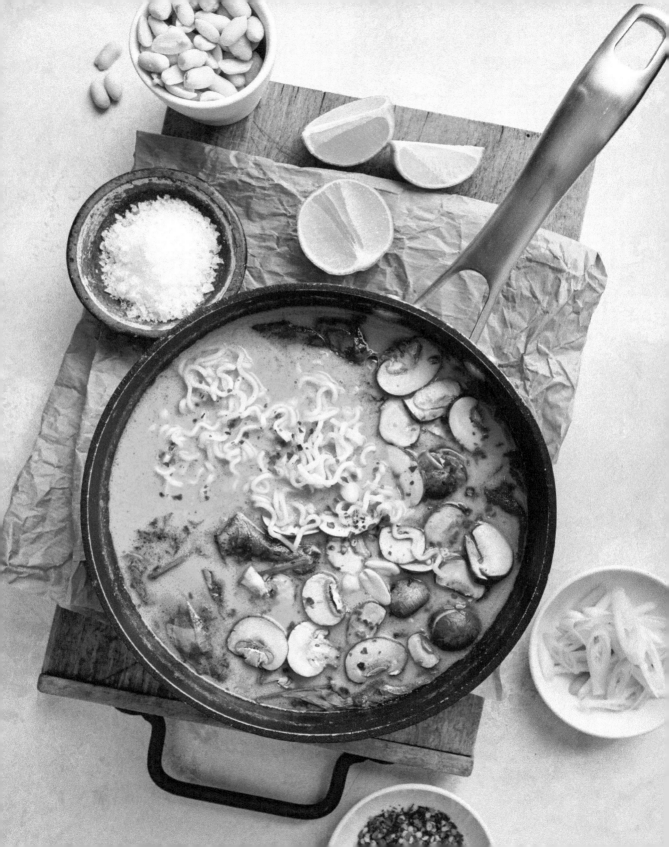

| Contents |

INTRODUCTION VIII

1 Chapter One:
Clean Eating Basics

19 Chapter Two:
The Meal Plans

49 Chapter Three:
Breakfast and Smoothies

73 Chapter Four:
Snacks and Sides

97 Chapter Five:
Soups and Salads

121 Chapter Six:
Vegetarian Mains

147 Chapter Seven:
Seafood

171 Chapter Eight:
Chicken

195 Chapter Nine:
Pork

219 Chapter Ten:
Beef and Lamb

247 Chapter Eleven:
Staples and Sauces

269 Chapter Twelve:
Desserts

COOKING TEMPERATURES 290

MEASUREMENT CONVERSIONS 291

RESOURCES 292

INDEX 293

| Introduction |

If you had told my parents when I was growing up that I would be a dietitian or that I would write a clean eating cookbook, they would have thought that you were talking about someone else's child. I was never particularly interested in food when I was younger. I had an appetite—and a sweet tooth—but my priorities were sports, playing with my dog, school, and being with my friends—anything but sitting still for an entire meal. Somehow, they suffered through my inability to sit still, my pickiness, and my love of chicken nuggets, and managed to introduce me to real food. I eventually came around not only to eating and enjoying good food but to cooking it as well. But it took moving away from home for me to realize the effect food had on my health, relationships, and overall well-being.

When I went away to college, I began to see the impact that food had on my health and on my athletic performance. As a collegiate swimmer with a picky palate and an overwhelming academic course load, I soon realized that the food I ate could affect my life for better (or worse). I was used to my mom cooking homemade meals every day—she made everything down to her marinara sauce (we called it "gravy") from scratch—so I took for granted what real, clean food was. As I picked my way through the offerings in the university dining hall, I started recognizing that when I ate whole foods—foods, like fruits and vegetables, that *are* ingredients and don't *have* ingredients—I felt better. On top of that, my ability to focus in the classroom and my performance in the pool improved.

The fact that my food choices had such a powerful effect on my health amazed me. I was even more surprised to find that this way of eating influenced both my overall lifestyle and my social life. When my friends wanted to hang out over dinner and drinks, I realized that being less picky made me a more enjoyable companion. Over the years, I've become a far more adventurous eater, and I've conducted some of my own individual experimentation on how different foods interact with me. For example, foods that contain gluten affect my digestion in a negative way, as do cashews and bananas, but a wide variety of real foods keep me energized, fuel my continued inability to sit still, help me sleep soundly, and allow me to partake in my favorite activities including swimming, CrossFit, hiking, and walking my dog.

I love sharing the joy of food with others because I want people to experience how good food can taste and how good it can make them feel. The problem is that many people get lost in the world of restrictions. They spend so much time worrying about what they can't have that they forget all the delicious things they can have. But clean eating is not about abiding by a strict set of rules. *Clean eating* is simply a term to describe a way of eating that incorporates more real food into your diet. It is one component of a healthy and balanced life, which also includes drinking plenty of water, engaging in activity, getting adequate sleep, and maintaining healthy relationships.

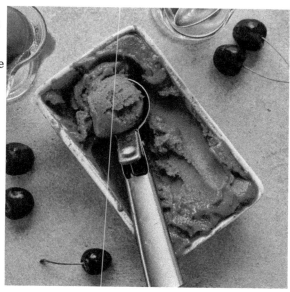

I tried to make this a complete book of clean eating by developing the broadest possible array of easy and delicious recipes. Among them, I have included some of my favorite go-tos, like French Toast Overnight Oats (page 55), Lamb Gyros (page 239), and Spaghetti Squash Primavera (page 140)—all tried-and-true recipes in my household.

This book also includes plenty of useful guidelines that will show you how to approach a clean eating lifestyle and how it can be effective no matter your ultimate goal or level of motivation. Eating clean is easy—it is simply the process of getting back to our roots and eating more whole foods and fewer processed foods.

The three meal plans in chapter 2 are meant to show you how you can put the recipes together in a way that will make your transition to clean eating easy and sustainable for the long term. The meal plans provide a framework to facilitate the achievement of your goals, but they can be modified to suit your preferences, to coordinate with what foods are in season, or to accommodate what might be on sale. Clean eating is meant to be a lifelong journey, not a "hit-it-and-quit-it" crash diet. There is no prize for being perfect; instead, focus on progress. Try one new recipe this week and then slowly add in others. Soon you'll be a clean eating culinary master.

Happy cooking!

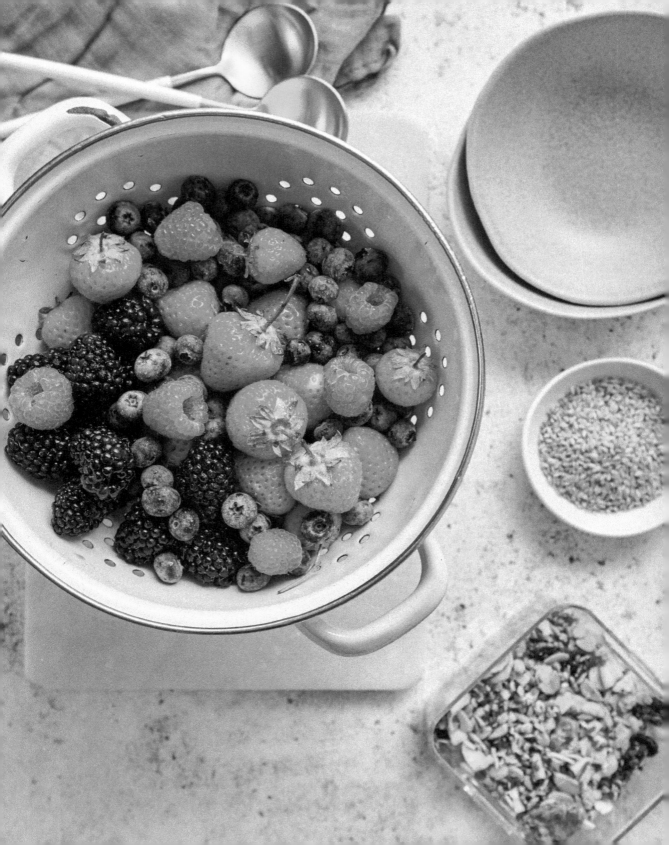

CHAPTER ONE

Clean Eating Basics

Clean eating is a broad term for eating food that is unprocessed; in other words, cooking and eating real food. It is not meant to be a restrictive diet or a limiting belief system. Clean eating encourages you to choose foods that not only taste good but also optimize your health and wellness. This chapter will help get you started with all of the basics of a clean eating lifestyle. The key is not perfection but making small steps over time that will help you achieve long-lasting results.

Why Eat Clean?

When most people think of the word *diet,* they think about it as a verb. They envision cutting back, restricting, going without, and setting limits in order to achieve a short-term goal. Thinking about *diet* as a verb and not a noun puts far too much emphasis on what you can't do, as opposed to what you can do. When I think about the word *diet,* I think about the big picture. Your diet is basically the *way* you eat, or what you eat and drink to fuel your life. It should not adversely affect your relationship with food, your body image, or your lifestyle.

This is where clean eating comes in. Why? Because it doesn't promote extremes, restrictions, or unhealthy relationships with food. It encourages a lifestyle approach for the long haul. This doesn't mean you can eat whatever you want, whenever you want, but it does mean you can enjoy the food you eat while fueling your activity and improving your health and wellness.

Clean eating, in my view, is nothing more than focusing on improving the quality of your diet while also striving for balance. The goal is to consume fewer processed foods and increase your intake of fruits, vegetables, and other healthy ingredients that support healthy living.

Processed foods are those that come in a box, bag, or package and have ingredient lists that contain chemicals and synthetic or artificial ingredients. It's not that you can't or shouldn't eat processed foods once in a while, but the majority of your diet should revolve around real foods like fruits, vegetables, meats, eggs, dairy, nuts, seeds, and legumes.

Let's think about why someone would want to eat clean. For some it's strictly about weight loss, but for most it's about building a healthy relationship with food in order to feel good inside and out. Some of the benefits of clean eating include improvements in immunity, quality and quantity of sleep, energy levels, mental clarity, athletic performance, sex drive, and overall wellness.

Eating clean can also ensure that you are giving your body the macro- and micronutrients it needs to reach its optimal health. Perhaps most importantly, clean eating is sustainable over the long term, because it emphasizes balance, rather than limitation or restriction. When integrated with movement and good sleep, clean eating can help you live a healthy, balanced life for years to come.

The Clean Eating Code

Clean eating is a lifestyle approach that promotes eating an unprocessed diet. It focuses on whole foods, minding portion sizes, and moving the body as it was intended. It's a simple approach to eating that fits easily into anyone's lifestyle and enhances overall health.

5 CORE CLEAN EATING PRINCIPLES

Some people think "clean eating" means eating food that is literally cleaned! While eating food that is not dirty is always a good idea, clean eating involves eating food that is natural and unprocessed and revolves around the following guidelines:

Choose whole foods

Eat whole foods that are as close to their natural state as possible. (i.e., a potato instead of a potato chip) and limit processed foods (those found in a box, bag, package, etc.).

Limit sugar

Limit foods with added sugar. This isn't the sugar you find naturally in fruit; it is the sugar added to a product to sweeten it. Sticking to whole foods helps reduce your overall added sugar intake.

Mind your portions

While quality is the main focus, the amount you eat is important, too. While everyone is different and thus portion sizes will differ person to person, a good rule of thumb is to think of the three macronutrients per meal as follows: protein as one or two deck(s) of cards, complex carbohydrates about the size of a tennis ball, and fat about the size of your thumb. From there, feel free to add in plenty of non-starchy vegetables, like greens, cauliflower, or peppers.

Drink plenty of water

Water is the best choice for hydrating your body. While there is a plethora of beverage options out there, many of them contain added sugar and artificial ingredients. Do yourself a favor and get your hydration from water and kick the sugar-sweetened beverages to the curb. Aim for eight glasses of water daily.

Move your body

Clean eating focuses not only on the food you put into your body but also your overall health. Your body was meant to move, and it loves activity. Make it a goal to engage in physical activity daily in order to build muscle and increase energy.

NUTRITIONAL GUIDELINES

It can be confusing to know where to start when it comes to clean eating, so I recommend keeping it simple. Here are a few things to keep in mind:

Read nutrition labels

Whole foods often don't have a label, so if you are eating more real foods, you don't have to worry. If you do see a label, look for minimal ingredients (fewer than five) and no added sugar or artificial ingredients.

Cook more and eat out less

From ingredients to portion sizes, you have far more control over what you are putting in your body when you make it at home. As much as possible, try to cook your own food—you may even find that you enjoy the process!

Plan ahead

There is a saying: "Fail to plan, plan to fail." With clean eating, planning ahead can save you time and effort at mealtime and can make all the difference in keeping you on track.

Listen to your body

Eat when you're hungry and stop when you're full. Trust your body—it will give you cues if you allow it to.

RECOMMENDED FOOD GROUPS

Clean eating is focused on striking a good balance between three macronutrients: protein, complex carbohydrates, and healthy fats. Here are some examples of each:

Protein: beans, beef, chicken, eggs, lamb, pork, turkey, seafood

Complex carbohydrates: fresh fruits and vegetables, whole grains

Healthy fats: full-fat dairy, nuts and seeds, oils (e.g., olive oil)

A balanced meal includes a good source of protein, a complex carbohydrate, and a healthy fat. If you divided up the plate, it would be about a quarter protein, a quarter carbs, half vegetables, and a spoonful of healthy fats. When having a snack, I like to aim for at least two of the three macronutrients, if not all of them.

Wellness Concerns

When considering a transition to clean eating, you may have some type of wellness concern in mind. Whether clearing up your skin, improving your gut health, getting a better night's sleep, or working to address a specific disease, nutrition is absolutely where you should turn for support. While there is no cure-all or specific diet that will fix all of your wellness concerns, it is possible that by improving your diet, you will also improve your quality of life, reduce chronic inflammation, and improve your overall energy levels.

INFLAMMATION

This word gets tossed around all the time. Is it good? Is it bad? Actually, it's a trick question; inflammation can be both good and bad. To better understand why inflammation occurs and how it affects the body, it can be helpful to separate it into two categories: acute inflammation and chronic inflammation.

Good inflammation, or acute inflammation, is what happens when you get a cut or an injury. Your body sends out helpers to respond to the injury in a timely manner in order to heal and repair that injury. The not-so-good inflammation, or chronic inflammation, is something like heart disease. This is when your body is in a constant state of inflammation and is constantly responding to perceived threats in the body.

Acute inflammation is what our bodies are made for. Chronic inflammation, on the other hand, can be due to a poor diet, or lifestyle and environmental factors. While diet can't fix or eliminate chronic inflammation, focusing on healthier real food options, including fruits, vegetables, grass-fed meats, and fish rich in omega-3 fatty acids, can help reduce chronic inflammation over time.

GUT HEALTH AND DIGESTION

As Hippocrates said long ago, "All disease starts in the gut." While that may not be 100 percent true, he was definitely on to something. If you don't have a healthy digestive system, it can be difficult to digest and absorb the nutrients you need from your food to achieve optimal health.

Food should make you feel good inside and out. If you notice that your digestion feels off, it's important to look closely at the possible reasons and to choose foods that keep your digestion running smoothly. Working with health professionals can help if you are struggling with what and how much to eat, as they can help you dig deeper into your personal concerns and give you advice tailored to your personal needs.

FATIGUE AND ENERGY

How great would it be if you constantly had energy like the Energizer bunny? Well, maybe you can. By eating fewer processed foods, less sugar, and more fiber, you can start to stabilize your blood sugar and improve your energy and mood. Certainly, getting a good night's sleep can't hurt either. Remember that diet is so much more than just the food you eat. Sleeping eight hours per night, engaging in daily physical activity, and reducing processed food and added sugar can help improve your overall energy and reduce fatigue.

Clean vs. Cleanse

When I talk about clean eating, I am talking about eating real foods—foods that are minimally processed. I am NOT talking about a restrictive diet or a fad diet or a cleanse. Fad diets come and go like bell-bottom jeans—sure, they stick around for a bit, but over time they just don't cut it.

I rarely, if ever, use the word *cleanse*, because your body has kidneys, a digestive system, and a liver that are meant to perform daily "cleanses." They protect you from toxins that enter the body due to diet and lifestyle, and they excrete anything your body doesn't want or need. If your body is not performing those functions, then it is a deeper issue that can't be solved by a five-day juice cleanse.

> **CLEAN:** eating real unprocessed food
> and focusing on a healthy lifestyle
> **VS.**
> **CLEANSE:** restricting food or taking
> supplements to "detox" the body

A cleanse often involves a short-term caloric restriction, pricey supplements, and probably a headache or two. Sure, you may lose weight in a week, but I guarantee you that it will not be sustainable or enjoyable. A clean eating approach is a far easier and more pleasurable way to maintain good health.

Clean Out and Stock Up

When starting out and adapting to a new way of eating, it's easy to want a black-and-white list of what to eat or what not to eat. Over time it will be easier to decipher which foods work best for your body and your lifestyle. The most important step is learning to turn over packages and read the label. Once you get in the habit of doing this, you can determine which foods to consume regularly and which foods to save for a special occasion or, better yet, make yourself.

When diving into a clean eating lifestyle, it's important to consider which foods may be best to focus on and which to limit or avoid as necessary. I'm not saying you should never eat processed food, but if you take a look at what you eat day to day and more than 50 percent is coming from a box, bag, or package, it might be time to look at the recommended food list and makes some easy, yet tasty, swaps.

RECOMMENDED FOODS

Instead of focusing on what you can't have, focus on the foods that you love from this list or the foods you are most curious about—and enjoy them!

The most important thing to consider is the quality of food you are eating. If you want to feel, look, and perform your best, then quality food is a good place to start. While some people think eating healthy is expensive, just remember your health is your wealth—and investing in it with healthy foods is worth it.

Let's take a look at the types of foods that you should be focusing on (see page 11 for a comprehensive list of foods to stock in your pantry and refrigerator):

Fruits and vegetables. Shop organic when you can and look for what's in season. Not sure? It's usually the fruits and vegetables that are in abundance in the grocery store, are the brightest in color, and that taste the best. But if you want to be certain, refer to the Seasonal Food Guide (seasonalfoodguide.org) to find out which foods are in season at a given time of year in your area.

Herbs and spices. Using herbs and spices can bring amazing flavor to any dish you make. Stock up on these and you'll be able to hit any recipe out of the park.

Healthy fats. When shopping for fats and oils, make sure you are picking unsaturated oils, like olive oil, that come in a dark glass jar. When looking for saturated fats like butter and coconut oil, look for butter from grass-fed cows and unrefined coconut oil.

Proteins. Quality is key here. If you can, shop local. Look for grass-fed (and grass-finished) meats, pasture-raised poultry and eggs, and wild game.

Legumes and whole grains. Look for single-ingredient legumes and whole grains—reading the label will help determine what is in a given product.

Dairy and dairy alternative products. When possible, stick to organic full-fat, unflavored dairy from grass-fed animals. While looking for dairy alternatives, read the label and look for those that have minimal ingredients and no added sugar.

Sweeteners. Not all sugar is bad, but it is especially important to control the quantity you use. Look for natural sweeteners like honey and maple syrup and use them sparingly.

FOODS TO MODERATE

It's important to recognize that there are no inherently bad foods, but rather foods that don't optimally fuel your health, athletic performance, or lifestyle. These are foods that should be limited to ensure long-term health and wellness. Look to limit the amount of artificial ingredients or sweeteners, chemicals, additives, and any other unfamiliar ingredients that seem less like a food and more like a tongue twister. A good rule of thumb is if it has more than five ingredients—or any questionable food ingredients—it is a processed food.

A note on sugar: Sugar, while delicious, is filled with empty calories, which tend to displace healthier food options in our diets. Eating too much sugar can sometimes make you crave more sugar, and that cycle is never-ending—you eat sugar, then you crave sugar, so you eat more, and so on. Natural sugar, like that found in fruits, is okay—but be mindful of the sugar added back to foods.

Listen to Your Body

In this day and age, it can be hard to trust your body. It seems like every influencer out there has a six-pack, and it can be easy to fall into the comparison trap. So, what is the secret to achieving optimal health? Listening to your OWN unique body! It's amazing what you can find out once you start listening to your body.

The goal is not to hyper-focus on every last gurgle your stomach makes but instead to focus on your energy, sleep, and digestion, as well as your hunger and satiety, in order to start figuring out what works best for you. You may find that when you eat nuts, you don't feel great but when you eat seeds, you feel amazing. Every body is unique and just because something works for one person does not mean it will work for you.

Because every body is so different, it's important to remember that you are uniquely you and you should not compare yourself and your diet to others. As I tell all my clients: "Eyes on your own plate!"

Stock Your Clean Kitchen

I always say if you stock a good pantry, fridge, and freezer, you're halfway there. So often we forget to meal plan, or we eat differently than we had envisioned for the week because of one thing or another. Planning ahead helps keep you on track. When meal prep doesn't go as planned, you burn the bacon (which happens to me all the time), or you run out of leftovers, a well-stocked kitchen will save you from the inevitable panic, ordering out, or relying on processed foods. This list will provide you with ideas about what kinds of things you might want to keep stocked in your kitchen and will provide a resource for the types of ingredients you will need to make the recipes in this book.

PANTRY

A well-stocked pantry can save you from having to do an extra grocery run during the week. I try to keep a few items in each category in my pantry at all times to ensure I can put together a quick meal. This is not an exhaustive list, nor do you have to buy every item listed. Instead focus on two or three items from each category (maybe a few more spices) and slowly stock up your pantry as you discover what you need and use the most. While many of these items have a decent shelf life, I'd recommend going through your pantry a few times per year or even monthly to make sure items are not expired or try to use them up before they do!

HEALTHY FATS

- Avocado
- Avocado oil
- Butter or ghee
- Coconut
- Coconut oil
- Flaxseed oil
- Nuts and nut butters: almonds, brazil nuts, cashews, hazelnuts, macadamias, peanuts, pecans, pistachios, walnuts, etc.
- Olives
- Olive oil
- Seeds: chia, flax, hemp, pepita, pumpkin, sesame, sunflower, etc.
- Sesame oil

BEANS AND LEGUMES

- Black beans
- Cannellini beans
- Chickpeas (Garbanzo beans)
- Kidney beans
- Lentils
- Lima beans
- Pinto beans
- Red beans
- Split peas

WHOLE GRAINS

- Barley
- Couscous
- Farro
- Millet
- Oats
- Quinoa
- Rice: arborio, basmati, brown, jasmine, white, etc.

HERBS AND SPICES

- Anise
- Basil
- Caraway
- Chili powder
- Cilantro
- Cinnamon
- Cumin
- Curry
- Dill
- Fennel
- Garam masala
- Garlic/garlic powder
- Ginger
- Lemongrass
- Marjoram
- Mint
- Nutmeg
- Onion powder
- Oregano
- Paprika
- Parsley
- Pepper
- Red pepper flakes
- Rosemary
- Sage
- Salt
- Thyme
- Turmeric

SWEETENERS

- Cane sugar
- Coconut sugar
- Dried fruit: cherries, cranberries, dates, figs, raisins, etc.
- Honey
- Maple syrup
- Molasses
- Pure vanilla extract

OTHER

- Baking powder
- Baking soda
- Coffee
- Flours/alternative flours: almond flour, coconut flour, cornstarch, arrowroot, tapioca starch, etc.
- Tea
- Unsweetened nut/seed butters: almond butter, peanut butter, sunflower seed butter, etc.

REFRIGERATOR AND FREEZER

The list that follows is a list of items that you can use by themselves or in the recipes found in this cookbook. By no means do you have to keep all of these on hand—that would be a lot of food to eat. Instead I'd recommend stocking up on a few of these items weekly to replenish your fresh fruits and vegetables and other perishable items. You might want to buy some frozen fruits and vegetables as they have a longer shelf life (a few months), so you can use them in a pinch.

FRUIT

- Apple
- Apricot
- Banana
- Berries: acai, blackberries, blueberries, raspberries, strawberries, etc.
- Cherries
- Dates
- Dragon fruit
- Figs
- Grapefruit
- Grapes
- Guava
- Kiwi
- Lemon
- Lime
- Mango
- Melons: cantaloupe, honeydew, watermelon, etc.
- Nectarine
- Oranges: blood orange, clementine, mandarin, navel, etc.
- Papaya
- Peach
- Pear
- Pineapple
- Plantain
- Plum
- Pomegranate
- Tangerine

VEGETABLES

- Artichoke
- Asparagus
- Bok choy
- Broccoli
- Brussels sprouts
- Cabbage
- Cauliflower
- Celery
- Corn
- Cucumber
- Eggplant
- Fennel
- Greens: chard, collard greens, kale, mustard greens, spinach, etc.
- Leeks
- Lettuce
- Mushrooms
- Onions
- Peppers
- Pumpkin
- Radishes
- Rhubarb
- Root vegetables: beets, carrots, parsnip, potatoes, yams, etc.
- Squash: acorn squash, butternut squash, cassava/yucca, delicata squash, spaghetti squash, etc.
- Tomatoes
- Zucchini

MEATS AND PROTEINS

- Beef
- Bison
- Eggs
- Fish: shellfish and freshwater finfish
- Lamb
- Poultry: chicken, turkey, duck, etc.
- Pork
- Tofu
- Wild game: boar, venison, etc.

DAIRY AND DAIRY ALTERNATIVE PRODUCTS

- Milk
- Cheese
- Cottage cheese
- Milk alternatives: almond, cashew, coconut, oat, rice, soy, etc.
- Yogurt/Greek yogurt

TOOLS AND EQUIPMENT

Having a well-equipped kitchen is a surefire way to make meal preparation and recipe execution a success. You don't need every item on this list, but as you begin to cook at home more often, you can also slowly build your kitchen to support your clean eating lifestyle. Here are some of my go-to kitchen tools and equipment.

Knife: Having a sharp knife and knowing how to use it is integral to efficient meal preparation. Not sure how to use it? Watch some YouTube videos, or sign up for a local knife skills class.

Cutting boards: A knife without a place to cut would be silly. I have three cutting boards so I can use two when cooking (one for meat and one for other ingredients) and one extra in case one of the others is dirty or someone is helping me prep.

Baking sheets: Sheet pan dinners can make getting food on the table a breeze and make cleanup even easier. All you need is one or two large sheet pans—just make sure they fit in your oven.

Food processor or blender: Having something to blend soups, smoothies, and other items can be helpful and a time-saver. You certainly don't need both, and if you don't have room to store one of these in your kitchen, consider getting an immersion blender.

Large cast iron skillet: A cast iron skillet is great for one-pan meals. It can be used on the stovetop or in the oven, and if it is seasoned properly, it is very easy to clean.

Baking dishes: I usually recommend investing in one 13-by-9-inch baking dish and one 8-by-8-inch baking dish to make casseroles and other dishes.

Slow cooker or pressure cooker: Once again, both are not necessary as they essentially do the same thing, but both can make meal prep and clean up relatively easy even for the beginner. Choose the one that fits your budget and your kitchen space.

Air fryer: This is definitely a nice-to-have kitchen appliance as it saves on time and cuts down on the oil when frying.

Coconut Oil

Ah, coconut oil, the latest and greatest health food that will solve all problems, including your bank account woes and relationship issues.

Just kidding! Coconut oil is not a superfood; it is simply a food. It is made up of mostly saturated fat, and when used in moderation, it is a healthy addition to a lot of recipes. Just do me a favor, don't brag about its superfood qualities, because giving any food that type of clout makes it a fad.

If you are looking for a dairy-free replacement for butter when you are cooking and baking, however, coconut oil can be a great swap to avoid any digestive distress.

About the Recipes

I hope that this cookbook gives you the knowledge and tools you need to adopt a clean eating lifestyle. The recipes are meant to be easy and are made using familiar ingredients. If you don't have something on hand, chances are you'll be able to swap it out for something else (such as broccoli for cauliflower). So, remember: Don't stress about the small stuff.

MEAL PLANS

The meal plans you'll find in chapter 2 (page 19) are provided as a guide to help you plan out your week using the recipes in this book. Meal planning can help set you up for success when trying to eat clean and fuel your body. It is not uncommon to leave meals for last minute and hope for the best. But when that happens, it is easy to eat whatever is fastest and easiest, which, unfortunately, is not always the healthiest. Use these meal plans to keep yourself on track. They will also help save you time during the week. There are three meal plans and each can help in different ways. Start by choosing the one that makes the most sense for your goals.

LABELS

The labels that appear on each recipe are meant to provide you with quick references so you can incorporate the recipes easily into your busy life. They will help you choose recipes based on the time you have available, the number of ingredients you might need, and your dietary preferences.

One-pot: These recipes use only one pot and make for easy cleanup.

5 ingredients or less: These recipes that contain five ingredients or less (not including some basic kitchen staples like spices and oil).

30 minutes or less: These recipes take less than 30 minutes to prepare and cook, start to finish.

Quick-prep: These recipes take 10 minutes or less to prepare.

Vegetarian: These recipes contain no animal meat products (although they may contain egg and dairy).

Nut-free: There are no peanuts or tree nuts in these recipes. (Coconut is technically a "tree nut" but does not fall in this category because it does not contain the same allergen.)

Dairy-free: These recipes contain no dairy.

Gluten-free: These recipes do use any ingredients that contain gluten.

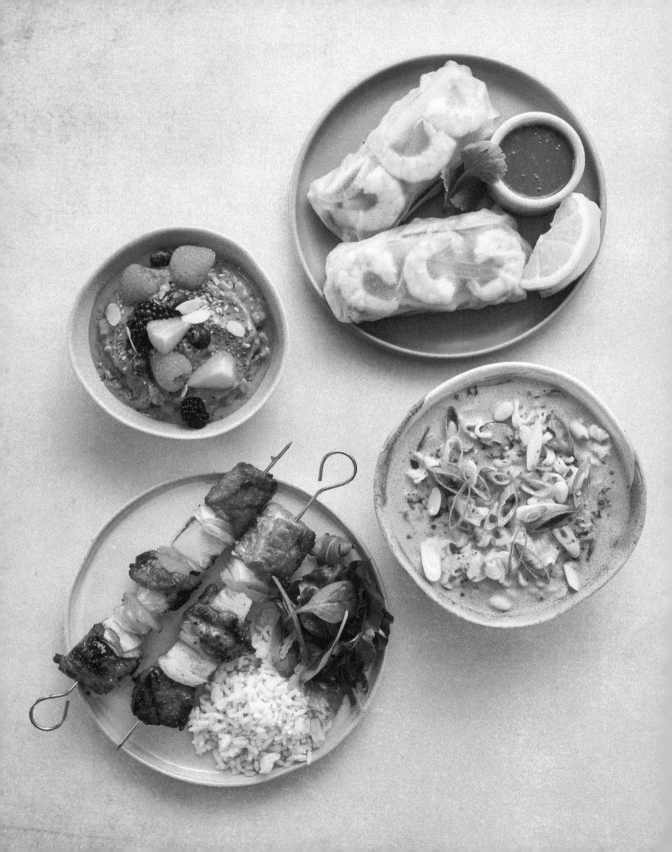

CHAPTER TWO

The Meal Plans

If you fail to plan, then you can plan to fail. While that might be extreme, I find that having a meal plan in place saves you time and worry during the week when you might not have much extra time. It also helps you make sure that you are getting a balance of protein, complex carbohydrates, and healthy fats, as well as plenty of fruits and vegetables so you can feel your best. These meal plans are easy to use for cooks of all experience levels. They are a great way to explore the recipes in this book, and they are customizable to your personal preferences. Feel free to follow the meal plans and the recipes to a tee or use them as inspiration.

Clean Eating 101 Plan

If you're new to clean eating, consider this your two-week introduction. This meal plan shows you how to plan clean, nutritionally balanced meals with recipes that are easy and approachable. Eating clean all week (or all the time) doesn't have to be complicated—it simply requires a little forethought. This plan gives you a great foundation for building a healthy, clean eating lifestyle.

While for some people leftovers may seem mundane, incorporating them into your meal plan is an easy way to keep your clean eating lifestyle on track and set yourself up for long-term success. If you find you are not too keen on leftovers, give the recipe a refresh by adding a different protein or new vegetables. If you are game for some batch cooking, try cooking things like rice and grains, hard-boiled eggs, soups, stews, and meats ahead of time, say on Saturday or Sunday, so you can spend more time during the week enjoying your meals and less time cooking.

WEEK 1:

	MEAL 1	MEAL 2	MEAL 3	SNACKS
MONDAY	Lemon Meringue Smoothie (page 51)	Strawberry–Goat Cheese Salad (page 110) and Skillet Garlic-Herb Steak (page 231)	Chicken Tortilla Soup (page 109)	Cinnamon Apple Chips (page 74), Chili-Lime Popcorn (page 76)
TUESDAY	PB and J Protein Smoothie (page 50)	Leftover Chicken Tortilla Soup (page 109)	Asian Lettuce Wraps with Hoisin Sauce (page 196)	Cinnamon Apple Chips (page 74), Chili-Lime Popcorn (page 76)
WEDNESDAY	Lemon Meringue Smoothie (page 51)	Leftover Strawberry–Goat Cheese Salad (page 110) and Leftover Skillet Garlic-Herb Steak (page 231)	Leftover Chicken Tortilla Soup (page 109)	Cinnamon Apple Chips (page 74), Chili-Lime Popcorn (page 76)
THURSDAY	PB and J Protein Smoothie (page 50)	Leftover Chicken Tortilla Soup (page 109)	Leftover Asian Lettuce Wraps with Hoisin Sauce (page 196)	Cinnamon Apple Chips (page 74), Chili-Lime Popcorn (page 76)
FRIDAY	Lemon Meringue Smoothie (page 51)	Orange-Beet-Arugula Salad (page 113) and 2 hard-boiled eggs	Hawaiian Pork Kebabs (page 197) and Avocado-Cucumber-Feta Salad (page 111)	Cinnamon Apple Chips (page 74), Chili-Lime Popcorn (page 76)
SATURDAY	Berry Berry Smoothie Bowl (page 53)	Deli turkey roll-ups with avocado, lettuce, and tomato	Burger Bowls (page 223)	Cinnamon Apple Chips (page 74), Chili-Lime Popcorn (page 76)
SUNDAY	Berry Berry Smoothie Bowl (page 53)	Leftover Avocado-Cucumber-Feta Salad (page 111) on toast and a hard-boiled egg	Leftover Hawaiian Pork Kebabs (page 197) over rice	Cinnamon Apple Chips (page 74), Chili-Lime Popcorn (page 76)

WEEKLY MEAL PREP

To make the most of the meal plans, set aside some time on the Sunday before the week begins to prepare as much as possible ahead of time. See page 25 for my philosophy on meal prepping; here are some things you can do to prepare for Clean Eating 101, Week 1:

Chicken Tortilla Soup: Make the Taco Seasoning (page 250). Chop vegetables and purée the chipotle and store (they can be stored together) in a covered container in the refrigerator overnight. On Monday morning put the ingredients in the slow cooker as directed in the recipe so that you can have dinner on the table by the evening.

Cinnamon Apple Chips: Make the entire recipe. Portion out into single servings and store in airtight containers for grab-and-go snacks during the week.

Chili-Lime Popcorn: Make the entire recipe and store in an airtight container or bag in the pantry until ready to eat.

Lemon Meringue Smoothie: Mix the yogurt, milk, and maple syrup together the night before you plan to have the smoothie, then combine with ice, lemon, and protein powder in the blender the next morning.

Skillet Garlic-Herb Steak: Make the entire recipe, slice and store in single portions in airtight containers in the refrigerator and add to salads at lunch.

Strawberry–Goat Cheese Salad: Make dressing separate from salad and store dressing in a separate container. Wait to dress the salad until ready to eat.

SHOPPING LIST

CANNED AND BOTTLED ITEMS

- Black beans,
  1 (15-ounce) can
- Chipotle peppers
  in adobo sauce,
  1 (7-ounce) can
- Diced tomatoes,
  1 (14.5-ounce) can

DAIRY AND EGGS

- Butter/ghee, 1 stick
  or ½ cup
- Cheddar cheese,
  shredded
  (8-ounce block)
- Eggs, large (1 dozen)
- Feta (8 ounces)
- Goat cheese
  (4 ounces)
- Greek yogurt, plain
  and unsweetened,
  1 (32-ounce) container
- Milk of choice
  (½ gallon)

FROZEN FOODS

- Corn, frozen,
  1 (16-ounce) bag
- Berries,
  frozen (5 cups)

MEAT

- Beef, ground (1 pound)
- Chicken breast
  (2 pounds)
- Pork loin, boneless
  (2 pounds)
- Pork, ground (1 pound)
- Steak, NY
  strip (1 pound)
- Turkey, deli (8 ounces)

PANTRY ITEMS

*Amounts only noted for some as ideally you would stock your pantry to have a
container of each of the following ingredients.*

- Apple cider vinegar
- Avocado oil
- Balsamic vinegar
- Chicken broth,
  1 (32-ounce) container
- Chili powder
- Cinnamon
- Corn tortillas (8)
- Cornstarch
- Cumin
- Dijon mustard
- Extra-virgin olive oil
- Garlic powder
- Honey
- Ketchup
- Maple syrup
- Onion powder
- Oregano

- Paprika
- Peanut butter, 1 (16-ounce) jar
- Pecans, halved (½ cup)
- Pepper
- Pickles
- Raspberry jelly
- Red pepper flakes
- Rosemary
- Salt
- Sesame oil
- Shelled walnuts, 1 (10-ounce) bag
- Soy sauce
- Sriracha
- Thyme
- Unsalted roasted peanuts (½ cup)
- Vanilla or unflavored protein powder
- White/brown rice (1 bag)
- Whole-grain bread (1 small loaf)
- Yellow mustard

PRODUCE

- Arugula (4 cups)
- Avocado (5)
- Beet (4)
- Bell pepper, color of choice (3)
- Butter lettuce (1 head)
- Carrot (1)
- Cucumber (3)
- Garlic (1 bulb)
- Ginger, fresh
- Green onions (1 bunch)
- Iceberg lettuce (1 head)
- Lemon (5)
- Mushrooms (8 ounces)
- Onion, red (2)
- Onion, yellow (2)
- Orange (1)
- Pepper, jalapeño (2)
- Pineapple (1)
- Spinach (4 cups)
- Strawberries (1 pint)
- Sweet potato (1 to 2)
- Tomato (2 to 3)

Built-In Prep

If you are relatively new to cooking at home, the idea of cooking ahead and doing meal prep can be overwhelming. However, once you get into the habit, you'll notice how your diet (i.e., the way you eat) becomes more of a lifestyle. Meal prep is not meant to cramp your style; instead, once you find what works for you, it will streamline your meal preparation and save time, so you can do all the things you love and feel your best while doing them.

Start by setting aside some time during the weekend (or during the week) to bulk prep your food. I love using Sunday afternoons as a time to make a few dishes for the week so I can spend my evenings enjoying my family and friends. During that time, prepare enough food so that you have leftovers for the week. Make extra servings of a dinner so that you can eat it again for lunch or dinner on a different day.

Have extra leftovers? Don't be afraid to freeze them. I recommend storing them in labeled single-serving portions.

WEEK 2:

	MEAL 1	MEAL 2	MEAL 3	SNACKS
MONDAY	Green Power Smoothie Bowl (page 54)	Greek Lamb Bowls with Turmeric Cauliflower Rice and Cucumber Salsa (page 243)	Pork and White Bean Stew (page 216)	Everything Bagel–Seasoned Hard-Boiled Eggs (page 81), celery sticks and Caramelized Onion and Carrot Hummus (page 84)
TUESDAY	French Toast Overnight Oats (page 55)	Leftover Pork and White Bean Stew (page 216)	Greek Lamb Bowls with Turmeric Cauliflower Rice and Cucumber Salsa (page 243)	Everything Bagel–Seasoned Hard-Boiled Eggs (page 81), celery sticks and Caramelized Onion and Carrot Hummus (page 84)
WEDNESDAY	Green Power Smoothie Bowl (page 54)	Waldorf Chicken Salad (page 175) over lettuce	Sheet Pan Chicken Fajitas (page 183)	Everything Bagel–Seasoned Hard-Boiled Eggs (page 81), celery sticks and Caramelized Onion and Carrot Hummus (page 84)
THURSDAY	Leftover French Toast Overnight Oats (page 55) and sliced banana	Deli turkey roll-ups with baby carrots and Easy Guacamole (page 83)	Leftover Sheet Pan Chicken Fajitas (page 183) over rice	Everything Bagel–Seasoned Hard-Boiled Eggs (page 81), celery sticks and Caramelized Onion and Carrot Hummus (page 84)
FRIDAY	Green Power Smoothie Bowl (page 54)	Leftover Waldorf Chicken Salad (page 175) in a wrap	One-Skillet Pepper Steak (page 230)	Everything Bagel–Seasoned Hard-Boiled Eggs (page 81), celery sticks and Caramelized Onion and Carrot Hummus (page 84)
SATURDAY	Green Eggs and Ham Frittata (page 64)	Leftover One-Skillet Pepper Steak (page 230)	Chicken Parmesan over Zoodles (page 192)	Everything Bagel–Seasoned Hard-Boiled Eggs (page 81), celery sticks and Caramelized Onion and Carrot Hummus (page 84)
SUNDAY	Leftover Green Eggs and Ham Frittata (page 64)	Leftover Chicken Parmesan over Zoodles (page 192) in a wrap	Easy Apple-Tuna Salad (page 169) and Garlic-Dijon Asparagus (page 87)	Everything Bagel–Seasoned Hard-Boiled Eggs (page 81), celery sticks and Caramelized Onion and Carrot Hummus (page 84)

WEEKLY MEAL PREP

On the Sunday before the week begins, prepare the following items:

French Toast Overnight Oats: Make the entire recipe and store in portion-sized airtight containers in the refrigerator until ready to eat.

Greek Lamb Bowls with Turmeric Cauliflower Rice and Cucumber Salsa: Prepare the entire recipe, but keep the lamb separate from the cauliflower rice and salsa. Combine when ready to eat.

Pork and White Bean Stew: Prepare the entire recipe and store in the refrigerator in a large sealed container until ready to eat.

Everything Bagel–Seasoned Hard-Boiled Eggs: Hard-boil as many eggs as you think you will need for the week. Store in an airtight container and refrigerate until ready to eat. Mix up the seasoning and keep it in a jar in the pantry until ready to use.

Caramelized Onion and Carrot Hummus: Prepare the recipe and store in an airtight container in the refrigerator until ready to eat.

SHOPPING LIST

CANNED AND BOTTLED ITEMS

- Cannellini beans, 1 (15-ounce) can
- Pumpkin purée, 1 (15-ounce) can
- Tomato paste, 1 (6-ounce) can
- Tuna, canned (10 ounces)
- White wine, dry (1 bottle)

DAIRY AND EGGS

- Almond milk (½ gallon)
- Eggs, large (1½ dozen)
- Feta cheese (4 ounces)
- Greek yogurt, plain and unsweetened, 1 (32-ounce) container
- Mozzarella, fresh (8 ounces)
- Parmesan, grated (1 cup)

FROZEN FOODS

- Spinach, frozen
  (6 ounces)

MEAT

- Bacon (1 pound)
- Chicken breast
  (5 pounds)
- Flank steak (1 pound)
- Lamb,
  ground (1 pound)
- Pork tenderloin
  (1 pound)
- Turkey, deli (8 ounces)

PANTRY ITEMS

- Apple cider vinegar
- Avocado oil
- Black pepper
- Bread crumbs
  (8 ounces)
- Broth (chicken
  or vegetable),
  1 (32-ounce)
  container
- Chia seeds
- Chili powder
- Cinnamon
- Cornstarch
- Cumin
- Dijon mustard
- Dill pickles
- Flax meal
- Garlic powder
- Ginger, fresh
- Hummus
- Maple syrup
- Marinara/pasta sauce,
  1 (24-ounce) jar
- Mayonnaise
- Oats, rolled (1 cup)
- Onion powder
- Oregano
- Paprika
- Parsley, fresh
- Poppy seeds
- Pumpkin seed butter,
  1 (8-ounce) jar
- Salt
- Sesame seeds
- Shelled walnuts
  (10 ounces)
- Soy sauce
- Turmeric
- Vanilla or unflavored
  protein powder
- White/brown rice
- Whole wheat
  wraps (8 wraps)

PRODUCE

- Apple (1)
- Asparagus (1 pound)
- Avocado (4)
- Banana (2)
- Bell pepper (7)
- Butter lettuce (1 head)
- Carrots, baby (1 bag)
- Cauliflower (1 head)

- Celery (1 head/bunch)
- Cucumber (1)
- Garlic (1 bulb)
- Grapes, red (1 bunch)
- Jalapeño (1)
- Kale (1 bunch)
- Kiwi (3)
- Lemon (3)

- Lime (2)
- Onion, red (3)
- Onion, yellow (3)
- Pear (1)
- Pineapple (1)
- Spinach, fresh (9 cups)
- Zucchini (2)

Wellness Plan

The Wellness Plan focuses on foods that are helpful for reducing inflammation and improving the quality of your regular diet. Eating quality real food (e.g., fresh fruit over canned fruit in syrup) can also help improve your digestion. When you are first focusing on improving the quality of the food in your diet, budget a little extra shopping time to compare your options in order to find quality ingredients that suit your taste and your pocketbook.

Many of the recipes in this plan are or can be made allergen-free (i.e., gluten-free, dairy-free, nut-free), which may be helpful in improving your overall health and digestion as well as other health ailments.

WEEK 1:

	MEAL 1	MEAL 2	MEAL 3	SNACKS
MONDAY	Freezer V-Egg-ie Burritos (page 70)	Broccoli-Walnut Salad with Dried Cherries (page 117) and chopped chicken	Lamb Lollipops with Chimichurri Sauce (page 245) over rice	Sliced bell peppers and Easy Guacamole (page 83), Almond Butter Energy Bites (page 86)
TUESDAY	Leftover Freezer V-Egg-ie Burritos (page 70)	Leftover Lamb Lollipops with Chimichurri Sauce (page 245)	Easy Stovetop Phở (page 100)	Sliced bell peppers and Easy Guacamole (page 83), Almond Butter Energy Bites (page 86)
WEDNESDAY	Leftover Freezer V-Egg-ie Burritos (page 70)	Easy Stovetop Phở (page 100)	Sheet Pan Sweet and Sour Chicken Rice Bowls (page 179)	Sliced bell peppers and Easy Guacamole (page 83), Almond Butter Energy Bites (page 86)
THURSDAY	French Toast Overnight Oats (page 55) and berries	Leftover Sheet Pan Sweet and Sour Chicken Rice Bowls (page 179)	Lemon Lentil Soup (page 107)	Sliced bell peppers and Easy Guacamole (page 83), Almond Butter Energy Bites (page 86)
FRIDAY	Leftover French Toast Overnight Oats (page 55) with berries	Leftover Lemon Lentil Soup (page 107)	Spinach Meatballs and Zucchini Noodles (page 233)	Sliced bell peppers and Easy Guacamole (page 83), Almond Butter Energy Bites (page 86)
SATURDAY	Southwest Eggs Benedict on Sweet Potato Toast (page 69)	Sesame Tofu and Brussels Sprouts Bowl (page 136)	Honey-Lime Salmon with Watermelon Salsa (page 164) and Crispy Garlic-Rosemary Potato Wedges (page 77)	Sliced bell peppers and Easy Guacamole (page 83), Almond Butter Energy Bites (page 86)
SUNDAY	Leftover Southwest Eggs Benedict on Sweet Potato Toast (page 69)	Leftover Sesame Tofu and Brussels Sprouts Bowl (page 136)	Leftover Spinach Meatballs and Zucchini Noodles (page 233)	Sliced bell peppers and Easy Guacamole (page 83), Almond Butter Energy Bites (page 86)

WEEKLY MEAL PREP

On the Sunday before the week begins, prepare the following items:

French Toast Overnight Oats: Make the entire recipe, and store in portioned-size airtight containers in the refrigerator until ready to eat.

Freezer V-Egg-ie Burritos: Make the entire recipe, then freeze per recipe directions.

Chimichurri Sauce: Make the Chimichurri Sauce for the lamb lollipops. Store in an airtight container in the refrigerator.

Easy Stovetop Phở: Make the broth, cover and refrigerate. Reheat on Tuesday in a large pot over medium heat and then add the noodles at the time of serving.

Almond Butter Energy Bites: Make the entire recipe and place in a bag or sealed container in the refrigerator. If you do not finish them within a week, place them in the freezer in a freezer-safe bag or sealed container.

SHOPPING LIST

CANNED AND BOTTLED ITEMS

- Pineapple, chunks, 1 (20-ounce) can
- Tomatoes, crushed, 1 (28-ounce) can
- Tomato paste, 1 (6-ounce) can

DAIRY AND EGGS

- Almond milk (½ gallon)
- Cheddar cheese (8-ounce block)
- Eggs, large (1½ dozen)
- Ghee, 1 (12-ounce) jar
- Parmesan, grated

MEAT

- Bacon (4 slices)
- Beef, ground and lean (1 pound)
- Chicken breast (3 pounds)
- Lamb, rib chops (1 pound)
- Salmon, 6 (4-ounce) fillets

PANTRY ITEMS

- Almond butter (1 cup)
- Apple cider vinegar
- Black pepper
- Broth, vegetable
- Brown sugar
- Cayenne
- Chia seeds
- Chocolate chips
- Cinnamon
- Cinnamon sticks
- Cornstarch
- Curry powder
- Dijon mustard
- Extra-virgin olive oil
- Fish sauce
- Flax meal
- Garlic powder
- Ginger, ground
- Honey
- Ketchup
- Lentils, dried (16 ounces)
- Maple syrup
- Mayonnaise
- Miso paste
- Oats, rolled (2 cups)
- Oregano
- Paprika
- Red pepper flakes
- Rice noodles, dried (7 ounces)
- Rice wine vinegar
- Salt
- Sesame seeds
- Soy sauce
- Sriracha
- Tofu, extra firm, 1 (16-ounce) block
- Turmeric
- Walnuts (4 ounces)
- White/brown rice
- Wraps, burrito size (4)

PRODUCE

- Avocado (1)
- Basil, fresh
- Bell pepper (5)
- Berries, fresh (1 pint)
- Broccoli (4 heads)
- Brussels sprouts (1 pound)
- Celery (2 stalks)
- Cilantro, fresh
- Cherries, dried and unsweetened (4 ounces)
- Garlic (2 to 3 bulbs)
- Jalapeño (1)
- Lemon (3)
- Lime (2)
- Mint, fresh
- Mushroom (8 ounces)
- Onion, red (2)
- Onion, yellow (5)
- Parsley, fresh
- Potatoes, russet (2 pounds)
- Rosemary, fresh
- Spinach, fresh (5 ounces)
- Sweet potato (3)
- Tomato (1)
- Watermelon, small (1)
- Zucchini (3)

WEEK 2:

	MEAL 1	MEAL 2	MEAL 3	SNACKS
MONDAY	Apple Breakfast Sausage Patties (page 61) and cantaloupe	Watermelon Gazpacho (page 98) and Paprika-Baked Chicken Thighs (page 180)	Sweet Potato Salmon Cakes (page 165) and Orange-Balsamic Brussels Sprouts (page 89)	Apple slices and Cookie Dough Dip (page 85), Sweet 'n' Spicy Nuts and Seeds (page 80)
TUESDAY	Leftover Apple Breakfast Sausage Patties (page 61) and cantaloupe	Leftover Sweet Potato Salmon Cakes (page 165) and Leftover Orange-Balsamic Brussels Sprouts (page 89)	Classic Minestrone (page 106)	Apple slices and Cookie Dough Dip (page 85), Sweet 'n' Spicy Nuts and Seeds (page 80)
WEDNESDAY	Leftover Apple Breakfast Sausage Patties (page 61) and cantaloupe	Leftover Watermelon Gazpacho (page 98) and Leftover Paprika-Baked Chicken Thighs (page 180)	BBQ Pulled Pork (page 206) and broccoli	Apple slices and Cookie Dough Dip (page 85), Sweet 'n' Spicy Nuts and Seeds (page 80)
THURSDAY	Pumpkin Spice Baked Oatmeal Bars (page 60) and Everything Bagel–Seasoned Hard-Boiled Eggs (page 81)	Leftover Classic Minestrone (page 106)	Leftover BBQ Pulled Pork (page 206) and Air-Fryer Sweet Potato Tots (page 94) and broccoli	Apple slices and Cookie Dough Dip (page 85), Sweet 'n' Spicy Nuts and Seeds (page 80)
FRIDAY	Leftover Pumpkin Spice Baked Oatmeal Bars (page 60) and Leftover Everything Bagel–Seasoned Hard-Boiled Eggs (page 81)	Egg Roll in a Bowl (page 178)	Mongolian Beef and Broccoli (page 229)	Apple slices and Cookie Dough Dip (page 85), Sweet 'n' Spicy Nuts and Seeds (page 80)
SATURDAY	Loaded Avocado Toast (page 65) and fresh berries	Leftover Mongolian Beef and Broccoli (page 229)	Grilled Sausage, Peppers, and Onions (page 201)	Apple slices and Cookie Dough Dip (page 85), Sweet 'n' Spicy Nuts and Seeds (page 80)
SUNDAY	Leftover Loaded Avocado Toast (page 65) and fresh berries	Leftover Egg Roll in a Bowl (page 178)	Leftover Grilled Sausage, Peppers, and Onions (page 201) over zoodles	Apple slices and Cookie Dough Dip (page 85), Sweet 'n' Spicy Nuts and Seeds (page 80)

WEEKLY MEAL PREP

On the Sunday before the week begins, prepare the following items:

Apple Breakfast Sausage Patties: Make the entire recipe. Divide into individual portions and store in the refrigerator in separate airtight containers so you can heat them up when you are ready to eat them.

Watermelon Gazpacho: Make the entire recipe. Refrigerate in a large covered bowl or sealed container until ready to eat.

Paprika-Baked Chicken Thighs: Make the entire recipe. Let it cool and cover it in baking dish or portion out into separate containers. Refrigerate and reheat in microwave when ready to eat.

Sweet Potato Salmon Cakes: Make the entire recipe. Refrigerate in an airtight container until ready to eat. Feel free to eat these cold or reheated.

Cookie Dough Dip: Make the entire recipe. Divide into 4 separate airtight containers in the refrigerator to grab and go for a quick snack.

Sweet 'n' Spicy Nuts and Seeds: Make on Sunday and store in airtight sealed containers in your pantry or refrigerator until ready to eat. Portion out into single servings for a quick grab-and-go snack.

SHOPPING LIST

CANNED AND BOTTLED ITEMS

- Cannellini beans, 1 (15-ounce) can
- Pumpkin purée, canned, 1 (15-ounce) can
- Salmon, canned in water, 2 (5-ounce) cans
- Tomato paste, 2 (6-ounce) cans
- Tomatoes, diced, 1 (14.5-ounce) can
- Tomatoes, diced, 1 (28-ounce) can

DAIRY AND EGGS

- Eggs, large (2 dozen)
- Ghee/butter
- Greek yogurt, plain and unsweetened, 1 (8-ounce) container
- Milk (½ gallon)

MEAT

- Chicken, ground (1 pound)
- Chicken thighs, boneless and skinless (2 pounds)
- Pork, boneless shoulder (3 to 4 pounds)
- Pork, ground (1 pound)
- Pork sausage links (1 pound)
- Steak, flank (1½ pounds)

PANTRY ITEMS

- Almond butter
- Almonds
- Apple cider vinegar
- Avocado oil
- Baking powder
- Balsamic vinegar
- Broth, vegetable
- Chili powder
- Chocolate chips
- Cinnamon
- Coconut oil
- Cornstarch
- Dijon mustard
- Extra-virgin olive oil
- Flax meal
- Flax seed
- Garlic powder
- Ginger, fresh
- Maple syrup
- Oats, rolled (2 cups)
- Onion powder
- Oregano
- Paprika
- Parsley
- Pasta, penne (1 pound, dry)
- Pepitas
- Pepper
- Poppy seeds
- Pure vanilla extract
- Red pepper flakes
- Rice vinegar
- Salt
- Sesame oil
- Sesame seeds
- Soy sauce
- Sriracha
- Thyme
- Walnuts, 1 (16-ounce) bag
- Whole-grain bread (1 small loaf)

PRODUCE

- Apple (6)
- Avocado (1)
- Bell pepper (3)
- Berries (1 pint)
- Broccoli (3 heads)
- Brussels sprouts (1 pound)
- Cabbage, green (1)
- Cantaloupe (1)
- Carrot (3)
- Cauliflower (1 head)
- Celery (1)

- Cilantro, fresh
- Cucumber (3)
- Garlic (2 bulbs)
- Lemon (1)
- Onion, green (1 bunch)

- Onion, red (1)
- Onion, yellow (5)
- Orange (2)
- Spinach, fresh (5 ounces)

- Sweet potato (2)
- Tomato (4)
- Watermelon (1 small)

Snacks

I love having an assortment of go-to snacks on hand for a pick-me-up between meals or when I know I'm going to be busy. I suggest stocking up on shelf-stable snacks like bars, nuts and seeds, and nut butters once per month and then restocking as needed week to week. If you leave snacking up to chance, it almost always results in grabbing whatever is easiest and most convenient, but not always healthiest. Additionally, in chapter 4 you will find easy recipes for make-ahead snacks, including Cinnamon Apple Chips (page 74), Caramelized Onion and Carrot Hummus (page 84), and Almond Butter Energy Bites (page 86), that will give you plenty of variety and keep you going during your busy week. Here are a few of my favorite grab-and-go snack ideas with no cooking required and suggested portion sizes, though I recommend that you listen to your body and reasonably adjust the portions in order to satisfy your hunger:

- 1 sliced apple with 2 tablespoons almond butter

- 2 to 3 celery stalks with 2 to 3 tablespoons hummus

- ½ sliced bell pepper with 2 to 3 tablespoons guacamole

- 1 tablespoon peanut butter and ½ cup blueberries on a rice cake

- 1 ounce deli turkey wrapped around 4 cucumber slices

- 1 cup plain unsweetened Greek yogurt with ¼ cup berries and 2 tablespoons walnuts

Healthy Lifestyle Plan

While I believe that everyone should find health and happiness in their own size and shape, there are some times when a person's goals include improving health and perhaps weight. Cooking at home and eating real food can help you not only reach your weight goals but feel your best when you are trying to reach your optimal health.

This meal plan is for anyone that is looking to improve their overall health and well-being or trying reach a certain weight. The recipes in this meal plan are more focused on fruits, vegetables, and leaner cuts of meat, but anyone can benefit from having their week planned out as it is in this plan. In this meal plan there is a bit more repetition in order to help you build routine and stay consistent. Being consistent and keeping things simple helps build healthy habits over the long term and sets you up for success in the short term.

A friendly reminder that hunger is not a badge of honor but instead a signal that your body is hungry, so if you find you are hungry on any of these meal plans, add in some healthy snacks or extra portions to ensure you are feeding and fueling your body appropriately.

WEEK 1:

	MEAL 1	MEAL 2	MEAL 3	SNACKS
MONDAY	Green Power Smoothie Bowl (page 54)	Greek Lamb Bowls with Turmeric Cauliflower Rice and Cucumber Salsa (page 243)	Spaghetti Squash Primavera (page 140) with Garlic-Parmesan Roasted Broccoli (page 88)	Cucumber slices and Tzatziki (page 261), Tropical Pineapple Fruit Leather (page 271)
TUESDAY	Chocolate Chip Cookie Dough Overnight Oats (page 57)	Leftover Greek Lamb Bowls with Turmeric Cauliflower Rice and Cucumber Salsa (page 243)	Leftover Spaghetti Squash Primavera and (page 140) and Leftover Garlic-Parmesan Roasted Broccoli (page 88)	Cucumber slices and Tzatziki (page 261), Tropical Pineapple Fruit Leather (page 271)
WEDNESDAY	Chocolate Chip Cookie Dough Overnight Oats (page 57) and ½ sliced banana	Beef Tacos in Lettuce (page 220) and Easy Guacamole (page 83)	Pork and White Bean Stew (page 216)	Cucumber slices and Tzatziki (page 261), Tropical Pineapple Fruit Leather (page 271)
THURSDAY	Chocolate Chip Cookie Dough Overnight Oats (page 57) and ½ sliced banana	Leftover Beef Tacos in Lettuce (page 220) and Easy Guacamole (page 83)	Leftover Pork and White Bean Stew (page 216)	Cucumber slices and Tzatziki (page 261), Tropical Pineapple Fruit Leather (page 271)
FRIDAY	Green Power Smoothie Bowl (page 54)	Leftover Pork and White Bean Stew (page 216)	Mediterranean Fish in Parchment (page 161) and steamed green beans	Cucumber slices and Tzatziki (page 261), Tropical Pineapple Fruit Leather (page 271)
SATURDAY	Green Shakshuka (page 67) and watermelon	Power Quinoa Bowl (page 135)	Chili-Stuffed Peppers (page 232) and Cilantro-Lime Cauliflower Rice (page 92)	Cucumber slices and Tzatziki (page 261), Tropical Pineapple Fruit Leather (page 271)
SUNDAY	Leftover Green Shakshuka (page 67) and watermelon	Leftover Power Quinoa Bowl (page 135)	Leftover Chili-Stuffed Peppers (page 232) and Cilantro-Lime Cauliflower Rice (page 92)	Cucumber slices and Tzatziki (page 261), Tropical Pineapple Fruit Leather (page 271)

WEEKLY MEAL PREP

On the Sunday before the week begins, prepare the following items:

Spaghetti Squash Primavera: Make the spaghetti squash on Sunday night and then finish preparing the primavera on Monday. Shred and store spaghetti squash in a sealed container in the refrigerator and reheat as needed.

Chocolate Chip Cookie Dough Overnight Oats: Make the entire recipe. Divide into individual portions and store in airtight containers in the refrigerator until ready to eat.

Greek Lamb Bowls with Turmeric Cauliflower Rice: Make the entire recipe but keep the lamb separate from the cauliflower rice. Store in airtight containers in the refrigerator. Combine and reheat when ready to eat.

Tzatziki: Make the entire recipe and store in the refrigerator in a sealed airtight container for the week.

Tropical Pineapple Fruit Leather: Make this over the weekend when you have a few hours to spare. Store in a bag in your pantry.

SHOPPING LIST

CANNED AND BOTTLED ITEMS

- Cannellini beans, 1 (15-ounce) can
- Green chiles, 1 (7-ounce) can
- Pumpkin purée, 1 (15-ounce) can
- Tomatoes, diced, 2 (14.5-ounce) cans
- Tomato paste, 1 (6-ounce) can
- White wine (½ cup, dry)

DAIRY AND EGGS

- Cheddar cheese, shredded (8 ounces)
- Eggs, large (2 dozen)
- Feta (20 ounces)
- Greek yogurt, plain and unsweetened, 1 (32-ounce) container
- Milk (1 pint)
- Parmesan cheese, grated, 1 (5-ounce) container

MEAT

- Bacon (1 pound)
- Beef, ground (2 pounds)
- Cod, 4 (6-ounce) fillets
- Lamb, ground (1 pound)
- Pork tenderloin (1 pound)

PANTRY ITEMS

- Almond butter
- Apple cider vinegar
- Balsamic vinegar
- Broth, chicken
- Capers
- Chili powder
- Chocolate chips
- Coconut sugar
- Cumin
- Extra-virgin olive oil
- Garlic powder
- Hummus
- Oats, rolled (3 cups)
- Onion powder
- Oregano
- Paprika
- Pepper
- Pumpkin seed butter (2 tablespoons)
- Pure vanilla extract
- Quinoa (1 cup dry)
- Red pepper flakes
- Salt
- Turmeric
- Vanilla or unflavored protein powder

PRODUCE

- Avocado (3)
- Banana (1 or 2)
- Basil, fresh
- Bell pepper (13)
- Broccoli (3 heads)
- Carrot (1)
- Cauliflower (1 head)
- Celery (1)
- Cucumber (1)
- Garlic (2 bulbs)
- Green beans (1 pound)
- Jalapeño (1)
- Kale (2 bunches)
- Kiwi (3)
- Lemon (4)
- Lettuce, romaine or butter (1 head)
- Lime (1)
- Mango (1)
- Mushrooms (4 ounces)
- Onion, red (1)
- Onion, yellow (6)
- Parsley, fresh
- Pineapple (2)
- Spaghetti squash (1)
- Spinach, fresh (2 pounds)
- Summer squash (1)
- Sweet potato (1)
- Tomatoes, grape/cherry (1 pint)
- Watermelon (1 small)

WEEK 2:

	MEAL 1	MEAL 2	MEAL 3	SNACKS
MONDAY	PB and J Protein Smoothie (page 50)	Chickpea Buddha Bowls (page 133)	Pork Fried Cauliflower Rice (page 209)	Chili-Spiced Fruit Cups (page 273), Crunchy Chickpeas (page 79)
TUESDAY	Sweet Potato Crust Quiche (page 68)	Leftover Chickpea Buddha Bowls (page 133)	Leftover Pork Fried Cauliflower Rice (page 209)	Chili-Spiced Fruit Cups (page 273), Crunchy Chickpeas (page 79)
WEDNESDAY	Leftover Sweet Potato Crust Quiche (page 68)	Leftover Pork Fried Cauliflower Rice (page 209)	Steak and Pepper Roll-Ups (page 228) and Air-Fryer Sweet Potato Tots (page 94)	Chili-Spiced Fruit Cups (page 273), Crunchy Chickpeas (page 79)
THURSDAY	Leftover Sweet Potato Crust Quiche (page 68)	Leftover Steak and Pepper Roll-Ups (page 228) and Air-Fryer Sweet Potato Tots (page 94)	Lamb Kofta Kababs (page 238) and Mashed Parmesan Cauliflower (page 91)	Chili-Spiced Fruit Cups (page 273), Crunchy Chickpeas (page 79)
FRIDAY	PB and J Protein Smoothie (page 50)	Leftover Lamb Kofta Kababs (page 238) and Leftover Mashed Parmesan Cauliflower (page 91)	Leftover Steak and Pepper Roll-Ups (page 228) over rice	Chili-Spiced Fruit Cups (page 273), Crunchy Chickpeas (page 79)
SATURDAY	Green Eggs and Ham Frittata (page 64)	BBQ Grilled Chicken (page 181) and Harvest Kale Salad with Goat Cheese and Dried Cranberries (page 118)	Salmon Tostada Salad (page 167)	Chili-Spiced Fruit Cups (page 273), Crunchy Chickpeas (page 79)
SUNDAY	Leftover Green Eggs and Ham Frittata (page 64)	Leftover Salmon Tostada Salad (page 167)	Leftover BBQ Grilled Chicken (page 181) and Harvest Kale Salad with Goat Cheese and Dried Cranberries (page 118)	Chili-Spiced Fruit Cups (page 273), Crunchy Chickpeas (page 79)

WEEKLY MEAL PREP

On the Sunday before the week begins, prepare the following items:

Sweet Potato Crust Quiche: Make the entire recipe. Let cool, slice into portions, and store in separate sealed containers in the refrigerator. Reheat when ready to eat.

Chickpea Buddha Bowls: Make the entire recipe, but do not pour the sauce over the bowl. Store the quinoa mixture in separate sealed containers in the refrigerator. Make the almond butter sauce, and store in separate small sealed containers in the refrigerator. Dress with the sauce when ready to eat.

Chili-Spiced Fruit Cups: Make the entire recipe and place in a large sealed container in the refrigerator until ready to eat. Alternatively, once prepared, store in individual portions for an easy grab-and-go snack option.

Crunchy Chickpeas: Make the entire recipe and store in an airtight container in the pantry.

SHOPPING LIST

CANNED AND BOTTLED ITEMS

- Chickpeas, 2 (15.5-ounce) cans
- Tomato, diced, 1 (14.5-ounce) can
- Tomato paste, 1 (6-ounce) can

DAIRY AND EGGS

- Eggs, large (2 dozen)
- Feta (8 ounces)
- Ghee/butter
- Goat cheese (4 ounces)
- Greek yogurt, plain and unsweetened, 1 (32-ounce) container
- Milk (½ gallon)
- Mozzarella (8-ounce block)
- Parmesan cheese, grated

FROZEN FOODS

- Berries, frozen (16 ounces)
- Peas, frozen, 1 (10-ounce) package
- Spinach, frozen, 1 (10-ounce) package

MEAT

- Bacon (4 slices)
- Beef, pan frying (1 pound)
- Chicken breast (1 pound)
- Lamb, ground (1 pound)
- Pork, ground (1 pound)
- Salmon, 4 (6-ounce) fillets

PANTRY ITEMS

- Almond butter
- Almonds
- Apple cider vinegar
- Avocado oil
- Basil
- Cayenne
- Chili powder
- Cinnamon
- Cooking oil spray
- Corn tortillas
- Cornstarch
- Cranberries, dried
- Cumin
- Dijon mustard
- Extra-virgin olive oil
- Garlic powder
- Ginger, fresh
- Honey
- Maple syrup
- Onion powder
- Paprika
- Peanut butter
- Pepitas
- Pepper
- Quinoa (10 ounces)
- Raspberry jelly
- Red pepper flakes
- Salt
- Sesame oil
- Sesame seeds
- Soy sauce
- Sriracha
- Turmeric
- Vanilla or unflavored protein powder
- Walnuts
- White/brown rice

PRODUCE

- Arugula (5-ounce package)
- Avocado (4)
- Bell pepper (3)
- Berries, frozen (16 ounces)
- Carrot (1)
- Cauliflower (2 heads)
- Cilantro, fresh
- Cucumber (1)
- Garlic (2 bulbs)
- Jalapeño (2)
- Kale (5 cups)
- Lemon (3)
- Lettuce, romaine hearts (12 ounces)
- Lime (3)
- Mango (2)
- Mint, fresh
- Onion, green (1 bunch)
- Onion, red (3)
- Onion, yellow (3)
- Pineapple (1)
- Strawberries (1 pint)
- Sweet potato (8)
- Watermelon (1 small)
- Zucchini (1)

Desserts

I am all in favor of treating yourself with some delicious desserts. However, I usually tell my clients that they need to figure out how these desserts fit into their lifestyle. What does that mean? It means that the kind and quantity of dessert must make sense for the individual and his or her goals.

Some people can have a small piece of chocolate daily and it keeps the sugar cravings away but satisfies the mind and body. For others having chocolate daily would open the floodgates, and they may soon be wanting desserts with every meal. While the desserts in this book are consistent with a healthy lifestyle and can even help keep you on track, it may not be in your best interest to eat desserts daily. Find what works for you and indulge as you need to enjoy your life, while also still keeping an eye toward your goals. Remember, balance is key.

A Clean Eating Lifestyle

This clean eating cookbook is meant to show you how to incorporate real food and home cooking into your life in an easy and delicious manner. It is not meant to be a crash diet, cleanse, or a fad. Instead this is a "forever" diet and is meant to be the way that you eat and enjoy food, not the way that you restrict it. While meal plans are helpful to get you started, get you back on track, or keep you on track, you do not need to follow them forever to see results in your health and wellness.

I love using meal planning as a tool to guide me and help me choose recipes that not only make my life easier and less stressful but also make me feel good and give me the energy I need to lead an active and engaged life. Your diet is nothing more than a way you nourish your body. You get to feed yourself, so eat food that is delicious and nutritious. Aside from that, recognize that your diet is more of a lifestyle and, as such, there are other factors like exercise, hydration, sleep, and stress management that can help complete your wellness circle.

EXERCISE

Moving your body is what it's there for! I recommend finding a way to move daily whether it's going for a walk or hike, biking, swimming, lifting weights, or doing yoga. Find ways to move your body that make you feel good and help improve your health. I find that diet and exercise go hand in hand, so move your body and nourish it on repeat.

WATER

While what you eat is important for your health, so is what you drink. Humans cannot live without water, so do not forget to drink a few glasses (if not more) daily. I find carrying a water bottle around with me helps me stay hydrated. A good level of hydration aids digestion and movement. It also improves sleep and boosts your energy levels. Drink up!

SHORTCUTS

I've been meal planning, prepping, and cooking for many years now, but since I've made many mistakes and learned the hard way, I figured I'd help you learn from my trials and tribulations. These are my top five go-to tips, tricks, and shortcuts to meal planning and prepping.

1. Cook once; eat twice (or more). Double a recipe or use a recipe that produces a larger number of servings so that you can have leftovers for the week. I recommend making recipes like Chicken Tortilla Soup (page 109), Easy Apple-Tuna Salad (page 169), and Spinach Meatballs and Zucchini Noodles (page 233), as they make for delicious leftovers.

2. Create a go-to recipe list. I have a list of 10 recipes that I return to regularly, like Sheet Pan Chicken Fajitas (page 183) and Chocolate Chip Cookie Dough Overnight Oats (page 57). I know how to make them, I know what ingredients I need, I know everyone will enjoy them, and I don't have to reinvent the wheel when I cook them.

3. Stock emergency food or meals. I always have back-up foods and meals in the fridge, freezer, and pantry for emergencies. I keep Freezer V-Egg-ie Burritos (page 70) and some other frozen meat and vegetables in my freezer at all times so I don't have to rely on fast food, just (homemade) freezer food. I also stock my pantry with nuts, seeds, canned fish, rice, beans, and pasta for easy snacks and meals.

4. Keep your kitchen appliances up to date. I love having a pressure cooker and air fryer so I can make recipes like Pressure Cooker Chicken Tikka Masala (page 189) and Air-Fryer Sweet Potato Tots (page 94) in a pinch.

5. Buy pre-made items with no shame. If you find that you hate shredding or dicing vegetables for the Apple-Cranberry Slaw (page 116), cooking and cubing chicken for recipes like the Waldorf Chicken Salad (page 175), or ricing cauliflower for the Cauliflower Pizza Crust (page 267), buy them pre-chopped, sliced, or riced so that you can get on with cooking and enjoying your food.

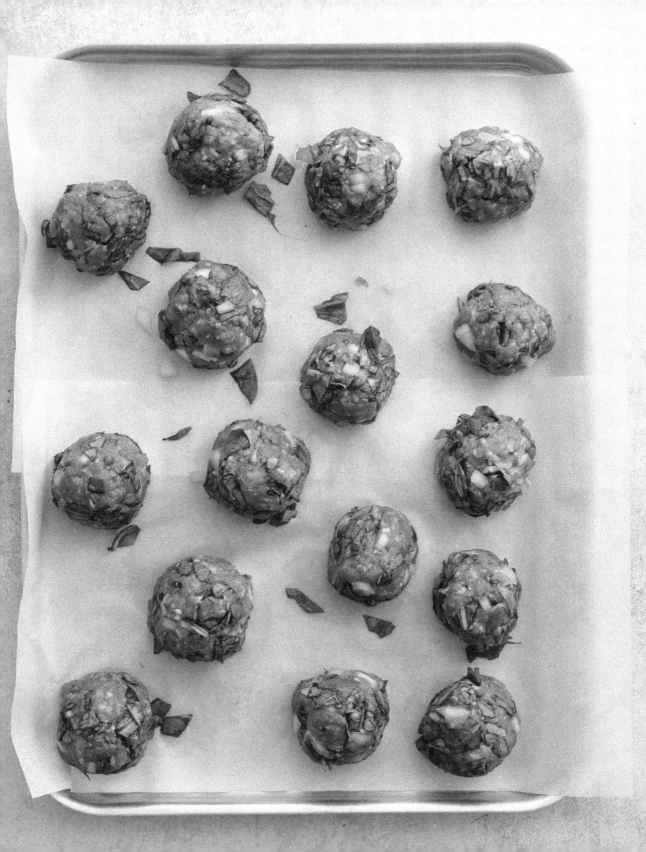

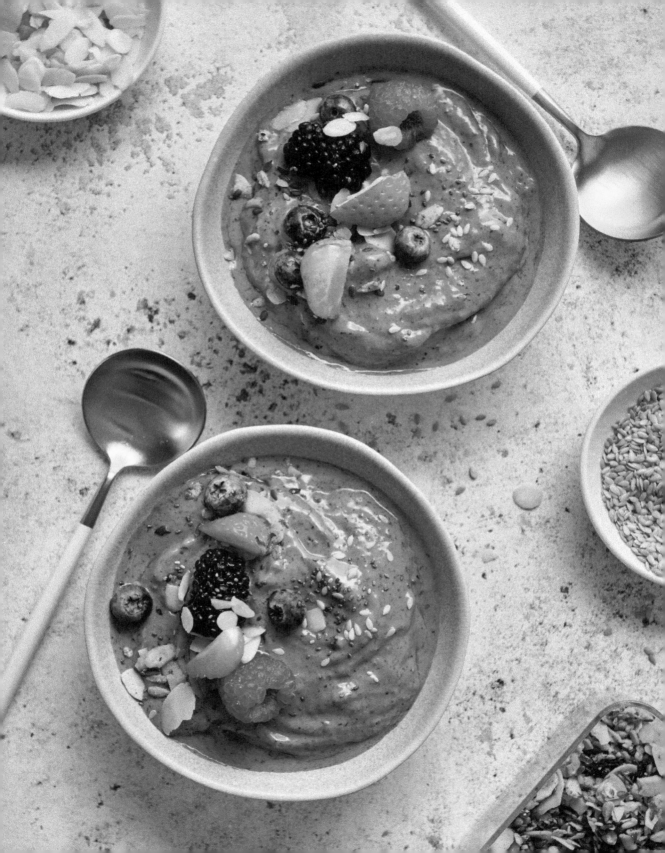

CHAPTER THREE

Breakfast and Smoothies

50 PB and J Protein Smoothie

51 Lemon Meringue Smoothie

52 Quick Vanilla Latte

53 Berry Berry Smoothie Bowl

54 Green Power Smoothie Bowl

55 French Toast Overnight Oats

56 Strawberry Shortcake Overnight Oats

57 Chocolate Chip Cookie Dough Overnight Oats

58 Blueberry-Oat Pancakes

59 Cinnamon Toast Waffles

60 Pumpkin Spice Baked Oatmeal Bars

61 Apple Breakfast Sausage Patties

62 High-Protein Egg Muffins

63 Bacon, Egg, and Cheese Sheet Pan Sandwiches

64 Green Eggs and Ham Frittata

65 Loaded Avocado Toast

67 Green Shakshuka

68 Sweet Potato Crust Quiche

69 Southwest Eggs Benedict on Sweet Potato Toast

70 Freezer V-Egg-ie Burritos

PB and J Protein Smoothie

SERVES: 1 / **PREP TIME:** 5 minutes

5 INGREDIENTS OR LESS, 30 MINUTES OR LESS, QUICK-PREP, VEGETARIAN, GLUTEN-FREE

If you love PB and J as much as I do, you'll love this breakfast shake. It's basically a peanut butter and jelly sandwich reimagined as a quick and easy breakfast smoothie. I lived off of peanut butter and jelly sandwiches as a kid, so this smoothie fills that void for me as an adult. If you like, you can add protein powder to make it a bit more filling. When you are looking for protein powder, pick one with minimal ingredients, like whey protein or egg white protein.

1 cup milk of choice

1 cup frozen berries

1 tablespoon smooth, unsweetened peanut butter

1 tablespoon raspberry jelly

1 scoop vanilla or unflavored protein powder (optional)

1. Place all of the ingredients in a blender and blend on high for 30 seconds or until smooth.

2. Enjoy immediately.

> **INGREDIENT TIP:** When shopping for jelly or jam, read the labels and choose brands that do not contain high-fructose corn syrup.

Per serving: Calories: 385; Total Fat: 17g; Saturated Fat: 6g; Cholesterol: 30mg; Sodium: 165mg; Carbohydrates: 47g; Fiber: 7g; Protein: 13g

Lemon Meringue Smoothie

SERVES: 1 / **PREP TIME:** 5 minutes

5 INGREDIENTS OR LESS, 30 MINUTES OR LESS, QUICK-PREP, VEGETARIAN, NUT-FREE, GLUTEN-FREE

When looking for breakfast ideas, everyone gets stuck sometimes, myself included. Smoothies are an easy way to add variety to your mornings without any fuss. While they are a quick and simple breakfast for a busy morning, they're also a great pre-workout snack or a satisfying dessert. The bright lemon flavor in this one is so refreshing—it tastes just like lemon meringue pie.

1½ cups ice

1 cup milk of choice (or water)

¾ cup plain unsweetened Greek yogurt

1 tablespoon maple syrup

Juice and zest of 1 lemon

1 scoop vanilla or unflavored protein powder (optional)

Place all of the ingredients in a blender and blend on high for 30 seconds or until smooth.

SUBSTITUTION TIP: Use your favorite milk or milk alternative in this smoothie; just opt for an unsweetened variety. Out of milk? Water will do the trick, too.

Per serving: Calories: 379; Total Fat: 18g; Saturated Fat: 12g; Cholesterol: 67mg; Sodium: 219mg; Carbohydrates: 41g; Fiber: 0g; Protein: 15g

Quick Vanilla Latte

SERVES: 1 / **PREP TIME:** 10 minutes

5 INGREDIENTS OR LESS, 30 MINUTES OR LESS, QUICK-PREP, VEGETARIAN, NUT-FREE, GLUTEN-FREE

I might be a coffee snob. I've been known to say, "If you don't like your coffee black, then you don't like coffee." But I make an exception for good lattes. If you find the right coffee and the right milk, you can drink these daily without getting bored. I also love that you do not need a frother, just some good arm muscles (and willpower) to froth up these bad boys. Enjoy with or without collagen (a type of flavorless protein).

4 ounces strong coffee (or 2 to 3 shots espresso)

¾ cup milk of choice

¼ teaspoon pure vanilla extract

1 scoop unflavored collagen peptides (optional)

1. Brew the coffee. Set aside, but keep warm.

2. Pour the milk and vanilla into a 2-cup glass jar (that has a lid, but leave lid off for now).

3. Microwave the milk on high for 2 minutes, checking every 30 seconds to see if hot enough (and to make sure that a film does not form the on top).

4. Remove the milk from the microwave, being careful not to burn yourself if the glass is hot. While the milk is still hot, but the glass is cool enough to handle safely, put the lid on the glass and shake vigorously for 30 seconds.

5. Carefully remove lid, add the coffee and collagen, if using. Replace the lid and shake for an additional 10 to 15 seconds.

INGREDIENT TIP: You can find collagen peptides at your local grocery, vitamin store, or through online at retailers that sell protein powders. Note that collagen is not vegetarian.

Per serving: Calories: 135; Total Fat: 6g; Saturated Fat: 4g; Cholesterol: 22mg; Sodium: 79mg; Carbohydrates: 9g; Fiber: 0g; Protein: 8g

Berry Berry Smoothie Bowl

SERVES: 1 / **PREP TIME:** 5 minutes

5 INGREDIENTS OR LESS, 30 MINUTES OR LESS, QUICK-PREP, VEGETARIAN, GLUTEN-FREE

I love the taste of bananas, but they make my stomach unhappy. Because of that, I have always steered clear of smoothie bowls. But I figured I might as well try one without bananas and see what happened. The result? Deliciousness in a bowl. It tastes just like dessert. I use any combination of fresh or frozen berries I happen to have on hand, including strawberries, raspberries, blueberries, or blackberries. And by all means, feel free to add a banana if you love them and miss the flavor.

1½ cups fresh or frozen berries

½ cup plain unsweetened Greek yogurt

½ cup milk of choice

2 tablespoons peanut butter (or nut or seed butter of choice)

1 scoop vanilla or unflavored protein powder (optional)

Ice (optional)

Berries, chia seeds, flax seeds, granola, sliced almonds, unsweetened shredded coconut, for topping (optional)

1. Place the berries, yogurt, milk, and peanut butter in a blender and blend on high for 30 seconds or until smooth.

2. Add the protein powder and ice, if desired, and blend until smooth.

3. Pour the smoothie into a medium bowl and sprinkle the toppings of your choice over the surface.

> **MAKE-AHEAD TIP:** Measure out all the ingredients and desired toppings the night before. In the morning, combine the ingredients in the blender, blend until smooth, and top with premeasured fruits, nuts, or seeds so you can get you out the door quickly.

Per serving: Calories: 495; Total Fat: 28g; Saturated Fat: 10g; Cholesterol: 40mg; Sodium: 277mg; Carbohydrates: 48g; Fiber: 11g; Protein: 17g

Green Power Smoothie Bowl

SERVES: 1 / **PREP TIME:** 5 minutes

30 MINUTES OR LESS, QUICK-PREP, VEGETARIAN, GLUTEN-FREE

Vegetables are not often the first thing people think of for breakfast, but it doesn't have to be that way. You just have to get creative sometimes. With this smoothie bowl, you can feel good about your day knowing you had vegetables with breakfast. The best part? You can't even tell that this bowl is made with spinach. It's amazing what a little fruit and avocado can do to sweeten and smooth out the flavor of the greens.

3 cups spinach

½ cup milk of choice

½ cup pineapple, chopped

½ cup puréed pumpkin

1 kiwi, peeled
   and chopped

¼ avocado, peeled
   and sliced

2 tablespoons pumpkin
   seed butter (or nut or
   seed butter of choice)

1 scoop vanilla or
   unflavored protein
   powder (optional)

Ice (optional)

Chia seeds, granola, hemp
   seeds, kiwi slices, sliced
   banana, unsweetened
   shredded coconut,
   walnuts, for topping
   (optional)

1. Place the spinach, milk, pineapple, pumpkin, kiwi, avocado, and pumpkin seed butter in a blender and blend on high until smooth.

2. Add the protein powder and ice, if desired, and blend until smooth.

3. Pour the smoothie into a medium bowl and top with the fruits, nuts, or seeds of your choice.

> **SUBSTITUTION NOTE:** Swap a medium banana for the pumpkin purée for a sweeter flavor.

Per serving: Calories: 454; Total Fat: 28g; Saturated Fat: 7g; Cholesterol: 15mg; Sodium: 178mg; Carbohydrates: 48g; Fiber: 13g; Protein: 19g

French Toast Overnight Oats

SERVES: 2 / PREP TIME: 5 minutes, plus 8 hours or overnight to chill

QUICK-PREP, VEGETARIAN, DAIRY-FREE, GLUTEN-FREE

Overnight oats are my jam. They are easy to throw together, and they make me look forward to the morning. After leaving them in the refrigerator overnight, they are the perfect consistency and you can grab them, along with some of your favorite toppings and head out the door. This cold version of oatmeal is incredibly refreshing, and nothing beats it for a fast and filling breakfast. With this for breakfast (which is ready to go when you are), there are no more excuses for giving in to that boring granola bar or unhealthy fast food.

1⅓ cups unsweetened almond milk

1 cup rolled oats

2 tablespoons flax meal

2 tablespoons maple syrup

2 teaspoons chia seeds

1½ teaspoons cinnamon

Fresh berries, maple syrup, or walnuts, for topping (optional)

1. In a medium bowl, combine all of the ingredients (except for the toppings) and mix well.

2. Evenly divide the oatmeal mixture into two 2-cup storage containers with lids.

3. Cover and refrigerate for 8 hours or overnight.

4. In the morning, remove the overnight oats from the refrigerator, add the toppings of your choice, and enjoy.

> **SUBSTITUTION NOTE:** You can swap out the almond milk for any other type of milk, if preferred.

Per serving: Calories: 272; Total Fat: 8g; Saturated Fat: 0g; Cholesterol: 0mg; Sodium: 109mg; Carbohydrates: 45g; Fiber: 8g; Protein: 8g

Strawberry Shortcake Overnight Oats

SERVES: 2 / **PREP TIME:** 5 minutes, plus 8 hours or overnight to chill
QUICK-PREP, VEGETARIAN, NUT-FREE, GLUTEN-FREE

I'm always looking for new ideas when it comes to overnight oats. I usually draw from what's in my pantry and refrigerator or simply what I'm craving. You never have to ask me twice if I want strawberry shortcake, so I decided to make a guilt-free version I could enjoy for breakfast.

1 cup milk

1 cup rolled oats

½ cup small-curd
cottage cheese

2 tablespoons honey

1 tablespoon chia seeds

2 teaspoons strawberry
jam or jelly (optional)

1 teaspoon pure
vanilla extract

1 cup sliced strawberries

1. In a medium bowl, combine the milk, oats, cottage cheese, honey, chia seeds, jam (if desired), and vanilla extract. Mix well.

2. Evenly divide the oatmeal mixture into two 2-cup storage containers with lids.

3. Cover and refrigerate for 8 hours or overnight.

4. In the morning, remove the overnight oats from the refrigerator and top each serving with ½ cup of freshly sliced strawberries.

INGREDIENT TIP: When shopping for jam or jelly, look for a variety that does not contain high-fructose corn syrup. Feel free to omit altogether if you prefer a less-sweet version of overnight oats.

Per serving: Calories: 405; Total Fat: 11g; Saturated Fat: 4g; Cholesterol: 27mg; Sodium: 289mg; Carbohydrates: 61g; Fiber: 8g; Protein: 17g

Chocolate Chip Cookie Dough Overnight Oats

SERVES: 2 / PREP TIME: 5 minutes, plus 8 hours or overnight to chill

QUICK-PREP, VEGETARIAN, GLUTEN-FREE

Who said you can't have cookies for breakfast? While I'm not recommending you go out and buy a box of cookies for your first meal of the day, you shouldn't settle for a boring, tasteless breakfast. I usually make my overnight oats in the nut- or seed-butter jars that are just about empty. The last bit of the nut butter gets incorporated into the oats and it's irresistible. This recipe will leave you wishing you could have breakfast for every meal.

1 cup rolled oats

¾ cup milk

½ cup plain unsweetened Greek yogurt

2 tablespoons Almond Butter (page 252)

2 tablespoons coconut sugar

2 tablespoons dark chocolate chips

1 teaspoon pure vanilla extract

Pinch salt

Coconut flakes, sliced almonds, or walnuts, for topping (optional)

1. In a medium bowl, combine all of the ingredients (except for the toppings) and mix well.

2. Evenly divide the oatmeal mixture into two 2-cup storage containers with lids.

3. Cover and refrigerate for 8 hours or overnight.

4. In the morning, remove the overnight oats from the refrigerator, add the toppings of your choice, and enjoy.

> **SUBSTITUTION TIP:** Nut and seed butters are interchangeable in this recipe, so use whatever you have on hand that has no added sugar. Some possible options include: peanut butter, cashew butter, sunflower seed butter, or pumpkin seed butter.

Per serving: Calories: 480; Total Fat: 23g; Saturated Fat: 8g; Cholesterol: 24mg; Sodium: 161mg; Carbohydrates: 60g; Fiber: 7g; Protein: 13g

Blueberry-Oat Pancakes

SERVES: 4 / PREP TIME: 10 minutes / COOK TIME: 10 minutes
30 MINUTES OR LESS, QUICK-PREP, VEGETARIAN, GLUTEN-FREE

These pancakes are my go-to pre-workout meal. They fill me up, energize me for a hard workout, and taste delicious. Feel free to add syrup or butter on top, but they are sweet enough for most people as is. You can also adjust the fillings to accommodate your preferences or what you have on hand. So if you feel like chocolate chips rather than blueberries, you can add those instead—or better yet, add them both.

2 eggs

1 cup plain unsweetened
   Greek yogurt

¼ cup maple syrup

½ cup milk of choice

1 teaspoon pure
   vanilla extract

1½ cups rolled oats

2 tablespoons flax meal

1 teaspoon
   baking powder

½ teaspoon cinnamon

Pinch salt

1 cup blueberries

Cooking oil spray

1. In a large bowl, whisk the eggs, yogurt, maple syrup, milk, and vanilla until frothy.

2. In a medium bowl, combine the oats, flax meal, baking powder, cinnamon, and salt and stir until well blended.

3. Pour the oat mixture into the wet ingredients and whisk until well combined.

4. Carefully fold the blueberries into the batter.

5. Heat a skillet or griddle over medium heat and coat the cooking surface with the cooking oil spray.

6. Working in batches, drop ¼ cup of the batter onto a hot skillet for each pancake. Cook for 2 to 3 minutes or until bubbles form on the surface of the pancake and begin to pop. Flip the pancake over and cook for another 60 to 90 seconds.

7. Remove from the heat, set aside, and repeat with the remaining batter.

> **MAKE-AHEAD TIP:** Make these ahead for the week for a convenient grab-and-go breakfast or snack. They will keep for 3 to 5 days in a sealed, airtight container in the refrigerator.

Per serving (2 to 3 pancakes): Calories: 316; Total Fat: 11g; Saturated Fat: 4g; Cholesterol: 109mg; Sodium: 130mg; Carbohydrates: 46g; Fiber: 5g; Protein: 11g

Cinnamon Toast Waffles

SERVES: 4 / **PREP TIME:** 10 minutes / **COOK TIME:** 15 minutes
30 MINUTES OR LESS, QUICK-PREP, VEGETARIAN, NUT-FREE

I LOVE waffles because when I have them it usually means it's the weekend—complete with a nice, slow start to my day, sleeping in, and relaxation. However, these can certainly be made ahead of time and frozen to enjoy during the week as well. For a gluten-free version of these waffles, you can make a 1-to-1 substitution of gluten-free flour for the wheat flour in this recipe.

Cooking oil spray

1 cup milk

3 large eggs

¼ cup coconut oil, melted

¼ cup coconut sugar, plus 2 tablespoons for topping (optional)

1 teaspoon pure vanilla extract

2 cups flour

2 teaspoons baking powder

1 teaspoon cinnamon, plus 1 teaspoon, for topping (optional)

Pinch salt

1. Coat a waffle iron with cooking oil spray and preheat for 3 to 5 minutes while preparing the waffle batter.

2. In a large bowl, whisk together the milk, eggs, coconut oil, ¼ cup sugar, and vanilla until frothy.

3. In a medium bowl, mix together the flour, baking powder, 1 teaspoon of cinnamon, and salt.

4. Pour the flour mixture into the milk mixture and whisk into a smooth batter.

5. Drop ¼ cup of batter into each side of the waffle iron.

6. If using, combine the remaining 1 teaspoon of cinnamon and 2 tablespoons of sugar in a small bowl and mix thoroughly. Close the waffle iron briefly, about 1 second, then reopen and sprinkle the waffles with a small amount (a little goes a long way!) of the cinnamon and sugar mixture.

7. Close the waffle iron and cook the waffles until they are cooked through, or per manufacturer instructions.

8. Top the waffles with fresh berries, yogurt, or maple syrup, and sprinkle with the cinnamon or sugar, if using.

Per serving (2 waffles): Calories: 461; Total Fat: 19g; Saturated Fat: 14g; Cholesterol: 147mg; Sodium: 121mg; Carbohydrates: 61g; Fiber: 2g; Protein: 13g

Pumpkin Spice Baked Oatmeal Bars

MAKES: 6 servings / **PREP TIME:** 10 minutes / **COOK TIME:** 45 minutes

QUICK-PREP, VEGETARIAN, GLUTEN-FREE

I'm not going to lie, I'm a fan of pumpkin anything, any time of year. I'm not a fan of overly sweet items, however, so these bars balance the savory taste of pumpkin with just a hint of maple-y sweetness. It doesn't have to be fall to enjoy these bars—but I won't stop you if you make them for an autumn-themed party or even for Thanksgiving. Pumpkin is not only tasty, but also full of vitamins and minerals—a win-win.

Cooking oil spray

2 cups rolled oats

1 teaspoon
baking powder

1 teaspoon cinnamon

Pinch salt

1 cup puréed pumpkin

¾ cup milk of choice

¼ cup maple syrup

1 large egg

1 teaspoon pure
vanilla extract

½ cup walnuts (optional)

1. Preheat the oven to 350°F and coat the inside of an 8-by-8-inch baking dish with cooking oil spray.

2. In a large bowl, mix together the oats, baking powder, cinnamon, and salt.

3. In a medium bowl, combine the pumpkin, milk, maple syrup, egg, and vanilla and stir until well blended and smooth.

4. Add the pumpkin mixture to the dry ingredients and stir until well combined.

5. Fold in the walnuts, if using.

6. Pour the batter into the prepared baking dish and bake in the oven for 45 minutes or until a knife inserted in the center comes out clean. Cut into 12 squares. Store in a sealed, airtight container in the refrigerator until ready to eat, or for up to 5 days.

INGREDIENT TIP: You can certainly buy pumpkin, roast it, and purée it yourself, but canned puréed pumpkin is easy to find and buy year-round. Make sure to read the label and pick one that has only one ingredient listed—pumpkin. Stay away from the similar-looking canned pumpkin pie filling, which is full of sugar.

Per serving (2 bars): Calories: 183; Total Fat: 4g; Saturated Fat: 1g; Cholesterol: 35mg; Sodium: 55mg; Carbohydrates: 32g; Fiber: 4g; Protein: 6g

Apple Breakfast Sausage Patties

SERVES: 4 / **PREP TIME:** 10 minutes / **COOK TIME:** 20 minutes

30 MINUTES OR LESS, QUICK-PREP, NUT-FREE, DAIRY-FREE, GLUTEN-FREE

Protein fills you up in the morning and keeps you going throughout the day, so these sausage patties are a staple for me. They are savory and sweet and pair well with toast and eggs. I sometimes make these ahead of time and freeze them so that I have some quick protein options for lunches or snacks. These are also great on the Bacon, Egg, and Cheese Sheet Pan Sandwiches (page 63).

2 to 3 tablespoons coconut oil, divided

½ cup minced apple

½ cup minced yellow onion

1 pound ground pork

1 teaspoon ground cinnamon

½ teaspoon garlic powder

½ teaspoon salt

¼ teaspoon ground black pepper

1. In a large skillet, heat 1 tablespoon of the oil over medium heat. Add the apple and the onion and sauté until soft, 3 to 5 minutes.

2. Meanwhile, in a medium bowl, mix ground pork with the cinnamon, garlic powder, salt, and black pepper. Set aside.

3. Remove the apples and onions from the heat and let cool for 5 minutes.

4. When cool, mix the apples and onions into pork mixture and form 12 even-size patties.

5. Heat 1 tablespoon of oil in the skillet over medium heat and add the patties in batches, cooking 4 to 5 minutes per side or until internal temperature reaches 160°F and the centers are no longer pink.

SUBSTITUTION NOTE: Use any ground meat (such as beef, bison, chicken, or turkey) in this recipe, as desired. You may need to use more or less oil to fry them, depending on the fat content of the meat. Leaner meats will require more oil.

Per serving (3 sausages): Calories: 376; Total Fat: 31g; Saturated Fat: 15g; Cholesterol: 82mg; Sodium: 355mg; Carbohydrates: 5g; Fiber: 1g; Protein: 19g

High-Protein Egg Muffins

SERVES: 6 / **PREP TIME:** 10 minutes / **COOK TIME:** 20 minutes
30 MINUTES OR LESS, QUICK-PREP, VEGETARIAN, NUT-FREE, GLUTEN-FREE

Egg muffins are what get me through stressful and busy weeks. I make a batch or two, freeze them, and then pull them out as needed to make sure that I have an easy and tasty option for breakfast. The best part is that you can vary the recipe by adding whatever fresh or frozen vegetables you have on hand, including broccoli, mushrooms, onions, or bell peppers.

Cooking oil spray

8 large eggs

½ cup plain unsweetened Greek yogurt

½ teaspoon salt

¼ teaspoon black pepper

½ cup Cheddar cheese, shredded

2 cups chopped raw vegetables

1. Preheat the oven to 350°F and coat the muffin cups of a 12-cup muffin tin with cooking oil spray.

2. In a large bowl, whisk the eggs, Greek yogurt, salt, and pepper until no large clumps are visible and the eggs are frothy.

3. Fold the cheese into the egg mixture and set aside.

4. Distribute the vegetables evenly among the muffin cups.

5. Pour about ¼ cup of the egg over the vegetables in each muffin cup.

6. Bake for 20 minutes or until cooked through.

> **SUBSTITUTION TIP:** Replace the yogurt with cottage cheese for a heartier flavor.

Per serving (2 muffins): Calories: 161; Total Fat: 11g; Saturated Fat: 5g; Cholesterol: 262mg; Sodium: 367mg; Carbohydrates: 3g; Fiber: 1g; Protein: 12g

Bacon, Egg, and Cheese Sheet Pan Sandwiches

SERVES: 6 / **PREP TIME:** 10 minutes / **COOK TIME:** 20 minutes
30 MINUTES OR LESS, QUICK-PREP

Bacon, egg, and cheese sandwiches were my favorite post-swim workout meal in college—when, of course, I never had time to make them and bought the fast-food versions. Making food at home can not only save money but also time in the long run. This dish is easy to make, delicious, and easy to customize to your liking—just add the toppings and spices that you most enjoy.

1 to 2 teaspoons bacon grease or oil of choice

12 large eggs

½ cup unsweetened almond milk

½ cup Cheddar cheese, shredded

¼ teaspoon ground black pepper

6 slices cooked bacon, crumbled

6 English muffins, sliced in half and toasted

Arugula, sliced avocado, sliced cheese, and sliced tomato, for topping (optional)

1. Preheat the oven to 400°F. Lightly coat a rimmed 18-by-13-inch baking sheet with bacon grease.

2. In a large bowl, whisk together the eggs, almond milk, cheese, and black pepper. Stir in the crumbled bacon.

3. Carefully pour the egg mixture into the baking sheet and then gently place the baking sheet in the oven. Bake for 15 to 20 minutes, or until the eggs in the center of the pan are cooked through.

4. Allow the eggs to cool then cut into 6 squares.

5. Make the sandwiches by placing the egg on top of half of a toasted English muffin. Add the toppings of your choice and top with the other half of the English muffin.

MAKE-AHEAD NOTE: You can make these ahead of time by freezing the cooked egg pieces inside an un-toasted English muffin, then, when ready to eat, microwave or toast the egg muffin and fill with toppings of your choice.

Per serving: Calories: 361; Total Fat: 18g; Saturated Fat: 7g; Cholesterol: 393mg; Sodium: 571mg; Carbohydrates: 25g; Fiber: 1g; Protein: 22g

Green Eggs and Ham Frittata

SERVES: 6 / **PREP TIME:** 10 minutes / **COOK TIME:** 25 minutes
QUICK-PREP, NUT-FREE, GLUTEN-FREE

Once in kindergarten or preschool, I remember that one day the snack theme was Green Eggs and Ham—and I refused to eat it. I'm not really sure why, maybe the green eggs alarmed me—but this adult version can be enjoyed without the fear of green food dye coming anywhere near the frittata.

6 large eggs

¼ cup Parmesan cheese, grated

¼ teaspoon black pepper

4 bacon slices

1 yellow onion, chopped

4 garlic cloves, minced

1 bell pepper, chopped

2 cups frozen chopped spinach or kale

1. Preheat the oven to 350°F.

2. In a medium bowl, whisk together the eggs, Parmesan cheese, and black pepper. Set aside

3. Heat an oven-safe skillet over medium heat.

4. Place the bacon in an oven-safe skillet and cook until crispy. Remove the bacon and place the slices on a paper towel–lined dish. Reserve 1 tablespoon of grease from the skillet. Safely dispose of any additional grease.

5. Return the reserved bacon grease to the skillet and heat it over medium heat. Add the onion and garlic and sauté for 2 to 3 minutes.

6. Add the bell pepper and spinach and cook until the spinach is heated through.

7. Pour the egg mixture over the vegetables and stir to combine so vegetables are spread out evenly.

8. Place the skillet in the oven and bake the frittata for 15 minutes, or until the center is cooked through.

9. Slice into 6 equal slices.

Per serving: Calories: 151; Total Fat: 8g; Saturated Fat: 3g; Cholesterol: 196mg; Sodium: 288mg; Carbohydrates: 8g; Fiber: 3g; Protein: 12g

Loaded Avocado Toast

SERVES: 2 / **PREP TIME:** 10 minutes / **COOK TIME:** 10 minutes
5 INGREDIENTS OR LESS, 30 MINUTES OR LESS, QUICK-PREP, VEGETARIAN, NUT-FREE, DAIRY-FREE

I have a reputation for putting an egg on everything. This avocado toast, however, needs and calls for an egg on top. Both the toast and the avocado are great soaker-uppers of the egg yolks, and once you finish you will be wishing for more, just as I do every time I have this dish. I can eat this for breakfast, lunch, or even dinner. It is one of my favorite go-to meals.

2 slices bread

½ avocado, smashed

1 tablespoon hemp or
  flax seed

2 slices tomato

2 Poached Eggs (page 248)

Salt

Pepper

Hot sauce (optional)

1. Toast the bread until golden brown.

2. Spread the smashed avocado evenly on the toast, sprinkle the seeds over the avocado, then press them into the avocado with the back of a fork.

3. Top each slice of toast with 1 slice of tomato and 1 poached egg.

4. Sprinkle salt and pepper and drizzle on hot sauce, if desired.

> **INGREDIENT TIP:** Buy avocados based on when you will use them. If you need them immediately, make sure you can press into the skin (not too far) with your thumb. If you need them to be ripe in a few days, buy ones that are hard so they won't be overripe when you need them.

Per serving: Calories: 288; Total Fat: 15g; Saturated Fat: 3g; Cholesterol: 211mg; Sodium: 323mg; Carbohydrates: 27g; Fiber: 9g; Protein: 15g

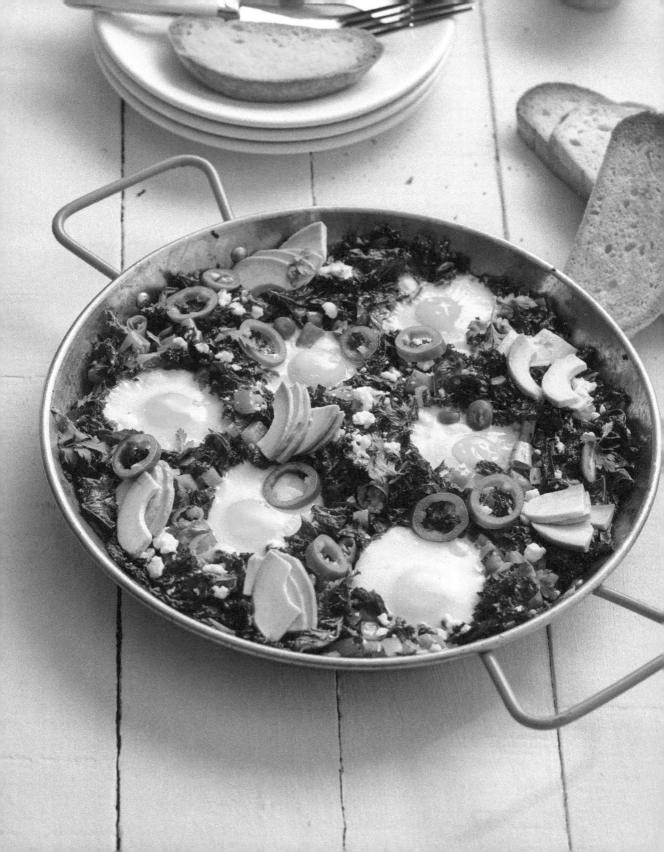

Green Shakshuka

SERVES: 6 / **PREP TIME:** 10 minutes / **COOK TIME:** 20 minutes
ONE-POT, 30 MINUTES OR LESS, QUICK-PREP, VEGETARIAN, NUT-FREE, GLUTEN-FREE

Shakshuka is a great recipe for a crowd. I make this when having friends over for brunch and it's always a hit. I usually make a traditional red shakshuka, but this green one is my new favorite variation. You can crack more eggs in it if you are using a large enough skillet. It's great on its own or served with toast.

1 tablespoon extra-virgin olive oil

1 yellow onion, chopped

1 green bell pepper, chopped

3 garlic cloves, minced

4 cups chopped kale

¼ cup fresh parsley, chopped

1 (7-ounce) can mild green chiles

6 large eggs

6 ounces feta, crumbled

1 avocado, sliced for topping

1 jalapeño, seeded and sliced in rings for topping

1. Preheat the oven to 375°F.

2. In a large oven-safe skillet, heat the oil over medium heat, then add the onion and sauté for 3 minutes, or until the onion starts to become translucent.

3. Add the green pepper and garlic and sauté for another 2 to 3 minutes.

4. Add the kale, parsley, and green chiles, stirring until the kale is wilted. Remove the skillet from the heat.

5. Make 6 wells in the pepper-and-onion mixture with a spatula.

6. Gently crack 1 egg into each well.

7. Place the skillet in the oven and bake for 10 minutes, or until the whites of the eggs are set and no longer translucent.

8. Serve with the crumbled feta, sliced avocado, and jalapeño rings on top.

> **SUBSTITUTION TIP:** If you don't have a cast iron or oven-safe skillet, transfer all of the ingredients to an oven-safe baking dish before step 5, then proceed with the recipe as directed.

Per serving: Calories: 261; Total Fat: 18g; Saturated Fat: 7g; Cholesterol: 211mg; Sodium: 499mg; Carbohydrates: 14g; Fiber: 5g; Protein: 13g

Sweet Potato Crust Quiche

SERVES: 6 / **PREP TIME:** 15 minutes / **COOK TIME:** 60 minutes

VEGETARIAN, NUT-FREE, GLUTEN-FREE

There are endless ways to make eggs, so when you think you're tired of making them, think again. This quiche is simple to make and even simpler to eat. When slicing the potatoes, make sure to use a sharp knife and slice evenly so that they are all cooked through at the same time.

FOR THE CRUST

Cooking oil spray

1 large (16- to 20-ounce) sweet potato, sliced into ⅛-inch slices

Salt

Pepper

FOR THE FILLING

1 tablespoon olive oil

1 small onion, chopped

2 garlic cloves, minced

1 bell pepper, chopped

6 large eggs

½ cup milk

2 teaspoons dried basil

Salt

Pepper

Red pepper flakes (optional)

½ cup shredded mozzarella cheese

1 cup chopped kale

TO MAKE THE CRUST

1. Preheat the oven to 350°F.

2. Spray the inside of a 9-inch round pan or pie dish with cooking oil spray. Place the sweet potatoes in the pan overlapping in tight concentric circles on the bottom and sides of pan. Sprinkle the potatoes with salt and pepper. Lightly coat the top of sweet potatoes with cooking oil spray.

3. Bake for 30 minutes or until tender. Note that the sweet potato will shrink somewhat.

TO MAKE THE FILLING

1. While the crust is cooking, heat the olive oil in a medium saucepan. Add the onion and garlic and cook for 1 minute, or until translucent. Add the bell pepper and cook for 3 to 4 minutes more, or until the bell pepper is tender. Turn heat to low.

2. In medium bowl, whisk together the eggs, milk, basil, salt, pepper, and red pepper flakes, if desired. Combine the egg mixture with the peppers and onions. Add the cheese and kale and stir.

3. Pour the egg mixture on top of the crust and bake for 30 minutes or until eggs are fully cooked. Slice into 6 pieces.

> **VARIATION TIP:** Change up the flavor by adding different vegetables or cheeses. Some combinations include: mushrooms and Gouda cheese or spinach with tomatoes and Cheddar cheese.

Per serving: Calories: 214; Total Fat: 10g; Saturated Fat: 3g; Cholesterol: 193mg; Sodium: 190mg; Carbohydrates: 21g; Fiber: 3g; Protein: 11g

Southwest Eggs Benedict on Sweet Potato Toast

SERVES: 4 / **PREP TIME:** 10 minutes / **COOK TIME:** 10 minutes

30 MINUTES OR LESS, QUICK-PREP, VEGETARIAN, NUT-FREE, DAIRY-FREE, GLUTEN-FREE

I love eggs, it's no lie. I usually save eggs Benedict for when I go out to brunch with friends, but when I found out how to make this easy no-cook version of hollandaise at home, I decided to try making it on my own. While I'll continue to order it when I go out to eat, now I can enjoy it from the comfort of my own home—and so can you.

FOR THE HOLLANDAISE

½ cup Homemade Mayo
   (page 254)

1 tablespoon lemon juice

1 teaspoon Dijon mustard

2 tablespoons Ghee
   (page 251), melted

¼ teaspoon salt, plus more
   for sweet potatoes

¼ teaspoon cayenne

Pinch pepper, plus more
   for sweet potatoes

FOR THE SWEET
   POTATO TOAST

1 to 2 sweet potatoes,
   sliced into four
   ½-inch slices

Olive oil

¼ cup guacamole or
   mashed avocado

1 tomato, sliced

4 Poached Eggs (page 248)

TO MAKE THE HOLLANDAISE

In a medium bowl, make the hollandaise by whisking together the mayonnaise, lemon juice, mustard, ghee, salt, cayenne, and pepper. Set aside.

TO MAKE THE SWEET POTATO TOAST

1. Put the sweet potato slices on a plate and heat them for 2 minutes in microwave, flipping halfway through cooking.

2. Remove and brush the sweet potatoes with olive oil, salt, and pepper, then toast in a toaster oven or under the broiler until soft on inside, about 5 minutes.

3. Assemble the sweet potato toast by topping each piece of sweet potato with 1 tablespoon of guacamole, 1 slice of tomato, 1 poached egg, and 1 to 2 tablespoons of hollandaise.

MAKE-AHEAD TIP: Make the hollandaise beforehand and keep stored in a sealed container in the refrigerator for up to a week.

Per serving: Calories: 378; Total Fat: 30g; Saturated Fat: 8g; Cholesterol: 241mg; Sodium: 468mg; Carbohydrates: 16g; Fiber: 3g; Protein: 8g

Freezer V-Egg-ie Burritos

SERVES: 4 / **PREP TIME:** 10 minutes / **COOK TIME:** 20 minutes
30 MINUTES OR LESS, QUICK-PREP, VEGETARIAN, NUT-FREE

Making food ahead of time for the week to come—or beyond—can ensure that you have healthy food on your plate at all times. When you are thinking of how you can set yourself up for success, these burritos are the perfect meal to make far in advance.

FOR THE VEGETABLES

1 tablespoon olive oil

4 garlic cloves, minced

1 yellow onion, chopped

1 bell pepper, chopped

1 medium sweet
  potato, diced

½ teaspoon paprika

½ teaspoon garlic powder

Salt

Pepper

FOR THE EGGS

8 eggs

Pinch paprika

Salt

Pepper

1 tablespoon water

1 cup shredded
  Cheddar cheese

FOR THE BURRITOS

4 large burrito wraps

TO MAKE THE VEGETABLES

1. In a large skillet, heat the oil over medium heat. Add the garlic, onion, bell pepper, and sweet potato and stir.

2. Cover and cook for 10 minutes, or until the potato is fork-tender. Add the paprika, garlic powder, salt, and pepper and stir so that all vegetables are evenly seasoned. Transfer the vegetables to a large bowl and set aside.

TO MAKE THE EGGS

1. In a medium bowl, whisk together the eggs, spices, and water until frothy.

2. Return the skillet to heat (add an extra teaspoon of oil if dry). Add the eggs to the skillet and stir constantly until they are just cooked. Stir in the cheese. Continue stirring until the cheese is melted. Remove from the heat.

TO MAKE THE BURRITOS

1. Prepare the burritos by spreading ¼ of the vegetables and ¼ of the eggs on each wrap. Fold the left and right sides of the wrap toward the middle, then (starting with end closest to you) roll the burrito up tightly.

2. To freeze, let the burritos cool to room temperature; wrap each burrito tightly with plastic wrap or parchment paper and then wrap again with aluminum foil. Place in the freezer and, when ready to eat, remove the burrito from both wraps and microwave for 60 seconds or until warm. Alternatively, you can warm the burrito in the oven or a toaster oven. Top with avocado and hot sauce.

INGREDIENT TIP: A flour tortilla works best for this as it tends to be more pliable and hold up better. However, if you prefer, you can find a gluten-free version as well—just make sure it's burrito size.

Per serving: Calories: 556; Total Fat: 29g; Saturated Fat: 11g; Cholesterol: 401mg; Sodium: 723mg; Carbohydrates: 49g; Fiber: 3g; Protein: 26g

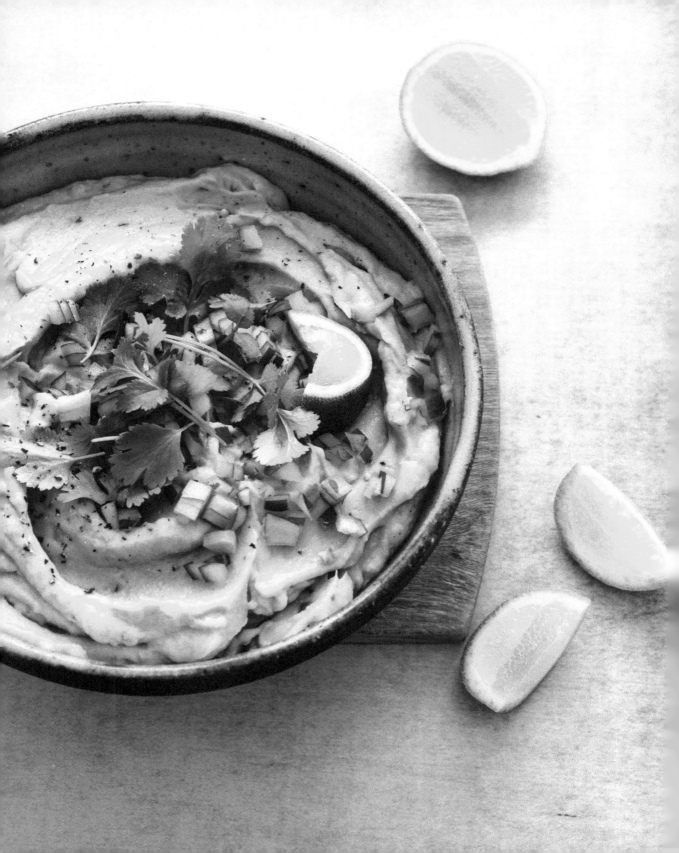

CHAPTER FOUR

Snacks and Sides

74 Cinnamon
    Apple Chips

75 Parmesan Crisps

76 Chili-Lime Popcorn

77 Crispy Garlic-
    Rosemary
    Potato Wedges

79 Crunchy Chickpeas

80 Sweet 'n' Spicy
    Nuts and Seeds

81 Everything Bagel–
    Seasoned Hard-
    Boiled Eggs

82 Strawberry-
    Jalapeño Salsa

83 Easy Guacamole

84 Caramelized Onion
    and Carrot Hummus

85 Cookie Dough Dip

86 Almond Butter
    Energy Bites

87 Garlic-Dijon
    Asparagus

88 Garlic-Parmesan
    Roasted Broccoli

89 Orange-Balsamic
    Brussels Sprouts

90 Buffalo
    Cauliflower Bites

91 Mashed Parmesan
    Cauliflower

92 Cilantro-Lime
    Cauliflower Rice

93 Turmeric Rice

94 Air-Fryer Sweet
    Potato Tots

Easy Guacamole, Page 83

Cinnamon Apple Chips

SERVES: 4 / **PREP TIME:** 10 minutes / **COOK TIME:** 3 to 4 hours
5 INGREDIENTS OR LESS, QUICK-PREP, VEGETARIAN, NUT-FREE, DAIRY-FREE, GLUTEN-FREE

Living in upstate New York means that there is a plethora of apples year-round. Sometimes I get sick of eating apples and applesauce, so I make apple chips to change up the texture. These are easy to make, but do take some time to cook, so make them while you have something else to keep you busy.

3 apples, cored and
  sliced thin

1 teaspoon cinnamon

1. Preheat the oven to 200°F. Line a baking sheet with parchment paper.

2. Toss the apples in a bowl with the cinnamon until evenly coated.

3. Place the apple slices in a single layer on the baking sheet. Bake for 1½ hours, then flip the apple slices and bake for an additional 1½ to 2 hours until the apples are crispy.

> **TECHNIQUE TIP:** To make the apples crispier, place a cooling rack on top of the baking sheet and place apples on top of cooling rack.

Per serving: Calories: 73; Total Fat: 0g; Saturated Fat: 0g; Cholesterol: 0mg; Sodium: 2mg; Carbohydrates: 19g; Fiber: 4g; Protein: 0g

Parmesan Crisps

MAKES: 8 crisps / **PREP TIME:** 5 minutes / **COOK TIME:** 5 minutes
ONE-POT, 5 INGREDIENTS OR LESS, 30 MINUTES OR LESS, QUICK-PREP, VEGETARIAN, NUT-FREE, GLUTEN-FREE

My mom used to make these as snacks for us when we were kids. I had no idea how fancy and ahead of her times she was. Now they sell crisps like this in the store. I suggest making them at home as an appetizer for yourself as you're cooking up dinner. They are delicious and take no time at all to make.

½ cup shredded
    Parmesan cheese

½ teaspoon black pepper

1. Preheat the oven to 400°F. Line a baking sheet with parchment paper.

2. Drop 1 tablespoon of cheese at a time on the baking sheet to form 8 small mounds, spacing each mound at least 1 inch apart. Sprinkle each mound of cheese with a pinch of pepper.

3. Press down on each mound gently with your hand.

4. Bake for 3 to 5 minutes or until crispy.

Per serving (1 crisp): Calories: 28; Total Fat: 2g; Saturated Fat: 1g; Cholesterol: 6mg; Sodium: 100mg; Carbohydrates: 0g; Fiber: 0g; Protein: 2g

Chili-Lime Popcorn

SERVES: 4 / **PREP TIME:** 5 minutes / **COOK TIME:** 5 minutes

5 INGREDIENTS OR LESS, 30 MINUTES OR LESS, QUICK-PREP, VEGETARIAN, NUT-FREE, DAIRY-FREE, GLUTEN-FREE

I used to put Old Bay spice on my popcorn and, while I don't do that much anymore, I am digging this new chili-lime combo on the popcorn. It gives some heat to an otherwise salty dish. Making popcorn on the stovetop is easy and takes only minutes. This is great for an appetizer, after-dinner snack, or as an accompaniment to a movie night.

3 tablespoons coconut oil

½ cup popcorn kernels

½ teaspoon chili powder

Juice of ½ lime

Pinch salt

Red pepper flakes
  (optional)

1. In a large pot, heat the oil over medium heat until glistening.

2. Test the heat by adding 2 to 3 kernels to the pan until one pops.

3. Add the remaining popcorn kernels, cover and cook until popping stops, shaking the pan intermittently to prevent burning.

4. Remove from the heat and transfer the popcorn to a large bowl. Toss the popcorn with chili powder, lime juice, salt, and red pepper flakes, if using.

VARIATION TIP: Make this with garlic powder, onion powder, or other spices of your choice to change up the taste.

Per serving: Calories: 165; Total Fat: 18g; Saturated Fat: 10g; Cholesterol: 0mg; Sodium: 42mg; Carbohydrates: 17g; Fiber: 5g; Protein: 2g

Crispy Garlic-Rosemary Potato Wedges

SERVES: 4 / **PREP TIME:** 10 minutes / **COOK TIME:** 35 minutes
5 INGREDIENTS OR LESS, QUICK-PREP, VEGETARIAN, NUT-FREE, DAIRY-FREE

Rosemary was meant for potatoes, I'm convinced. While I love it on many other foods, I find myself time and time again dressing my potatoes with rosemary and garlic. These are a great side dish for any meat dish or even a change up from normal fries with a burger.

2 pounds russet potatoes, washed and cut into wedges

2 tablespoons olive oil

3 garlic cloves, minced

½ teaspoon salt

¼ teaspoon pepper

2 tablespoons fresh rosemary

1. Preheat the oven to 425°F. Line one or two baking sheets with parchment paper.

2. In a large bowl, toss the potatoes with the olive oil, garlic, salt, pepper, and rosemary.

3. Spread the potatoes evenly on the baking sheet(s) in a single layer. Bake for 35 minutes turning halfway through.

> **VARIATION TIP:** If you have an air fryer, you can make these in batches. Cook them at 400°F for about 15 minutes per batch.

Per serving: Calories: 233; Total Fat: 7g; Saturated Fat: 1g; Cholesterol: 0mg; Sodium: 291mg; Carbohydrates: 41g; Fiber: 3g; Protein: 5g

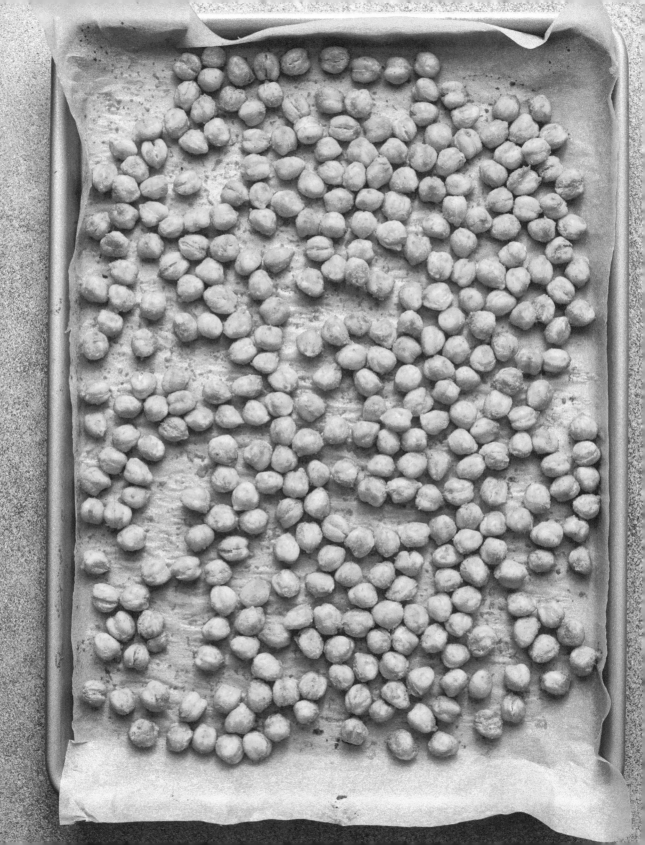

Crunchy Chickpeas

SERVES: 6 / **PREP TIME:** 5 minutes / **COOK TIME:** 45 minutes

5 INGREDIENTS OR LESS, QUICK-PREP, VEGETARIAN, NUT-FREE, DAIRY-FREE, GLUTEN-FREE

I once had crunchy chickpeas at an expo I attended, and I was immediately hooked. It's a crunchy snack that you can have on its own or use as a topping for things like quinoa bowls or salads. I keep a jar of these in my pantry, but they never last long, because I'm constantly sneaking a taste.

1 (15.5-ounce) can chickpeas, drained, rinsed, and dried

1 tablespoon olive oil

½ teaspoon salt

½ teaspoon paprika

¼ teaspoon onion powder

¼ teaspoon garlic powder

Pinch black pepper

1. Preheat the oven to 350°F. Line a baking sheet with parchment paper.

2. Make sure the chickpeas are thoroughly dried. Discard any skins that come off during drying.

3. In a medium bowl, toss the chickpeas with the oil and salt.

4. Spread the chickpeas on the baking sheet in a single layer. Bake for 45 minutes or until crispy.

5. Remove the chickpeas from the oven and transfer to a medium bowl. Toss the chickpeas with the paprika, onion powder, garlic powder, and pepper until well coated. Enjoy!

> **VARIATION TIP:** Toss these in cinnamon and sugar instead of the other spices for a sweeter snack.

Per serving: Calories: 100; Total Fat: 4g; Saturated Fat: 0g; Cholesterol: 0mg; Sodium: 197mg; Carbohydrates: 13g; Fiber: 4g; Protein: 4g

Sweet 'n' Spicy Nuts and Seeds

SERVES: 8 / **PREP TIME:** 5 minutes / **COOK TIME:** 25 minutes
30 MINUTES OR LESS, QUICK-PREP, VEGETARIAN, GLUTEN-FREE

I find unflavored nuts and seeds to be boring and not all that enjoyable to eat. I developed this nuts and seeds recipe with the thought that they could be used as a snack all by themselves or as a part of a dish. They aren't too sweet or too spicy but a nice balance of both.

1½ cups walnuts

1½ cups almonds

1 cup pepitas

¼ cup maple syrup

1 tablespoon butter or Ghee (page 251), melted

1 teaspoon paprika

1 teaspoon salt

1 teaspoon cinnamon

1. Preheat the oven to 350°F. Line a baking sheet with parchment paper.

2. In a large bowl, mix together all of the ingredients until the nuts and seeds are coated with the butter and spices.

3. Spread the nuts and seeds on the baking sheet in a single layer. Bake for 20 minutes or until golden brown.

4. Remove from the oven and let the nuts and seeds cool for about 5 minutes. Store in a sealed container in the refrigerator for up to 1 week.

> **SUBSTITUTION TIP:** Make with any combination of nuts and seeds that you like; just maintain the volume (4 cups) to ensure that there is enough butter and spices to cover.

Per serving (½ cup): Calories: 405; Total Fat: 35g; Saturated Fat: 4g; Cholesterol: 4mg; Sodium: 355mg; Carbohydrates: 16g; Fiber: 6g; Protein: 14g

Everything Bagel–Seasoned Hard-Boiled Eggs

SERVES: 6 / **PREP TIME:** 5 minutes / **COOK TIME:** 15 minutes, plus 10 minutes in an ice bath to cool
30 MINUTES OR LESS, QUICK-PREP, VEGETARIAN, DAIRY-FREE, NUT-FREE, GLUTEN-FREE

Hard-boiled eggs are a great snack to have on hand. I cook a batch over the weekend so that they are available for quick snacks or breakfasts whenever I need them during the week. Also, this everything bagel seasoning makes them a bit more interesting and less bland. You can even use this seasoning on other things like scrambled eggs, popcorn, and vegetables if you find you like it.

6 large eggs

1 tablespoon
   sesame seeds

2 teaspoons poppy seeds

1 teaspoon garlic powder

1 teaspoon onion powder

1 teaspoon sea salt

1. In a large stockpot, cover the eggs with 1 inch of water and bring the water to a boil over high heat.

2. Once the water is boiling, cover the pot and remove from the heat. Let the pot sit, covered, for 12 minutes.

3. Meanwhile, in a small bowl, mix together the sesame seeds, poppy seeds, garlic powder, onion powder, and salt. Set aside.

4. Remove the eggs from the water and place in an ice water bath (a bowl with ice and cold water) for 10 minutes to cool.

5. Peel the eggs and dip them in everything bagel seasoning.

> **VARIATION TIP:** If you have a pressure cooker, pour 1 cup of water in the bottom, then place a trivet over the water. Place the eggs on the trivet. Seal the pressure cooker and cook the eggs on manual for 8 minutes. Quick release, then place the eggs in an ice bath for 10 minutes.

Per serving: Calories: 88; Total Fat: 6g; Saturated Fat: 2g; Cholesterol: 186mg; Sodium: 459mg; Carbohydrates: 2g; Fiber: 0g; Protein: 7g

Strawberry-Jalapeño Salsa

SERVES: 8 / **PREP TIME:** 5 minutes

ONE-POT, 5 INGREDIENTS OR LESS, 30 MINUTES OR LESS, QUICK-PREP, VEGETARIAN, NUT-FREE, DAIRY-FREE, GLUTEN-FREE

When strawberries are in season (late spring and early summer), I cannot get enough of them. Who am I kidding? I can't get enough of them all year long. I decided this year to see what kinds of fun and creative recipes I could make with strawberries. I was looking at salsa next to a pint of strawberries and wondered what strawberry salsa would taste like. The verdict? An absolutely delicious mix of spicy and sweet flavors.

1 pint strawberries, chopped, stems removed

½ cup diced red onion

1 jalapeño, seeded and diced

2 tablespoons cilantro, chopped

1 lime, juiced and zested

½ teaspoon salt

½ teaspoon maple syrup (optional)

In a medium bowl, combine all of the ingredients. Chill, covered, in the refrigerator for 2 hours or until ready to serve.

> **INGREDIENT TIP:** If you are a daredevil and like spicy food, leave the seeds in from the jalapeños to turn up the heat.

Per serving: Calories: 20; Total Fat: 0g; Saturated Fat: 0g; Cholesterol: 0mg; Sodium: 146mg; Carbohydrates: 5g; Fiber: 1g; Protein: <1g

Easy Guacamole

SERVES: 6 / **PREP TIME:** 5 minutes

ONE-POT, 5 INGREDIENTS OR LESS, 30 MINUTES OR LESS, QUICK-PREP, VEGETARIAN, NUT-FREE, DAIRY-FREE, GLUTEN-FREE

Everybody loves a good guacamole. Serve it at a party and I guarantee it's the first dish to go. Why? Because freshly made guacamole is the perfect balance of creamy, salty, and spicy. I usually have to double or triple this recipe to ensure that everyone gets enough. You can use it as a dip with vegetables or chips or on top of a burger or salad. Or, if you're like me, just eat it with a spoon.

¼ cup diced red onion

1 jalapeño, seeded and diced

Juice of 2 limes

½ teaspoon salt

¼ teaspoon black pepper

3 avocados, pitted and peel removed

1. In a large bowl, mix together the onion, jalapeño, lime juice, salt, and pepper.

2. Add the avocados. With the back of a fork, mash the avocados with the onion-and-jalapeño mixture until the avocado is relatively smooth and the ingredients are well combined.

3. Taste and add additional salt or pepper, if desired.

> **INGREDIENT TIP:** Try garnishing your guacamole with a little bit of cilantro for some added flavor and color.

> **VARIATION TIP:** Put all of the ingredients in a food processor and blend to make a smoother guacamole.

Per serving: Calories: 151; Total Fat: 13g; Saturated Fat: 2g; Cholesterol: 0mg; Sodium: 201mg; Carbohydrates: 8g; Fiber: 6g; Protein: 2g

Caramelized Onion and Carrot Hummus

MAKES: 10 to 12 servings / **PREP TIME:** 10 minutes / **COOK TIME:** 15 minutes
5 INGREDIENTS OR LESS, 30 MINUTES OR LESS, QUICK-PREP, VEGETARIAN, NUT-FREE, DAIRY-FREE, GLUTEN-FREE

When it comes to snacks, hummus is a shoo-in for me. It's easy to make and even easier to eat. I personally like to eat hummus with sliced carrots, bell peppers, and celery, or on a salad or sandwich. This hummus veers from a traditional garlic or roasted red pepper hummus, but it's just as tasty and will give new life to your snacks, salads, and sandwiches.

¼ cup, plus 1 teaspoon olive oil, divided

1 yellow onion, sliced

1 large carrot, chopped

1 (15-ounce) can chickpeas, drained and rinsed

Juice of 1 lemon

Salt

Pepper

1. In a large skillet, heat 1 teaspoon of the olive oil over medium heat. Add the onion, stirring frequently until caramelized, or 10 to 15 minutes.

2. Transfer the caramelized onion to a food processor or blender and add the carrot, chickpeas, lemon juice, the remaining ¼ cup olive oil, salt, and pepper. Pulse until the hummus is smooth.

3. Serve with sliced vegetables.

VARIATION TIP: If you don't have time for the caramelized onion, omit it and just go with carrot hummus.

Per serving: Calories: 107; Total Fat: 7g; Saturated Fat: 1g; Cholesterol: 0mg; Sodium: 7mg; Carbohydrates: 10g; Fiber: 3g; Protein: 3g

Cookie Dough Dip

SERVES: 4 / **PREP TIME:** 5 minutes

ONE-POT, 5 INGREDIENTS OR LESS, 30 MINUTES OR LESS, QUICK-PREP, VEGETARIAN, GLUTEN-FREE

Greek yogurt is one of my staple snacks. It's versatile, satisfying, and a good base for both savory and sweet recipes. This cookie dough is great on its own but is also good as a side or a dip. I prefer to dip cut up apple slices in it but feel free to use berries, graham crackers, or pretzels to enjoy the dip.

1 cup plain unsweetened Greek yogurt

¼ cup Almond Butter (page 252)

1 tablespoon maple syrup

½ teaspoon pure vanilla extract

Pinch of salt

¼ cup chocolate chips

Fruit for dipping (optional)

1. In a large bowl, use a hand mixer to mix together the Greek yogurt, almond butter, maple syrup, vanilla, and salt until smooth.

2. Fold in the chocolate chips.

3. Enjoy with fruit, vegetables, or by itself.

> **INGREDIENT NOTE:** It may be necessary to melt almond butter for 30 to 60 seconds in the microwave to make the mixing easier.

Per serving: Calories: 238; Total Fat: 17g; Saturated Fat: 6g; Cholesterol: 17mg; Sodium: 89mg; Carbohydrates: 20g; Fiber: 2g; Protein: 6g

Almond Butter Energy Bites

SERVES: 6 / **PREP TIME:** 5 minutes

ONE-POT, 5 INGREDIENTS OR LESS, 30 MINUTES OR LESS, QUICK-PREP, VEGETARIAN, DAIRY-FREE, GLUTEN-FREE

When I started working at a gym, I realized I needed to find a way to pack more convenient snacks. These protein balls were just the thing to keep me satisfied while I was constantly on my feet. They are also a great way to make friends. I make these all the time for parties to share with others because people love any excuse to eat nut butter.

1 cup Almond Butter
  (page 252)
1 cup rolled oats
¼ cup flax meal
¼ cup maple syrup
½ cup chocolate chips

1. In a large bowl, use a large spatula or hand mixer to mix together the almond butter, oats, flax meal, and maple syrup.

2. Fold in the chocolate chips.

3. Roll the dough into 18 golf ball–size balls. Store in a sealed, airtight container in the refrigerator for up to 1 week or in the freezer for up to 1 month.

> **SUBSTITUTION TIP:** Use any type of nut/seed butter, preferably unsweetened.

Per serving (3 bites): Calories: 456; Total Fat: 32g; Saturated Fat: 5g; Cholesterol: 5mg; Sodium: 19mg; Carbohydrates: 40g; Fiber: 6g; Protein: 10g

Garlic-Dijon Asparagus

SERVES: 4 / **PREP TIME:** 10 minutes / **COOK TIME:** 30 minutes
5 INGREDIENTS OR LESS, QUICK-PREP, VEGETARIAN, NUT-FREE, DAIRY-FREE, GLUTEN-FREE

Take your asparagus to the next level with this recipe. I love asparagus, especially in the spring when it's in season. The nice part is you can eat asparagus raw. However, by roasting it, you are just changing the texture and melding flavors together, so don't worry how long you cook it, just make sure you don't burn it.

Cooking oil spray
1 tablespoon olive oil
1 tablespoon Dijon mustard
Juice of ½ lemon
3 garlic cloves, minced
¼ teaspoon salt
¼ teaspoon black pepper
1 pound asparagus, trimmed

1. Preheat the oven to 400°F. Line a baking sheet with aluminum foil and spray the foil with cooking oil spray.

2. In a medium bowl, whisk together the olive oil, mustard, lemon juice, garlic, salt, and pepper.

3. Add the asparagus and gently toss to coat.

4. Lay the asparagus on the baking sheet in a single layer. Roast for 20 to 30 minutes, or until crispy.

> **TECHNIQUE TIP:** If you have a cookie cooling rack, place that over a lined baking sheet and cook the asparagus on top of the rack for a crispier asparagus.

Per serving: Calories: 65; Total Fat: 4g; Saturated Fat: 1g; Cholesterol: 0mg; Sodium: 238mg; Carbohydrates: 6g; Fiber: 2g; Protein: 3g

Garlic-Parmesan Roasted Broccoli

SERVES: 4 / **PREP TIME:** 10 minutes / **COOK TIME:** 30 minutes

ONE-POT, 5 INGREDIENTS OR LESS, QUICK-PREP, VEGETARIAN, NUT-FREE, GLUTEN-FREE

I hear so many people say they only like cheesy broccoli. I'm guessing they mean broccoli that is smothered in a cheese sauce. I developed this recipe with that idea in mind, but I also wanted you to actually see the broccoli and enjoy the bold taste it has to offer. This recipe has enough Parmesan to give the broccoli a little bit of a salty and creamy flavor, but it is not doused in a heavy sauce.

3 heads broccoli, chopped

4 garlic cloves, minced

¼ cup Parmesan cheese, grated

2 tablespoons olive oil

Salt

Pepper

Red pepper flakes (optional)

1. Preheat the oven to 400°F. Line a baking sheet with parchment paper.

2. On the lined baking sheet, mix all of the ingredients together so the broccoli is evenly coated.

3. Spread out the broccoli evenly and bake for 30 minutes, or until crispy.

Per serving: Calories: 221; Total Fat: 10g; Saturated Fat: 2g; Cholesterol: 5mg; Sodium: 240mg; Carbohydrates: 25g; Fiber: 14g; Protein: 16g

Orange-Balsamic Brussels Sprouts

SERVES: 4 / **PREP TIME:** 5 minutes / **COOK TIME:** 30 minutes

5 INGREDIENTS OR LESS, QUICK-PREP, VEGETARIAN, NUT-FREE, DAIRY-FREE, GLUTEN-FREE

When I was growing up, I—like many kids— thought I hated Brussels sprouts. Maybe it's because they are green or that they look like a brain, but either way, I had no idea what I was missing. Once you start roasting and seasoning your Brussels sprouts correctly, they'll become a staple in your household.

1 pound Brussels sprouts, trimmed and halved

2 teaspoons olive oil

Salt

Pepper

Zest and juice of 1 small orange

3 tablespoons balsamic vinegar

1 tablespoon maple syrup

1. Preheat the oven to 400°F. Line a baking sheet with parchment paper.

2. Toss the Brussels sprouts on the baking sheet with the olive oil, salt, and pepper.

3. Roast for 20 to 30 minutes, or until crispy.

4. Meanwhile, in a small saucepan, combine the orange zest, orange juice, balsamic vinegar, and maple syrup and simmer until thickened, about 5 minutes.

5. Once the Brussels sprouts are done, transfer them to a medium bowl and toss them in orange balsamic glaze. Serve.

> **VARIATION TIP:** Add ¼ cup of walnuts at step 5 for an extra crunch.

Per serving: Calories: 99; Total Fat: 3g; Saturated Fat: 0g; Cholesterol: 0mg; Sodium: 33mg; Carbohydrates: 18g; Fiber: 5g; Protein: 4g

Buffalo Cauliflower Bites

SERVES: 4 / **PREP TIME:** 10 minutes / **COOK TIME:** 30 minutes

5 INGREDIENTS OR LESS, QUICK-PREP, VEGETARIAN, NUT-FREE

The nice thing about cauliflower is that it takes on the flavor of whatever you pair it with. In this case, when you pair it with buffalo sauce, it tastes just like your favorite wings but with vegetables instead of chicken. The blue cheese on the end of this was done on a whim because I had some on hand and couldn't resist pairing it with hot sauce. Feel free to sprinkle some sliced green onions on top, too.

½ cup water

½ cup flour

1 teaspoon dried parsley

2 teaspoons garlic powder

1 head
   cauliflower, chopped

⅔ cup hot sauce

¼ cup blue cheese
   crumbles (optional)

Pepper

1. Preheat the oven to 450°F. Line a baking sheet with parchment paper.

2. In large bowl, mix together the water, flour, parsley, and garlic powder.

3. Toss the cauliflower in the flour mixture to coat.

4. Place the cauliflower on a baking sheet in a single layer. Bake for 10 minutes, then flip over. Bake for 5 to 10 minutes more.

5. Remove the cauliflower from the oven and pour the hot sauce over the cauliflower evenly. Return the cauliflower to the oven to bake for an additional 8 to 10 minutes.

6. If desired, top the cauliflower with blue cheese and broil for 1 to 2 minutes. Sprinkle with pepper.

SUBSTITUTION TIP: For a gluten-free version of this dish, you can make a 1-to-1 substitution of gluten-free flour for the wheat flour in this recipe.

Per serving: Calories: 131; Total Fat: 0g; Saturated Fat: 0g; Cholesterol: 0mg; Sodium: 3724mg; Carbohydrates: 19g; Fiber: 4g; Protein: 5g

Mashed Parmesan Cauliflower

SERVES: 4 / **PREP TIME:** 5 minutes / **COOK TIME:** 20 minutes
ONE-POT, 5 INGREDIENTS OR LESS, 30 MINUTES OR LESS, QUICK-PREP, VEGETARIAN, NUT-FREE, GLUTEN-FREE

If you are someone who wants to add more vegetables to your diet but can't figure out how to do so, add in some cauliflower. It is an incredibly versatile vegetable. Feel free to add the spices of your choice to make this dish your own.

1 head
cauliflower, chopped

⅓ cup Easy Broth
(page 253) or water

⅓ cup shredded
Parmesan cheese

1 tablespoon Ghee
(page 251) or butter

2 garlic cloves, minced

¼ teaspoon pepper

Chives (optional)

1. In a large stockpot, combine the cauliflower and the broth and bring to a boil. Reduce the heat to low, cover and simmer for 10 to 15 minutes.

2. Add the cheese, ghee, garlic, pepper, and chives, if using. Use an immersion blender on high for 30 seconds, or until the cauliflower has a creamy consistency similar to mashed potatoes. Alternatively, if you don't have an immersion blender, blend in a blender or food processor in batches as needed.

Per serving: Calories: 98; Total Fat: 5g; Saturated Fat: 3g; Cholesterol: 12mg; Sodium: 161mg; Carbohydrates: 9g; Fiber: 4g; Protein: 5g

Cilantro-Lime Cauliflower Rice

SERVES: 4 / **PREP TIME:** 5 minutes / **COOK TIME:** 10 minutes

5 INGREDIENTS OR LESS, 30 MINUTES OR LESS, QUICK-PREP, VEGETARIAN, NUT-FREE, DAIRY-FREE, GLUTEN-FREE

I often get bored with rice, and cauliflower rice is just the thing to fix that. I'm not going to lie, I sometimes buy pre-riced cauliflower from the produce or frozen foods aisle to save time and, of course, cleanup. I encourage you to do what works best for you.

1 head cauliflower, chopped

1 tablespoon olive oil

Juice of 1 lime

¼ cup cilantro, chopped

Salt

1. Place the cauliflower in a food processor and pulse until the cauliflower is in small, rice-like pieces. Alternatively, if you do not have a food processor, mince the cauliflower.

2. In a large skillet, heat the oil over medium heat. Add the cauliflower and sauté for 3 to 5 minutes.

3. Remove the cauliflower from the heat and add the lime, cilantro, and salt.

Per serving: Calories: 70; Total Fat: 4g; Saturated Fat: 0g; Cholesterol: 0mg; Sodium: 43mg; Carbohydrates: 8g; Fiber: 4g; Protein: 3g

Turmeric Rice

SERVES: 4 / **PREP TIME:** 5 minutes / **COOK TIME:** 30 minutes
ONE-POT, 5 INGREDIENTS OR LESS, QUICK-PREP, VEGETARIAN, NUT-FREE, DAIRY-FREE, GLUTEN-FREE

A few years ago, I had turmeric rice for the first time when I was out to eat at a Mediterranean restaurant. It was so good that I had to figure out how to make it myself. Turns out it's not hard at all; you make the rice and then simply add the spices to it. Serve this lovely, fragrant rice when you want to take your meal up a notch.

1 cup long-grain white rice

2 cups Easy Broth (page 253) or water

2 teaspoons ground turmeric

1 teaspoon olive oil

½ teaspoon salt

1. Put the rice in a medium saucepan and cover with broth.

2. Bring the rice to a boil over high heat. Once it is at a full boil, reduce the heat to low, cover, and cook for 20 minutes.

3. Remove the rice from the heat and let it rest for 10 minutes.

4. Fluff the rice with a fork and gently mix in the turmeric, olive oil, and salt.

MAKE-AHEAD TIP: Make this rice ahead of time in a pressure cooker or rice cooker and then mix in oil and spices when you are ready to eat.

Per serving: Calories: 192; Total Fat: 1g; Saturated Fat: 0g; Cholesterol: 0mg; Sodium: 364mg; Carbohydrates: 40g; Fiber: 2g; Protein: 4g

Air-Fryer Sweet Potato Tots

SERVES: 4 / **PREP TIME:** 5 minutes / **COOK TIME:** 25 minutes

5 INGREDIENTS OR LESS, 30 MINUTES OR LESS, QUICK PREP, VEGETARIAN, NUT-FREE, DAIRY-FREE, GLUTEN-FREE

I love sweet potatoes and probably eat them most days of the week. These tots are a treat and are crispy on the outside and soft on the inside. They are just the right amount of sweet and can be paired with any dinner or maybe even dessert. Honestly, they're so good that it's hard to get them to the dinner table, because I end up eating them as I make them.

Cooking oil spray

1 (10- to 12-ounce) sweet potato, peeled

1 teaspoon cornstarch (or more as needed)

½ teaspoon cinnamon, plus 1 teaspoon (optional)

Pinch salt

1 to 2 tablespoons coconut sugar (optional)

1. Preheat the air fryer for 2 to 3 minutes at 400°F. Spray the bottom of the air-fryer insert with cooking oil spray.

2. Meanwhile, wrap the sweet potato in a damp paper towel and cook it in the microwave on high for 4 to 5 minutes until soft. Remove and let cool.

3. Using a cheese grater (or grater attachment on food processor), grate the sweet potato into a large bowl.

4. Add the cornstarch and ½ teaspoon of cinnamon to grated sweet potato and stir to combine.

5. Form the sweet potato mixture into thumb-size tots.

6. In a small dish, combine 1 teaspoon of cinnamon and the sugar, if using. Roll each tot in the cinnamon and sugar.

7. Working in batches, place the tots in the bottom of the basket of the air fryer and cook for 15 minutes, shaking the basket halfway through.

VARIATION TIP: Don't have an air fryer? That's okay, you can bake these in the oven on a baking sheet lined with parchment paper for 15 to 20 minutes, or until crispy on the outside (you may also need to broil for 1 to 2 minutes at the end).

Per serving: Calories: 64; Total Fat: 0g; Saturated Fat: 0g; Cholesterol: 0mg; Sodium: 78mg; Carbohydrates: 15g; Fiber: 2g; Protein: 1g

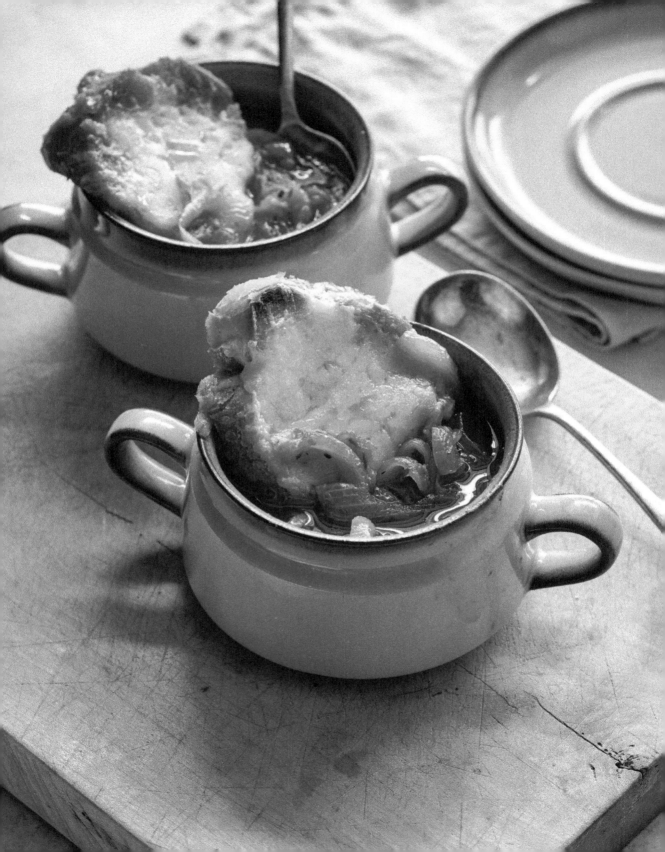

CHAPTER FIVE

Soups and Salads

98 Watermelon Gazpacho

99 Simple French Onion Soup

100 Easy Stovetop Phở

101 Creamy Garlic Cauliflower Soup

102 Homemade Cream of Mushroom Soup

104 Loaded Baked Potato Soup

105 Roasted Red Pepper Soup and Ricotta Cheeseballs

106 Classic Minestrone

107 Lemon Lentil Soup

108 Crab Bisque

109 Chicken Tortilla Soup

110 Strawberry–Goat Cheese Salad

111 Avocado-Cucumber-Feta Salad

113 Orange-Beet-Arugula Salad

114 Chopped Caprese Salad

115 Mexican Street Corn Salad

116 Apple-Cranberry Slaw

117 Broccoli-Walnut Salad with Dried Cherries

118 Harvest Kale Salad with Goat Cheese and Dried Cranberries

119 Quinoa Tabbouleh

Watermelon Gazpacho

SERVES: 4 / PREP TIME: 10 minutes

30 MINUTES OR LESS, QUICK-PREP, VEGETARIAN, NUT-FREE, DAIRY-FREE, GLUTEN-FREE

When watermelon is in season, it is the most refreshing fruit there is, probably because it is mostly made of water. This gazpacho, a cold soup, is not only easy to make but also easy to eat. It can be served as a side dish on a warm summer evening or can be the main attraction of a nice refreshing lunch. Try topping it with some crumbled feta cheese.

4 cups watermelon, cubed

1 small red onion, chopped

1 cucumber, chopped

2 tomatoes, chopped

1 red or green bell pepper, chopped

4 garlic cloves, smashed

1 tablespoon apple cider vinegar

Salt

Pepper

Chopped avocado, chopped cilantro, chopped cucumber, chopped tomato, and sliced jalapeño, for topping (optional)

1. Put all of the ingredients (except the toppings) into a blender and blend on high for 30 to 60 seconds, pulsing to get all ingredients blended evenly.

2. Pour the gazpacho into a large bowl, cover, and chill for 30 minutes, or until ready to serve.

3. Garnish with toppings of your choice.

> **SUBSTITUTION TIP:** If you don't have apple cider vinegar, you can use white vinegar, lemon juice, or lime juice.

Per serving: Calories: 87; Total Fat: 1g; Saturated Fat: 0g; Cholesterol: 0mg; Sodium: 11mg; Carbohydrates: 21g; Fiber: 3g; Protein: 3g

Simple French Onion Soup

SERVES: 4 / **PREP TIME:** 10 minutes / **COOK TIME:** 45 minutes

QUICK PREP, VEGETARIAN, NUT-FREE

I don't know about you, but I've always loved ordering French onion soup when I go out to eat because it seems like such a hard dish to make at home. But here's the thing: it's surprisingly easy. The most important thing is to make sure you don't burn the onions. Otherwise, it's fairly straightforward, not to mention delicious.

2 tablespoons Ghee (page 251) or butter

4 large sweet onions, peeled and sliced

4 garlic cloves, minced

1 teaspoon dried thyme

¼ teaspoon black pepper

¼ teaspoon salt

6 cups vegetable broth, divided

4 slices day-old bread

4 slices Swiss cheese

1. In a large stockpot, melt the ghee over medium heat. Add the onions, garlic, thyme, pepper, and salt, and cook, stirring occasionally, until the onions are caramelized, about 25 minutes.

2. Add 1 cup of broth to the stockpot and swirl it around to remove any stuck-on onions. Simmer for 2 to 3 minutes.

3. Add the remaining broth and bring the soup to a simmer for 15 minutes.

4. In the oven, broil the bread for 1 minute. Remove the bread from the oven and set aside.

5. Pour the soup into four oven-safe bowls and top each with a slice of toasted bread and a slice of cheese.

6. Place the bowls on a baking sheet for easy handling and carefully slide the baking sheet into the oven. Broil until the cheese is golden and melted, about 1 minute. Carefully remove the sheet pan from the oven. Serve.

> **VARIATION TIP:** If you want to add a layer of flavor, use 1 cup of red wine in place of the 1 cup of broth in step 2 to remove any onions stuck to the side or bottom of the pot.

Per serving: Calories: 367; Total Fat: 17g; Saturated Fat: 10g; Cholesterol: 41mg; Sodium: 1804mg; Carbohydrates: 42g; Fiber: 8g; Protein: 16g

Easy Stovetop Phở

SERVES: 4 / **PREP TIME:** 10 minutes / **COOK TIME:** 35 minutes
ONE-POT, QUICK-PREP, NUT-FREE, DAIRY-FREE

I think my favorite part about cooking phở with friends is that everyone can adapt it to their own specific tastes based on which toppings they use. Feel free to fill your phở with toppings galore or just eat it as is.

1 tablespoon olive oil

1 onion, sliced

5 garlic cloves, peeled and smashed

5 slices fresh ginger, dime size

6 cups vegetable broth

2 cups water

¼ cup soy sauce

1 tablespoon maple syrup

1 tablespoon rice wine vinegar

1 tablespoon fish sauce

1 teaspoon ground black pepper

2 cinnamon sticks

1 tablespoon Sriracha or Gochujang (page 258)

8 ounces mushrooms, sliced

4 cups broccoli florets, chopped

7 ounces dried rice noodles

Salt

Pepper

Cilantro, basil leaves, lime wedges, pea shoots, shredded chicken, sliced green onions, or sliced jalapeños, for topping (optional)

1. In a large stockpot, heat the oil over medium heat. Add the onion, garlic, and ginger and sauté for 3 minutes.

2. Pour in the broth, water, soy sauce, maple syrup, vinegar, and fish sauce. Then, whisk in the pepper, cinnamon, and Sriracha. Bring the soup to a boil.

3. Reduce the heat to low and simmer for 30 minutes.

4. Remove the soup from the heat and strain the broth through a thin mesh strainer. Discard the solids.

5. Return the strained broth to the pot and return it to a simmer. Add the mushrooms, broccoli, and rice noodles and cook for 3 to 5 minutes. You will have to press the noodles down so they become wet and then they will begin to soften and fit in the pot.

6. Taste the broth and add salt and pepper as needed. Divide the phở evenly among four bowls and garnish with toppings of your choice.

> **SUBSTITUTION TIP:** If you don't have fish sauce, either omit it or use extra soy sauce instead.

Per serving: Calories: 293; Total Fat: 5g; Saturated Fat: 1g; Cholesterol: 0mg; Sodium: 2759mg; Carbohydrates: 56g; Fiber: 5g; Protein: 9g

Creamy Garlic Cauliflower Soup

SERVES: 4 / **PREP TIME:** 10 minutes / **COOK TIME:** 20 minutes
ONE-POT, 30 MINUTES OR LESS, QUICK-PREP, VEGETARIAN, NUT-FREE, GLUTEN-FREE

Garlic is a flavor that reminds me of home. It is the first flavor I smell when I begin cooking most of my meals. It's so delightfully aromatic and can make or break many dishes. Garlic, in my opinion, is the star of the show, and frankly if you want to use more than 5 cloves in this recipe, I won't judge you.

2 tablespoons olive oil

1 small yellow onion, chopped

5 garlic cloves, crushed

1 large head cauliflower, chopped

4 cups vegetable broth

1½ cups shredded Cheddar cheese

¼ cup chopped fresh parsley

1 teaspoon salt

½ teaspoon pepper

Red pepper flakes

⅓ cup heavy cream (optional)

Crumbled bacon, Crunchy Chickpeas (page 79), sliced green onion, for topping (optional)

1. In a large stockpot, heat the oil over medium heat. Add the onion and garlic and cook until fragrant, about 3 minutes.

2. Add the cauliflower and cook for 5 minutes more.

3. Pour in the broth and bring the soup to a simmer, turn the heat down, and cook for 10 minutes, or until the cauliflower is soft.

4. Using an immersion blender, blend the soup until smooth. (Alternatively, pour the soup into a blender, blend until smooth, then return the soup to the pot.)

5. Remove from the heat and add the Cheddar cheese, parsley, salt, pepper, and red pepper flakes. Whisk in heavy cream, if using.

6. Garnish with toppings of your choice.

INGREDIENT TIP: If you don't like an extra kick, leave out the red pepper flakes. On the flip side if you love spice, feel free to spice it up with more.

Per serving: Calories: 307; Total Fat: 21g; Saturated Fat: 9g; Cholesterol: 45mg; Sodium: 1858mg; Carbohydrates: 17g; Fiber: 6g; Protein: 15g

Homemade Cream of Mushroom Soup

SERVES: 6 / **PREP TIME:** 10 minutes / **COOK TIME:** 40 minutes
ONE-POT, QUICK-PREP, VEGETARIAN, NUT-FREE, GLUTEN-FREE

I cannot stand soup from a can; I know that probably makes me sound ridiculous but it's true. When you learn how easy and rewarding it is to make soup on your own, you may never go back. This cream of mushroom soup is so hearty and comforting on its own and makes for a great snow day (or any day) treat. You can make this soup with any variety of mushroom you choose. Experiment and find the ones you like best. And try throwing in some crumbled bacon to make it even more delicious.

2 tablespoons extra-virgin olive oil, divided

1 small sweet onion, chopped

4 garlic cloves, minced

24 ounces mushrooms, washed and sliced

1½ cups vegetable broth (or water)

1½ cups milk

1 teaspoon salt

1 tablespoon fresh rosemary

1 teaspoon dried parsley

¼ teaspoon ground black pepper

1. In a large stockpot or Dutch oven, heat the oil over medium heat. Add the onion and sauté for 3 minutes. Add the garlic and sauté for 3 minutes more, or until the onion becomes translucent.

2. Add the mushrooms and stir to coat in olive oil. Sauté for 5 minutes or until mushrooms give off their juice.

3. Reserve 1 cup of mushrooms and set aside.

4. Add the broth and the milk, as well as the salt, rosemary, parsley, and pepper. Increase the heat to high and whisk continuously while the liquid comes to a boil. Then, reduce the heat to low and simmer for 15 minutes.

5. Use an immersion blender to purée the soup (or pour the soup into a blender and purée, then return the puréed soup to the pot).

6. Add the reserved mushrooms back to pot, and bring back to a simmer for 10 minutes, stirring every few minutes.

> **INGREDIENT TIP:** To make this soup dairy-free, use coconut or almond milk instead of cow's milk.

Per serving: Calories: 114; Total Fat: 7g; Saturated Fat: 2g; Cholesterol: 7mg; Sodium: 654mg; Carbohydrates: 9g; Fiber: 2g; Protein: 6g

Loaded Baked Potato Soup

SERVES: 4 / **PREP TIME:** 10 minutes / **COOK TIME:** 35 minutes
ONE-POT, QUICK-PREP, NUT-FREE, GLUTEN-FREE

I don't know about you, but I love loaded baked potatoes. I love them so much, in fact, that one day I got the idea that a soup that tasted like a loaded baked potato would probably be the most comforting meal I could imagine. I'll let you decide if I'm right or not.

4 bacon slices, chopped

1 yellow onion, chopped

4 garlic cloves, minced

2 large russet potatoes, peeled and cut to a 1-inch dice

1 teaspoon garlic powder

1 teaspoon onion powder

2 cups chicken or vegetable broth

2 cups full-fat milk

1 tablespoon Ghee (page 251) or butter

1 cup shredded Cheddar cheese

Sliced green onions (optional)

Salt

Pepper

1. In a large stockpot, cook the bacon over medium heat, stirring until crispy and cooked through.

2. Remove the bacon from the pot and set aside on a paper towel–lined dish.

3. Reserve 2 tablespoons of bacon grease in the pot, and safely discard any remaining grease. Return the reserved bacon grease to the pot and heat it over medium heat.

4. Add the onion and cook for 2 minutes, then add the garlic and potatoes and cook for 2 minutes more.

5. Add the garlic powder and the onion powder.

6. Pour the broth and milk over the vegetables and stir to combine.

7. Bring the soup to a boil, then reduce the heat to low and simmer for 20 minutes, or until the potatoes are fork-tender.

8. You may at this point purée the soup using an immersion blender, or leave it chunky, if you prefer.

9. Stir in the ghee, cheese, bacon, green onions (if using), salt, and pepper.

> **VARIATION:** Make this with sweet potatoes instead for a sweeter soup. Top with Sweet 'n' Spicy Nuts and Seeds (page 80) instead of the cheese and green onions.

Per serving: Calories: 430; Total Fat: 20g; Saturated Fat: 11g; Cholesterol: 65mg; Sodium: 886mg; Carbohydrates: 44g; Fiber: 3g; Protein: 20g

Roasted Red Pepper Soup and Ricotta Cheeseballs

SERVES: 4 / **PREP TIME:** 10 minutes / **COOK TIME:** 30 minutes
QUICK-PREP, VEGETARIAN, NUT-FREE

When I was completing my internship to become a dietitian, my fellow interns and I were asked if we could be any vegetable, what would we be and why? I answered that I would be a roasted red pepper because I'm sweet but also a little spicy. That being said, I do love roasted red peppers and could eat them by the handful. This soup fills that need for me and is paired with ricotta cheese dumplings to boot. I dare you to eat just one bowl.

FOR THE SOUP

1 tablespoon olive oil

1 yellow onion, chopped

4 garlic cloves, chopped

1 large carrot, chopped

1 (12-ounce) jar roasted red peppers, drained

1 (28-ounce) can crushed tomatoes

4 cups vegetable broth

½ cup fresh basil

½ teaspoon onion powder

Pinch red pepper flakes

Salt

Pepper

FOR THE RICOTTA CHEESEBALLS

1 cup full-fat ricotta

1 cup grated Parmesan cheese

½ cup flour

1 large egg

TO MAKE THE SOUP

1. In a large stockpot, heat the oil over medium heat.

2. Add the onion, garlic, and carrot and sauté for 3 to 4 minutes, or until the onion starts to turn translucent.

3. Add the red peppers, tomatoes, broth, basil, onion powder, and red pepper flakes. Stir to combine, then bring to a simmer.

4. Purée the soup using an immersion blender. (Alternatively, pour batches of soup into a blender or food processor and purée on high for 30 seconds, then, after all of the soup is puréed, return it to the pot.) Reduce the heat to low and simmer for 10 minutes to allow the flavors to blend. Season with salt and pepper.

TO MAKE THE RICOTTA CHEESEBALLS

1. In a medium bowl, mix the ricotta with the Parmesan, flour, and egg until a dough forms.

2. Roll the ricotta mixture into ping-pong–size balls. Gently place the ricotta balls in the soup and allow the soup to simmer for 5 to 10 minutes more.

Per serving: Calories: 438; Total Fat: 19g; Saturated Fat: 11g; Cholesterol: 66mg; Sodium: 2234mg; Carbohydrates: 40g; Fiber: 6g; Protein: 25g

Classic Minestrone

SERVES: 4 / **PREP TIME:** 10 minutes / **COOK TIME:** 30 minutes
ONE-POT, QUICK-PREP, VEGETARIAN, NUT-FREE

I love that minestrone is full of vegetables. It's a great way to get a nutrient and fiber boost without feeling like you are skimping on flavor or texture. This soup is great on its own or with pasta—it's up to you to decide on the finishing touches.

1 tablespoon olive oil

1 yellow onion, chopped

1 large carrot, chopped

1 celery stalk, chopped

4 garlic cloves, minced

4 cups vegetable broth

¼ cup tomato paste

1 (28-ounce) can diced tomatoes

1 (15-ounce) can cannellini beans, drained and rinsed

2 cups chopped spinach

2 teaspoons oregano

1 teaspoon thyme

Salt

Pepper

Freshly grated Parmesan

4 cups cooked pasta (optional)

1. In a large stockpot, heat the oil over medium heat. Add the onion, carrot, and celery and sauté for 3 to 5 minutes.

2. Add the garlic and sauté for 1 minute more.

3. Pour in the vegetable broth, then add the tomato paste, diced tomatoes, and beans. Bring the soup to a simmer.

4. Stir in the spinach, oregano, thyme, salt, and pepper, then reduce to the heat to low and cook for 20 minutes.

5. Add the Parmesan and cooked pasta, if desired.

INGREDIENT TIP: You can cook the pasta—I like small shells, orecchiette, or elbows—in the minestrone but may need to add an extra 1 to 2 cups water. Bring the minestrone to a boil, then add the pasta and continue to boil until cooked, about 8 minutes.

Per serving: Calories: 251; Total Fat: 5g; Saturated Fat: 1g; Cholesterol: 0mg; Sodium: 1759mg; Carbohydrates: 42g; Fiber: 11g; Protein: 11g

Lemon Lentil Soup

SERVES: 4 / **PREP TIME:** 10 minutes / **COOK TIME:** 25 minutes
ONE-POT, QUICK-PREP, VEGETARIAN, NUT-FREE, DAIRY-FREE, GLUTEN-FREE

So often people think they need fat, salt, or sugar to make something taste good. But a splash of lemon juice or a bit of lemon zest can be a terrific—and healthy—addition to many recipes. Try adding lemon to some of your favorite dishes, and you'll notice it not only brightens the dish but also draws out the flavor. This soup is no different; the lemon puts a new twist on an old favorite.

1 tablespoon olive oil

1 yellow onion, chopped

2 celery stalks, chopped

4 garlic cloves, minced

4 cups vegetable broth

2 cups water

1½ cups lentils

1 teaspoon curry powder

1 teaspoon turmeric

¼ teaspoon cayenne

Juice and zest of 1 lemon

Salt

Pepper

1. In a large stockpot, heat the oil over medium heat. Add the onion and celery and sauté for 3 minutes, then add the garlic and sauté for 1 minute more, or until the garlic is fragrant.

2. Stir in the broth, water, lentils, curry powder, turmeric, and cayenne until combined. Bring the soup to a boil.

3. Reduce the heat to low, cover, and cook for 15 minutes, stirring occasionally, until the lentils are tender.

4. Using an immersion blender, purée the soup until smooth. (Alternatively, pour batches of the soup into a blender or food processer and blend until smooth, then, after all of the soup is puréed, return the soup to the pot.)

5. Add the lemon juice and zest. Season with salt and pepper.

SUBSTITUTION NOTE: If you don't have vegetable broth, feel free to use Easy Broth (page 253) or store-bought chicken or beef broth in its place.

Per serving: Calories: 297; Total Fat: 5g; Saturated Fat: 1g; Cholesterol: 0mg; Sodium: 977mg; Carbohydrates: 47g; Fiber: 21g; Protein: 19g

Crab Bisque

SERVES: 4 / **PREP TIME:** 10 minutes / **COOK TIME:** 30 minutes
ONE-POT, QUICK-PREP, NUT-FREE, DAIRY-FREE, GLUTEN-FREE

I grew up in Maryland, so you could say that I hold crab near and dear to my heart. The underlying ingredients in this bisque bring out the delicate sweetness of the crab without overpowering it. As an added bonus, this bisque is completely dairy-free. So even though it may seem indulgent, it is in fact a healthy meal.

2 tablespoons avocado oil

1 small red
onion, chopped

2 celery stalks, chopped

4 garlic cloves, minced

1 cup dry white wine

4 cups vegetable or
fish broth

2 tablespoons
tomato paste

1 (14-ounce) can diced
tomatoes

1 cup full-fat coconut milk

1 pound crab claw meat,
drained and checked
for shells

½ teaspoon salt

½ teaspoon
cayenne pepper

¼ teaspoon black pepper

¼ teaspoon celery salt

1. In a medium stockpot, heat the oil over medium heat. Add the onion and sauté for about 3 minutes. Add the celery and garlic and cook for 2 to 3 minutes more. Add the wine and let it simmer for 30 seconds.

2. Pour in the broth, then stir in the tomato paste, tomatoes, and coconut milk.

3. Simmer for 10 minutes, then using an immersion blender, blend on high for 30 seconds until smooth. (Alternatively, pour batches of the soup into a blender or food processer and blend until smooth, then, after all of the soup is puréed, return the soup to the pot.)

4. Add the crab, salt, cayenne, black pepper, and celery salt, and simmer for an additional 10 minutes.

> **SUBSTITUTION TIP:** If you prefer a dairy option, use cow's milk in place of coconut milk and butter in place of avocado oil.

Per serving: Calories: 359; Total Fat: 20g; Saturated Fat: 9g; Cholesterol: 113mg; Sodium: 1668mg; Carbohydrates: 9g; Fiber: 1g; Protein: 25g

Chicken Tortilla Soup

SERVES: 8 / **PREP TIME:** 10 minutes / **COOK TIME:** 6 to 8 hours
ONE-POT, QUICK-PREP, NUT-FREE, DAIRY-FREE, GLUTEN-FREE

I love fix-it-and-forget-it meals. They are easy to prep and make enough food for several meals during the week. There is nothing better than coming home from work to a dinner that is ready for you to eat. My husband requests this soup all the time, because it's easy for him to heat up when I'm away. For dinner, we often pour this soup over rice to make it more filling and to soak up all the juices.

1½ to 2 pounds
chicken breast

4 cups chicken broth

1 yellow onion, diced

2 jalapeño peppers,
seeded and diced

1 green bell
pepper, chopped

2 chipotle peppers (from
a can of chipotles
in adobo) with
½ tablespoon adobo
sauce, puréed

1 (15-ounce) can
black beans, drained
and rinsed

1 (16-ounce) bag frozen
corn kernels

1 (14-ounce) can diced
tomatoes

1½ tablespoons Taco
Seasoning (page 250)

8 corn tortillas, sliced thin
(for garnish)

1 avocado, sliced (for
garnish)

1. Place all of the ingredients, except the corn tortillas and avocado, in a slow cooker and cook on low for 6 to 8 hours (or on high for 4 to 6 hours).

2. Remove the chicken from the pot. Shred the chicken with two forks, then place it back in the soup and stir. Serve topped with sliced corn tortilla strips and avocado slices.

> **SUBSTITUTION TIP:** If you don't already have taco seasoning made up, you can use 2 teaspoons chili powder, 2 teaspoons garlic powder, and ½ teaspoon cayenne powder.

Per serving: Calories: 294; Total Fat: 7g; Saturated Fat: 1g; Cholesterol: 51mg; Sodium: 730mg; Carbohydrates: 38g; Fiber: 8g; Protein: 25g

Strawberry–Goat Cheese Salad

SERVES: 4 / PREP TIME: 10 minutes

ONE-POT, 30 MINUTES OR LESS, QUICK-PREP, VEGETARIAN, GLUTEN-FREE

The combination of strawberries and goat cheese is undeniably delicious. While I could focus on the flavor all day, the nutritive power of this salad is pretty great, too. Strawberries are filled with vitamins and minerals to help keep you fueled and feeling your best. They are sweet without being overly so and they are surprisingly filling.

8 strawberries, sliced

4 ounces goat cheese, crumbled

½ cup sliced red onion

4 cups spinach

½ cup pecan halves

1 cucumber, diced

Maple Vinaigrette (page 260)

1. In a large bowl, combine all of the ingredients except for the dressing and lightly toss, being careful not to let all of the strawberries and nuts sink to the bottom.

2. Dress with maple vinaigrette and enjoy.

> **MAKE-AHEAD TIP:** If you are making this salad ahead of time for lunches or dinners, skip step 2 and wait to dress each individual serving until right before you are ready to eat.

Per serving: Calories: 229; Total Fat: 19g; Saturated Fat: 7g; Cholesterol: 22mg; Sodium: 172mg; Carbohydrates: 9g; Fiber: 4g; Protein: 9g

Avocado-Cucumber-Feta Salad

SERVES: 4 / **PREP TIME:** 5 minutes

ONE-POT, 5 INGREDIENTS OR LESS, 30 MINUTES OR LESS, QUICK-PREP, VEGETARIAN, NUT-FREE, GLUTEN-FREE

This green salad is quick to make and can be served as a side dish or even as a snack. The salt and feta cheese really bring out the flavors of both the avocado and the cucumbers and make it irresistible. I make this salad and throw it on top of greens to make it more robust, but feel free to just eat it as is.

2 avocados, chopped

2 English
  cucumbers, chopped

4 ounces feta cheese,
  crumbled

1 tablespoon olive oil

2 tablespoons lemon juice

½ teaspoon salt

¼ teaspoon pepper

Pinch red pepper flakes
  (optional)

In a large bowl, combine all of the ingredients and refrigerate until ready to serve.

MAKE-AHEAD TIP: Mix up the dressing (olive oil, lemon juice, salt, pepper, and red pepper flakes) separately ahead of time and then toss with freshly chopped cucumber and avocado along with the crumbled feta when ready to eat.

Per serving: Calories: 274; Total Fat: 23g; Saturated Fat: 7g; Cholesterol: 25mg; Sodium: 615mg; Carbohydrates: 14g; Fiber: 6g; Protein: 7g

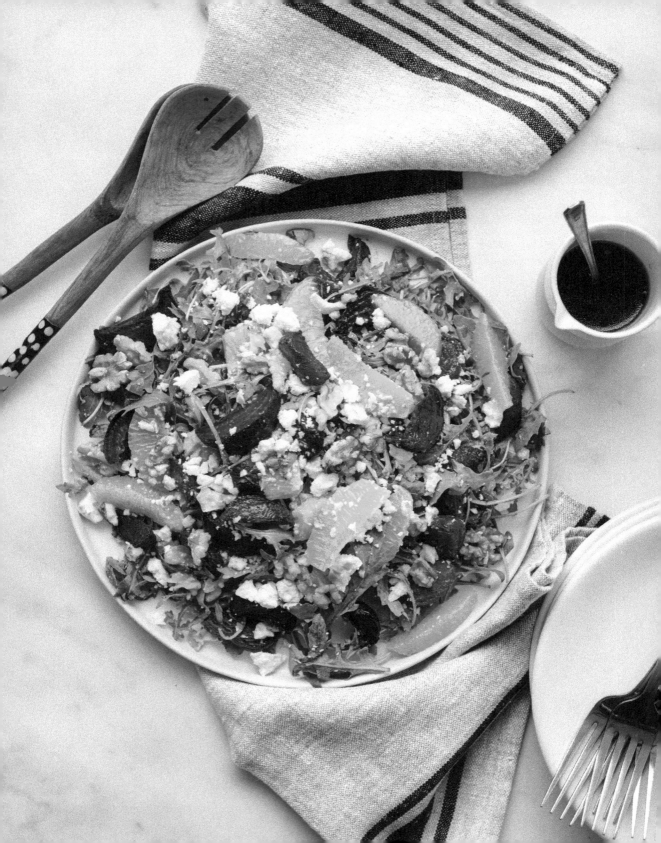

Orange-Beet-Arugula Salad

SERVES: 6 / **PREP TIME:** 15 minutes / **COOK TIME:** 30 minutes
VEGETARIAN, GLUTEN-FREE

This colorful salad can be eaten as is or, for a more substantial meal, can be topped with the protein of your choice. It is also an attention-grabbing side salad at a party or gathering. The oranges add a lovely bright balance to the earthiness of the beets and the peppery-kick of the arugula. With the creamy feta to pull it all together, this recipe is salad heaven.

FOR THE SALAD

4 beets, peeled and chopped

⅔ cup walnuts, chopped

3 ounces feta, crumbled

1 orange, peeled and sliced in rounds

4 cups arugula

FOR THE DRESSING

¼ cup olive oil

2 tablespoons balsamic vinegar

1 tablespoon honey

Salt

Pepper

1. Preheat the oven to 400°F. Line a baking sheet with parchment paper.

2. Spread the beets on the baking sheet in a single layer and bake for 30 minutes, or until fork-tender.

3. Meanwhile, in a small bowl, whisk together all of the ingredients for dressing. Set aside.

4. In a large bowl, combine the walnuts, feta, orange, arugula, and cooked beets.

5. Pour the dressing over the salad and toss, being careful not to let all of the beets, oranges, and walnuts sink to the bottom.

> **VARIATION TIP:** If you are short on time, use peeled and shredded raw beets instead of cooked beets. Or buy pre-cooked beets, chop them, and add to the salad.

Per serving: Calories: 253; Total Fat: 21g; Saturated Fat: 4g; Cholesterol: 13mg; Sodium: 206mg; Carbohydrates: 14g; Fiber: 3g; Protein: 5g

Chopped Caprese Salad

SERVES: 8 / **PREP TIME:** 10 minutes / **COOK TIME:** 10 minutes
30 MINUTES OR LESS, QUICK-PREP, VEGETARIAN, NUT-FREE, GLUTEN-FREE

I'm Italian so it's no surprise that I had to add a caprese salad to the mix. I love the mixture of tomatoes, mozzarella, and basil and thought making it into a chopped version would make it more realistic for your busy life. In this version, instead of worrying about presentation, you can focus on the flavors. If you want to make it ahead of time, chop the tomatoes, mozzarella, and basil and keep them separate in sealed containers in the refrigerator. Mix them together and dress them right before you are ready to eat so you won't have any wilting or soggy ingredients.

10 vine-ripened
    tomatoes, chopped
8 ounces buffalo
    mozzarella, chopped
½ cup basil, chopped
½ teaspoon salt
¼ teaspoon pepper
2 teaspoons olive oil
½ cup balsamic vinegar
2 tablespoons honey

1. In a large bowl, mix together the tomatoes, mozzarella, basil, salt, and pepper. Drizzle with the olive oil and set aside.

2. In a small saucepan, heat the balsamic vinegar and honey over medium-high heat until simmering, reduce the heat to low and simmer for 5 to 10 minutes, or until thickened. Remove from the heat and let cool for 5 minutes.

3. Pour the balsamic glaze over the salad and refrigerate until ready to serve.

> **VARIATION TIP:** You can make this like a traditional caprese salad by slicing the tomatoes and placing the slices on a platter. Top each slice of tomato with a slice of mozzarella and a leaf of basil. Dress with olive oil and the balsamic glaze. Season with salt and pepper.

Per serving: Calories: 127; Total Fat: 6g; Saturated Fat: 3g; Cholesterol: 15mg; Sodium: 189mg; Carbohydrates: 14g; Fiber: 2g; Protein: 7g

Mexican Street Corn Salad

SERVES: 6 / **PREP TIME:** 5 minutes

30 MINUTES OR LESS, QUICK-PREP, VEGETARIAN, NUT-FREE, GLUTEN-FREE

I love corn on the cob but it's not always convenient to eat, and it can be a pain to get all the strands out of your teeth. This salad gives you the sweet taste of corn without the hassle. It is easy to make, and the flavor gets better the more you let the salad sit and marinate. I make it ahead of time and then eat it either with my meals or serve it as an appetizer or salad at parties.

FOR THE SALAD

3 cups fresh or frozen corn kernels

2 medium vine-ripened tomatoes, diced

1 medium avocado, diced

1 red bell pepper, diced

½ cup red onion, chopped

FOR THE DRESSING

2 tablespoons plain unsweetened Greek yogurt

½ cup crumbled Cotija cheese

2 tablespoons lime juice (juice of 1 to 2 limes)

2 tablespoons cilantro

½ teaspoon paprika

¼ teaspoon salt

¼ teaspoon pepper

¼ teaspoon garlic powder

¼ teaspoon cumin

TO MAKE THE SALAD

In a large bowl, mix together the corn, tomatoes, avocado, bell pepper, and onion.

TO MAKE THE DRESSING

1. In a small bowl, combine the yogurt, cheese, lime juice, cilantro, paprika, salt, pepper, garlic powder, and cumin. Mix well.

2. Pour the yogurt dressing over the corn salad and stir to coat evenly.

3. Enjoy immediately or refrigerate in a covered container for 3 to 4 days.

SUBSTITUTION TIP: You can also use fresh corn on the cob, just grill or boil 3 to 4 ears of corn, then use a knife cut the kernels from the cob.

Per serving: Calories: 184; Total Fat: 9g; Saturated Fat: 3g; Cholesterol: 8mg; Sodium: 209mg; Carbohydrates: 22g; Fiber: 5g; Protein: 7g

Apple-Cranberry Slaw

SERVES: 8 / **PREP TIME:** 1 hour

ONE-POT, VEGETARIAN, GLUTEN-FREE

A slaw is the perfect crunchy side dish to go with whatever is on your plate. This one is filled with food you can feel good about. It's a great make-ahead option for the week, as the taste gets even better over time.

2 apples, cored and cut
   into matchsticks

½ head green cabbage,
   sliced thin

2 carrots, shredded

½ red onion, sliced thin

1 cup dried cranberries

1 cup sliced almonds

1 cup plain unsweetened
   Greek yogurt

1 tablespoon olive oil

1 tablespoon apple
   cider vinegar

1 tablespoon honey

½ teaspoon salt

¼ teaspoon pepper

In a large bowl, combine all of the ingredients. Mix well. Refrigerate, covered, for at least 1 hour before serving.

> **SUBSTITUTION TIP:** If you prefer, you can substitute Homemade Mayo (page 254) for the Greek yogurt.

Per serving: Calories: 214; Total Fat: 10g; Saturated Fat: 2g; Cholesterol: 6mg; Sodium: 190mg; Carbohydrates: 29g; Fiber: 5g; Protein: 5g

Broccoli-Walnut Salad with Dried Cherries

SERVES: 8 / **PREP TIME:** 10 minutes

30 MINUTES OR LESS, QUICK-PREP, DAIRY-FREE, GLUTEN-FREE

I used to hate broccoli so much that I used to try to feed it to my dog. My dog also hated broccoli, so the joke was on me. This broccoli salad, however, is now one of my favorite salads. Broccoli doesn't have to be boring. Dress it up with ingredients like walnuts and dried cherries, and all of a sudden broccoli steals the show.

FOR THE SALAD

2 pounds broccoli
    florets, chopped

½ cup red onion, minced

½ cup walnuts, chopped

½ cup dried unsweetened
    cherries, minced

4 slices Crispy Baked
    Bacon (page 198)

FOR THE DRESSING

½ cup extra-virgin olive oil

1 tablespoon apple
    cider vinegar

1 tablespoon
    Dijon mustard

2 tablespoons
    maple syrup

¼ teaspoon salt

¼ teaspoon black pepper

TO MAKE THE SALAD

In a large bowl, mix together the broccoli, onion, walnuts, cherries, and bacon.

TO MAKE THE DRESSING

1. In a small bowl, whisk the olive oil, vinegar, mustard, maple syrup, salt, and pepper.

2. Pour the dressing over the salad and stir to coat all of the ingredients evenly.

> **MAKE-AHEAD TIP:** Make this the night before so that the flavor of the dressing has time to set in. It is a great make-ahead dish for a lunches, parties, or potlucks.

Per serving: Calories: 266; Total Fat: 20g; Saturated Fat: 3g; Cholesterol: 5mg; Sodium: 222mg; Carbohydrates: 18g; Fiber: 5g; Protein: 7g

Harvest Kale Salad with Goat Cheese and Dried Cranberries

SERVES: 8 / **PREP TIME:** 10 minutes / **COOK TIME:** 10 minutes
30 MINUTES OR LESS, QUICK-PREP, VEGETARIAN, GLUTEN-FREE

Kale can be a polarizing green. At first glance it looks tasty, but once you get your hands on it, you realize it is a rather tough green. Instead of trying to chew your way through it, learn how to massage kale to make it an enjoyable experience. All it takes is a little oil and a little acid as well as your hands to help break down the kale so you can fully enjoy its flavor and texture.

2 teaspoons olive oil

4 cups sweet potato or butternut squash, peeled and cut to a ½-inch dice

Salt

Pepper

4 cups chopped kale

¾ cup Maple Vinaigrette (page 260)

4 ounces goat cheese, crumbled

½ cup Sweet 'n' Spicy Nuts and Seeds (page 80)

½ cup dried cranberries

1. In a large skillet, heat the oil over medium heat.

2. Add the sweet potato and cover for 10 minutes, or until fork-tender. Remove from the heat, season the potatoes with salt and pepper, and set aside.

3. Meanwhile, use your hands to massage the kale with the maple vinaigrette for 1 to 2 minutes.

4. Toss the kale with the goat cheese, nuts and seeds, dried cranberries, and cooked sweet potato.

> **VARIATION TIP:** If you don't have time to make the vinaigrette, massage the kale with 1 tablespoon each of olive oil and lemon juice until slightly wilted. Add any dressing of choice to add desired flavor.

Per serving: Calories: 357; Total Fat: 20g; Saturated Fat: 5g; Cholesterol: 12mg; Sodium: 240mg; Carbohydrates: 38g; Fiber: 4g; Protein: 7g

Quinoa Tabbouleh

SERVES: 8 / **PREP TIME:** 10 minutes / **COOK TIME:** 25 minutes
QUICK-PREP, VEGETARIAN, NUT-FREE, GLUTEN-FREE

Quinoa is a higher protein grain, which means it can help keep you full longer. The problem with quinoa is that many people don't know how to make it. I'll let you in on a secret: It's just like making rice. All you have to do is place it in a saucepan with water to cover, bring it to a boil, put a lid on the pan, reduce the heat, and cook on low for 15 to 20 minutes. It's that simple!

1 cup uncooked quinoa

2 cups water

8 ounces cherry tomatoes, quartered

1 cucumber, chopped

1 cup chopped roasted red peppers

4 ounces feta cheese, crumbled

½ cup diced red onion

Juice of 1 lemon

1 tablespoon olive oil

¼ cup parsley fresh, chopped

Salt

Pepper

1. In a medium saucepan, add the quinoa and water and bring to a boil. Cover, reduce the heat to low, and cook for 15 minutes, or until all of the water has been absorbed. Fluff with a fork.

2. In a large bowl, combine the cooked quinoa with the remaining ingredients and mix well.

3. Refrigerate until ready to serve.

MAKE-AHEAD TIP: Make the quinoa ahead of time and refrigerate it in a sealed, airtight container until ready to make the salad or for up to 3 days.

SUBSTITUTION TIP: If you don't have quinoa on hand, try using brown rice, but note that the cooking time will increase since brown rice takes about 20 to 25 minutes longer to cook than quinoa.

Per serving: Calories: 161; Total Fat: 6g; Saturated Fat: 2g; Cholesterol: 13mg; Sodium: 224mg; Carbohydrates: 21g; Fiber: 3g; Protein: 6g

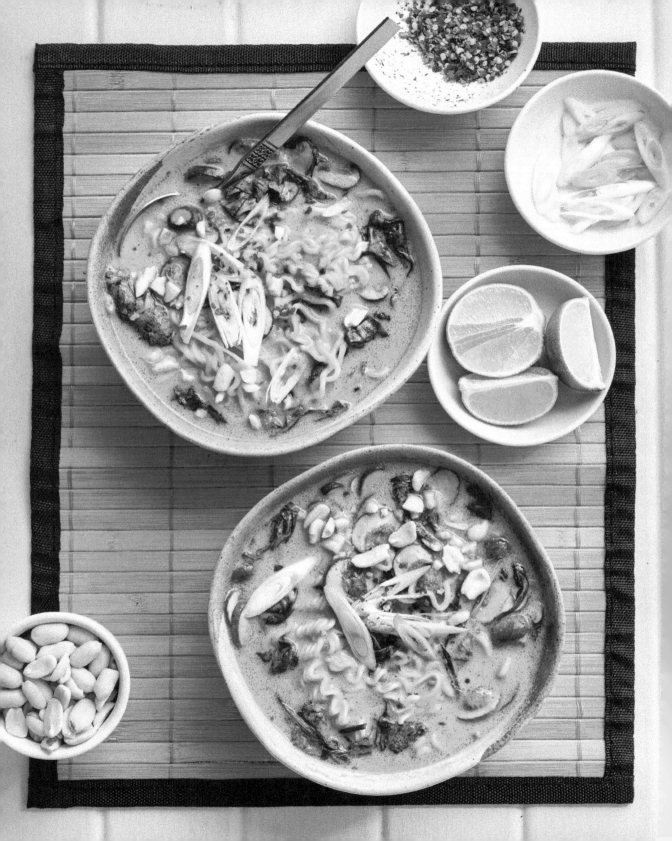

CHAPTER SIX

Vegetarian Mains

122 Portobello Tacos

123 Sweet-and-Sour Eggplant

124 Sheet Pan Eggplant Parmesan

125 Pesto-Baked Cauliflower Steaks

126 Cauliflower Curry

127 Thai Peanut Ramen

128 Roasted Veggie Hummus Panini

129 Beet Burger

130 Tex-Mex Veggie Burger

131 Vegetarian Black Bean Enchiladas

132 Chickpea Tofu Marsala

133 Chickpea Buddha Bowls

135 Power Quinoa Bowl

136 Sesame Tofu and Brussels Sprouts Bowl

138 Grape Leaf Pilaf

139 Vegetable Risotto

140 Spaghetti Squash Primavera

141 Five-Ingredient Veggie Lasagna

142 High Protein Pressure Cooker Mac & Cheese

143 Butternut Squash Mac & Cheese

144 Butternut Squash, Mushroom, and Goat Cheese Cauliflower Pizza

145 Easy Homemade Falafel

Thai Peanut Ramen, Page 127

Portobello Tacos

SERVES: 4 / **PREP TIME:** 10 minutes / **COOK TIME:** 20 minutes
30 MINUTES OR LESS, QUICK-PREP, VEGETARIAN, NUT-FREE, GLUTEN-FREE

Mushrooms get a bad reputation, but I find it's just because they aren't seasoned properly or are often overcooked. Portobellos are meaty enough for this to be a filling meal in its own right. But for those who might be skeptical, I recommend adding some sort of cooked meat like shredded chicken to the mix so you can ease yourself into it.

1 tablespoon olive oil

1 tablespoon Taco Seasoning (page 250)

2 portobello mushroom caps, sliced

2 bell peppers, sliced

1 small red onion, sliced

¼ cup Cotija cheese, crumbled

Juice of 1 lime

8 corn tortillas

2 cups shredded iceberg or romaine lettuce

1 avocado, sliced

1. Preheat the oven to 400°F. Line a baking sheet with parchment paper.

2. In a large bowl, combine the oil and taco seasoning with the mushrooms, peppers, and onion. Toss so that the vegetables are thoroughly coated with the oil and seasoning.

3. Spread the vegetables on baking sheet in a single layer and cook for 20 minutes, or until softened.

4. Remove the vegetables from the oven, then sprinkle with the cheese and lime juice.

5. Divide the vegetable filling among the 8 tortillas and top with the lettuce and avocado.

> **INGREDIENT TIP:** Corn tortillas are best when warmed up first. If you have a gas stovetop, light a burner on the lowest setting and use tongs to place each tortilla over heat for 10 seconds per side. Otherwise, wrap tortillas in a damp paper towels on a plate and microwave for 30 to 60 seconds, or until warm.

Per serving (2 corn tortillas with filling): Calories: 286; Total Fat: 14g; Saturated Fat: 3g; Cholesterol: 7mg; Sodium: 145mg; Carbohydrates: 37g; Fiber: 9g; Protein: 8g

Sweet-and-Sour Eggplant

SERVES: 6 / **PREP TIME:** 10 minutes / **COOK TIME:** 15 minutes
ONE-POT, 30 MINUTES OR LESS, QUICK-PREP, VEGETARIAN, NUT-FREE, DAIRY-FREE

This is a recipe that's outside of the box even for me. It is sweet and spicy and a new way to enjoy eggplant. The nice thing about eggplant is that it holds up well to sauces, and this recipe is no exception. Serve this dish over rice so that the rice can soak up any extra sauce, because it is so good that you don't want to miss out on any of it.

1 tablespoon olive oil

½ yellow onion, diced

3 garlic cloves, minced

1 head broccoli, diced

1 to 2 eggplants, cut to a
   1-inch dice

1 teaspoon fresh
   grated ginger

1 cup Sweet-and-Sour Sauce
   (page 262)

Salt

Pepper

1. In a large skillet, heat the oil over medium heat. Add the onion and garlic and cook for 3 to 5 minutes, or until the onion is translucent. Then add the broccoli and sauté until tender.

2. Add the eggplant and grated ginger to the pan and cook until the eggplant softens, about 5 minutes.

3. Add the sweet-and-sour sauce to the skillet and stir. Bring to a simmer and let cook for 5 minutes, or until the sauce has thickened.

> **SUBSTITUTION TIP:** If you don't have sweet-and-sour sauce ready to go, use a couple of tablespoons each of maple syrup, Sriracha, and soy sauce.

Per serving: Calories: 133; Total Fat: 3g; Saturated Fat: <1g; Cholesterol: 0mg; Sodium: 355mg; Carbohydrates: 29g; Fiber: 5g; Protein: 4g

Sheet Pan Eggplant Parmesan

SERVES: 4 / **PREP TIME:** 10 minutes / **COOK TIME:** 25 minutes

QUICK-PREP, VEGETARIAN, NUT-FREE, GLUTEN-FREE

When I think of eggplant parmesan, I think of a very greasy dish from a classic Italian restaurant that I would go to in college. I didn't particularly love how greasy that dish was, but I liked the basic ingredients. So I developed a recipe that is more about the eggplant than the oil. Enjoy this dish on its own or with a side salad.

1 medium eggplant, cut in 8 (¼-inch) slices

2 tablespoons olive oil

Salt

Pepper

2 cups Homemade Marinara Sauce (page 266) or tomato sauce

8 ounces mozzarella, cut into 8 slices

½ cup shredded Parmesan

½ teaspoon dried basil

1. Preheat the oven to 400°F. Line a baking sheet with parchment paper.

2. Place the eggplant slices on the baking sheet in a single layer and brush them with olive oil on both sides. Season the eggplant with salt and pepper.

3. Bake for 15 minutes.

4. Remove the eggplant from the oven and top each slice with ¼ cup marinara sauce and a slice of mozzarella, then return the baking sheet to the oven and bake for an additional 5 minutes, until the cheese is melted.

5. Meanwhile, in a small bowl, mix the Parmesan with the basil.

6. Remove the eggplant from the oven and sprinkle each slice with the Parmesan and basil mixture. Turn the oven to broil and return the baking sheet to the top rack of the oven. Broil for 1 to 2 minutes.

> **VARIATION TIP:** For a more traditional eggplant parmesan, add 1 cup of bread crumbs into the Parmesan and basil mixture and broil for a minute or two longer, or until the bread crumbs and cheese are golden.

Per serving (2 eggplants): Calories: 225; Total Fat: 15g; Saturated Fat: 7g; Cholesterol: 31mg; Sodium: 332mg; Carbohydrates: 10g; Fiber: 4g; Protein: 11g

Pesto-Baked Cauliflower Steaks

SERVES: 4 / **PREP TIME:** 5 minutes / **COOK TIME:** 30 minutes

ONE-POT, 5 INGREDIENTS OR LESS, QUICK-PREP, VEGETARIAN, DAIRY-FREE, GLUTEN-FREE

While these cauliflower "steaks" have absolutely no meat in them, they do resemble steaks in the way that they are cooked because of how thick you leave them. The pesto gives a nice herb-and-nut flavor to the cauliflower. Feel free to make your own pesto or use your favorite pesto from the market to save time.

2 heads cauliflower, stems removed and sliced into 1-inch steaks/slices

¾ cup Spinach-Walnut Pesto (page 265)

1. Preheat the oven to 400°F. Line a baking sheet with parchment paper.

2. Place the cauliflower steaks on the baking sheet in a single layer. (You may need more than one baking sheet.)

3. Brush half of the pesto on top of steaks and bake for 15 minutes.

4. Flip the steaks and brush on remaining half of the pesto over them and bake for 15 minutes more.

5. Turn the oven to broil and broil for 1 to 2 minutes, or until as crisp as desired.

> **VARIATION TIP:** Garnish with some chopped walnuts for a more exciting texture.

Per serving: Calories: 316; Total Fat: 26g; Saturated Fat: 4g; Cholesterol: 3mg; Sodium: 393mg; Carbohydrates: 39g; Fiber: 8g; Protein: 9g

Cauliflower Curry

SERVES: 4 / **PREP TIME:** 10 minutes / **COOK TIME:** 20 minutes
ONE-POT, 30 MINUTES OR LESS, QUICK-PREP, VEGETARIAN, NUT-FREE, DAIRY-FREE, GLUTEN-FREE

Cauliflower is a meaty, filling vegetable that pairs well with a wide variety of flavors. Cauliflower itself is not all that overpowering, which means it's great for something as strong as curry flavor. This one-pot meal is easy to make and is full of amazing flavors.

1 tablespoon olive oil

1 yellow onion, chopped

3 garlic cloves, minced

1 jalapeño, seeded and diced

1 large head cauliflower, cut into florets

1 (13.5-ounce) can full-fat coconut milk

1 (28-ounce) can diced tomatoes

1 tablespoon curry powder

1 teaspoon cumin

½ teaspoon cinnamon

½ teaspoon turmeric

¼ cup fresh parsley, chopped (optional)

1. In a large stockpot, heat the oil over medium heat. When the oil is shimmering, add the onion and cook for 2 minutes. Then, add the garlic and jalapeño and cook for an additional 2 to 3 minutes.

2. Stir in the cauliflower and sauté for 2 minutes.

3. Pour in the coconut milk, then add the diced tomatoes, curry powder, cumin, cinnamon, and turmeric. Stir.

4. Simmer the curry for 10 minutes, or until the cauliflower is softened. Garnish with the parsley, if using.

Per serving: Calories: 317; Total Fat: 21g; Saturated Fat: 15g; Cholesterol: 0mg; Sodium: 410mg; Carbohydrates: 28g; Fiber: 13g; Protein: 8g

Thai Peanut Ramen

SERVES: 6 / **PREP TIME:** 10 minutes / **COOK TIME:** 20 minutes

ONE-POT, 30 MINUTES OR LESS, QUICK-PREP, VEGETARIAN, DAIRY-FREE

This dish is all about the peanut butter, which makes the broth rich and savory. The nice thing about ramen is the noodles take no time at all to cook. If you want to use this as a make-ahead meal, make the broth ahead of time and then make a quick batch of noodles while you are reheating the broth. Put the cooked noodles into the broth at the same time as you add the spinach and cook just long enough for the spinach to wilt.

1 tablespoon avocado oil

1 tablespoon fresh ginger, minced

3 garlic cloves, minced

2 tablespoons red curry paste

4 cups vegetable broth

1 (13.5-ounce) can coconut milk

⅔ cup unsweetened peanut butter

2 tablespoons soy sauce

2 tablespoons maple syrup

Juice of 1 lime

8 ounces mushrooms, sliced

10 to 12 ounces dry ramen noodles

4 cups baby spinach

Green onions, peanuts, red pepper flakes, for topping (optional)

1. In a large stockpot, heat the oil over medium heat. Add the ginger and garlic and sauté for 3 minutes. Add the curry paste and stir.

2. Pour in the broth and the coconut milk, then add the peanut butter, soy sauce, maple syrup, and lime juice. Whisk to combine.

3. Add the mushrooms and simmer for 10 minutes.

4. Add the ramen noodles and cook until soft, then add the spinach and cook until wilted. Remove the ramen from the heat and serve with an assortment of topping choices.

> **SUBSTITUTION TIP:** Try Almond Butter (page 252) instead of peanut butter for something different. If you can't have gluten, use gluten-free noodles in place of regular noodles.

Per serving: Calories: 537: Total Fat: 30g; Saturated Fat: 13g; Cholesterol: 0mg; Sodium: 1,501mg; Carbohydrates: 53g; Fiber: 11g; Protein: 15g

Roasted Veggie Hummus Panini

MAKES: 4 sandwiches / **PREP TIME:** 10 minutes / **COOK TIME:** 15 minutes
ONE-POT, 30 MINUTES OR LESS, QUICK-PREP, VEGETARIAN, NUT-FREE

Who doesn't love a sandwich, am I right? I love that this sandwich is full of vegetables and packs a punch of flavor. You can certainly add more protein in the form of an egg, turkey, or chicken, but it's already robust. I love the combination of hummus and vegetables. If you have other vegetables on hand that you like to roast, throw them in as well.

1 eggplant, sliced lengthwise (ends removed)

1 yellow squash, sliced lengthwise (ends removed)

1 red bell pepper, sliced

2 tablespoons olive oil, divided

½ teaspoon salt, divided

½ teaspoon pepper, divided

5 garlic cloves, minced

¼ cup hummus

2 ounces goat cheese

8 slices bread, toasted (unless using panini press)

1. Preheat the oven to 450°F. Line a baking sheet with aluminum foil.

2. Place the eggplant, squash, and bell pepper on the baking sheet in a single layer. Brush the surface of the vegetables with the oil, using about 1 tablespoon. Sprinkle half of the salt and pepper over the vegetables.

3. Sprinkle the garlic over the vegetables and roast for 10 minutes. Remove the vegetables from the oven and flip them over. Brush the surface of vegetables with the remaining oil and season with the remaining salt and pepper. Return the vegetables to the oven and cook for 5 minutes.

4. Remove the vegetables from the oven and let cool for 5 minutes.

5. Spread 1 tablespoon of hummus on each slice of bread, then assemble each sandwich using a quarter of the vegetables and ½ ounce of goat cheese.

6. If you have a panini press, press the sandwich; otherwise, eat as is.

Per serving: Calories: 412; Total Fat: 16g; Saturated Fat: 4g; Cholesterol: 11mg; Sodium: 771mg; Carbohydrates: 59g; Fiber: 15g; Protein: 19g

Beet Burger

SERVES: 8 / **PREP TIME:** 10 minutes / **COOK TIME:** 60 minutes

QUICK-PREP, VEGETARIAN, NUT-FREE, DAIRY-FREE

Beets are a hearty root vegetable and the star of this unique recipe. I love the meaty texture and hearty flavor of this burger. The patty mixture is a bit wet when you put it on the baking sheet, but don't worry, they bind and cook up just fine. You can pair these burgers with your favorite toppings, and they are great with a side of Air-Fryer Sweet Potato Tots (page 94).

2 to 3 medium beets, peeled and grated

1 cup rolled oats

¼ cup flax meal

1 large egg

1 (14-ounce) can black beans, drained and rinsed

½ cup roughly chopped yellow onion

2 garlic cloves, peeled and smashed

½ teaspoon salt

¼ teaspoon black pepper

8 hamburger buns

Avocado, lettuce, pickled onion, and tomato, for topping (optional)

1. Preheat the oven to 350°F. Line baking sheet with parchment paper.

2. Shred the beets with a food processor shredding attachment.

3. Remove the shredding attachment and insert the food processor's regular blade. Add the oats, flax meal, egg, black beans, onion, garlic, salt, and pepper to the beets in the bowl of the food processor. Process for 30 seconds, then scrape down the sides of the bowl. Continue to pulse until well combined.

4. Form the patty mixture into 8 patties and place them on the baking sheet. Bake for 25 minutes. Remove from the oven, flip each patty over, then return the baking sheet to the oven and cook for an additional 25 to 30 minutes, or until the outside is slightly golden brown.

5. Serve on a bun with your choice of toppings.

> **VARIATION TIP:** Try these with melted goat cheese and caramelized onions on top.

Per serving: Calories: 300; Total Fat: 4g; Saturated Fat: <1g; Cholesterol: 23mg; Sodium: 469mg; Carbohydrates: 54g; Fiber: 6g; Protein: 11g

Tex-Mex Veggie Burger

SERVES: 8 / **PREP TIME:** 10 minutes / **COOK TIME:** 50 minutes
QUICK-PREP, VEGETARIAN, DAIRY-FREE

These burgers pack a nice spicy (but not too spicy) punch. They may look like chocolate chip cookies when they come out of the oven, but they are an entirely different sort of treat. They have the texture of a burger and the flavor of your favorite Tex-Mex dish. Pair this with some pepper jack cheese, avocado, and maybe some salsa, and you'll have a new favorite burger dish.

1 tablespoon olive oil

1 small red onion, chopped

1 carrot, chopped

1 celery stalk, chopped

2 garlic cloves

1 (15-ounce) can black beans, drained and rinsed

8 ounces mushrooms, roughly chopped

½ cup walnuts

1 tablespoon flax meal

1 large egg

1 tablespoon soy sauce

1 teaspoon chili powder

1 teaspoon cumin

Salt

Pepper

Cooking oil spray

8 hamburger buns (optional)

Lettuce, salsa, sliced avocado, sliced cheese, or tomatoes, for topping (optional)

1. Preheat the oven to 400°F. Line a baking sheet with parchment paper.

2. In a large skillet, heat the oil over medium heat. Add the onion, carrot, celery, and garlic, and sauté for 10 minutes to soften.

3. Transfer the sautéed vegetables to a food processor fit with regular blade. Add the black beans, mushrooms, walnuts, flax meal, egg, soy sauce, chili powder, cumin, salt, and pepper to the food processor and pulse for 30 seconds, then process until smooth, about 30 seconds more.

4. Spray the parchment paper-lined baking sheet with cooking oil spray. Scoop the black bean patty mixture onto the parchment paper, forming 8 patties (the patty mixture will be wet, but that is fine).

5. Spray the top of each patty lightly with cooking oil spray.

6. Bake for 20 minutes. Remove the baking sheet from the oven and gently flip the patties and cook for another 15 minutes. Then turn the oven to broil and broil on high for 2 to 3 minutes or until the outside is crispy.

7. Serve with or without a bun. Garnish with the toppings of your choice.

Per serving: Calories: 135; Total Fat: 7g; Saturated Fat: 1g; Cholesterol: 23mg; Sodium: 140mg; Carbohydrates: 13g; Fiber: 4g; Protein: 6g

Vegetarian Black Bean Enchiladas

SERVES: 6 / **PREP TIME:** 20 minutes / **COOK TIME:** 40 minutes
VEGETARIAN, NUT-FREE, DAIRY-FREE, GLUTEN-FREE

You will get your hands dirty making this dish, but I promise you the mess is worth the end result. You may need two baking dishes for this recipe in order to spread out the sauce and tortillas.

1½ cups Enchilada Sauce (page 263), divided

1 tablespoon avocado oil

1 small red onion, chopped

3 garlic cloves, minced

1 red bell pepper, chopped

1 (15-ounce) can black beans, drained and rinsed

1 cup frozen corn kernels

8 ounces mushrooms, sliced

1 tablespoon Taco Seasoning (page 250)

18 corn tortillas

Cilantro-Lime Cauliflower Rice (page 92)

1 cup shredded Cheddar cheese

avocados, cilantro, and limes, for topping (optional)

1. Preheat the oven to 350°F. Put ¼ cup of the enchilada sauce in the bottom of a 13-by-9-inch baking dish and spread the sauce out so it covers the bottom of the dish.

2. In a large skillet, heat the oil over medium heat. Add the onion and garlic and sauté for 2 to 3 minutes, or until the onion starts to turn translucent. Add the bell pepper, black beans, and corn to the skillet and sauté for 2 to 3 minutes.

3. Add the mushrooms and Taco Seasoning and sauté for 2 to 3 minutes.

4. Assemble enchiladas by filling each corn tortilla with about ¼ cup each cauliflower rice and black bean mixture. Roll up each enchilada and place it seam-side down in baking dish.

5. Top enchiladas with the remaining sauce and cheese.

6. Bake for 25 minutes, cover the baking dish with aluminum foil, and bake for 25 minutes more. Remove the foil and bake for 3 to 5 minutes more, or until the cheese is melted.

7. Garnish as desired and serve.

Per serving (3 enchiladas): Calories: 428; Total Fat: 19g; Saturated Fat: 5g; Cholesterol: 17mg; Sodium: 497mg; Carbohydrates: 56g; Fiber: 11g; Protein: 14g

Chickpea Tofu Marsala

SERVES: 4 / **PREP TIME:** 10 minutes, plus 2 hours to press tofu (optional, see tip) / **COOK TIME:** 20 minutes
VEGETARIAN, NUT-FREE, GLUTEN-FREE

I love a good Italian dish and while I often make this with chicken (see chapter 8, page 186) I think this tofu dish is a great alternative. If you can, I highly recommend that you take the time to press your tofu first (see tip) so that it has the chance to soak up as much of the flavor of the dish as possible. You can certainly omit that step but just know it may be a bit more watery and the tofu may absorb less flavor.

¼ cup cornstarch, for dredging, plus 1 tablespoon

16 ounces extra-firm tofu, cut into 8 slices and pressed (see tip)

1 tablespoon olive oil

2 cups sliced mushrooms

1 yellow onion, sliced

1 teaspoon thyme

1 teaspoon oregano

3 garlic cloves, minced

¼ cup Marsala wine

2 cups vegetable broth

1 (15.5-ounce) can chickpeas, drained and rinsed

2 tablespoons butter or Ghee (page 251)

Salt

Pepper

1. Place ¼ cup of cornstarch in a shallow bowl. Dredge the tofu in the cornstarch, shaking any excess back into the bowl.

2. In a large skillet, heat the oil over medium heat until sizzling (but not brown). Sauté the tofu until it is brown on both sides, 2 to 3 minutes per side. Remove the tofu from the skillet and set aside.

3. Add the mushrooms, onion, thyme, and oregano, and sauté for 2 to 3 minutes. Add the garlic and sauté for 1 minute more.

4. Pour in the Marsala and simmer for 3 minutes.

5. Add the remaining 1 tablespoon of cornstarch and mix well. Stir in the broth and the chickpeas.

6. Whisk in the butter and let simmer for 3 to 5 minutes, or until sauce thickens. Add the tofu to the sauce, gently pressing down so it becomes completely immersed.

7. Remove from the heat and serve over rice or pasta.

INGREDIENT TIP: To press the water out of the tofu, unwrap the tofu and slice it into 8 slices. Line a baking sheet with paper towels. Place the tofu slices on the paper towels and cover with another layer of paper towels. Place cutting boards over the top layer of paper towels and rest a weight (like a tea kettle) on top of the cutting boards. Press the tofu for at least 2 hours.

Per serving: Calories: 417; Total Fat: 17g; Saturated Fat: 5g; Cholesterol: 15mg; Sodium: 541mg; Carbohydrates: 42g; Fiber: 8g; Protein: 19g

Chickpea Buddha Bowls

SERVES: 4 / **PREP TIME:** 10 minutes / **COOK TIME:** 15 minutes
30 MINUTES OR LESS, QUICK-PREP, VEGETARIAN, DAIRY-FREE, GLUTEN-FREE

I love bowls because they are so versatile. This chickpea bowl is a classic for me and easy to prep on the weekends. Feel free to make this Buddha bowl your own and fill it with ingredients that excite you. It makes for a delicious lunch or dinner. Feel free to top it with a protein of your choice as well to bulk it up.

FOR THE ALMOND BUTTER SAUCE

¼ cup Almond Butter (page 252)

1 tablespoon maple syrup

½ teaspoon cinnamon

1 teaspoon lemon juice

Water (as necessary for thinning)

FOR THE BOWLS

2 sweet potatoes, cut to a ½-inch dice

2 teaspoons olive oil

1 (15-ounce) can chickpeas, drained and rinsed

½ teaspoon turmeric

1 teaspoon paprika

½ teaspoon salt

¼ teaspoon black pepper

1 teaspoon sesame seeds

6 cups arugula

1 cup cooked quinoa

1 red onion, chopped

1 avocado, sliced

TO MAKE THE ALMOND BUTTER SAUCE

Whisk together all of the ingredients for the sauce and set aside.

TO MAKE THE BOWLS

1. Toss the chopped sweet potatoes in the oil. Place them in a large skillet and cook over medium heat for 3 to 5 minutes. Cover and continue to cook on medium-low for 10 minutes, or until fork-tender. Transfer the potatoes to a large bowl.

2. Add the chickpeas, turmeric, paprika, salt, pepper, and sesame seeds to the sweet potatoes and thoroughly toss.

3. In four large serving bowls, assemble the ingredients. For each bowl include 1½ cups arugula, ¼ cup quinoa, ¼ of the sweet potato and chickpea mixture, ¼ of the red onion, ¼ of the avocado, and finish with ¼ of the almond butter sauce.

MAKE-AHEAD TIP: Assemble the bowls without the sauce and keep them in the refrigerator in four covered containers. Make the sauce ahead of time and add it to the individual serving just before you are ready to eat.

Per serving: Calories: 492; Total Fat: 22g; Saturated Fat: 2g; Cholesterol: 0mg; Sodium: 319mg; Carbohydrates: 65g; Fiber: 15g; Protein: 15g

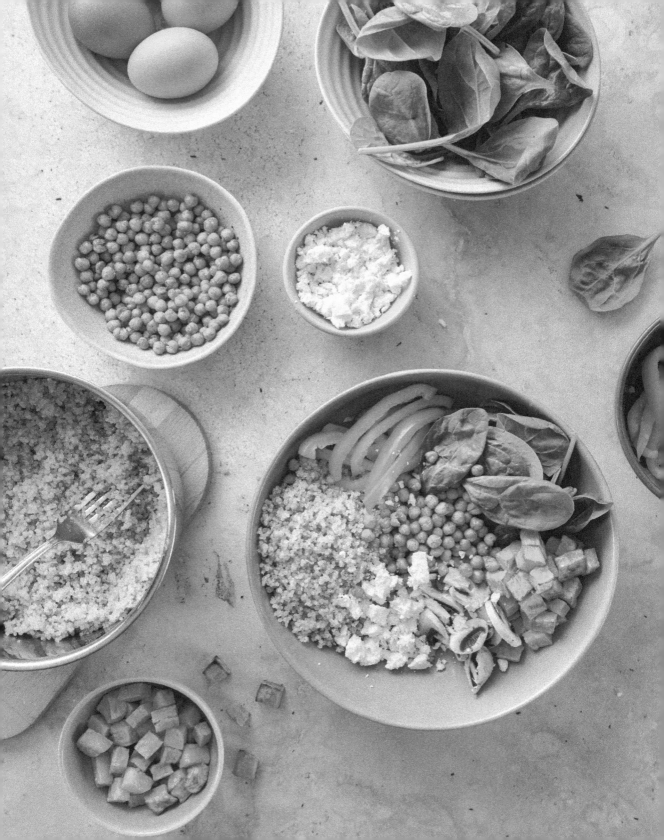

Power Quinoa Bowl

SERVES: 4 / **PREP TIME:** 10 minutes / **COOK TIME:** 30 minutes
QUICK-PREP, VEGETARIAN, NUT-FREE, GLUTEN-FREE

I gain inspiration for recipes from all around me. This one comes from a restaurant I stopped in for lunch one day. I loved how vibrant the bowl was, not to mention that it was delicious and incredibly filling. The quinoa adds volume to the bowl, and the egg—however you like it: hard-boiled, fried, over-easy—is like a savory icing on top.

1 cup uncooked quinoa

2 cups water

1 sweet potato, cut to a
 ½-inch dice

1 tablespoon olive oil

8 cups spinach

2 ounces feta, crumbled

1 red bell pepper, sliced

4 ounces mushrooms,
 sliced

4 eggs, cooked to your liking

1 avocado, sliced

Caramelized Onion and
 Carrot Hummus (page 84)
 (optional)

Crunchy Chickpeas (page 79)
 (optional)

Lemon juice (optional)

Balsamic vinegar (optional)

1. Preheat the oven to 400°F. Line a baking sheet with parchment paper.

2. In a medium saucepan, combine the quinoa and the water and bring to a boil. Cover and reduce the heat to low. Cook for 15 minutes. Remove from the heat and fluff with a fork.

3. Meanwhile, toss the sweet potatoes in olive oil and spread them out on the baking sheet in a single layer. Roast for 30 minutes.

4. In four large serving bowls, assemble the ingredients. For each bowl include 2 cups of spinach, ¾ cup cooked quinoa, ¼ cup sweet potato, ½ ounce feta, ¼ red bell pepper, 1 ounce mushrooms, 1 egg, and ¼ of the sliced avocado. Add 2 tablespoons of the hummus and chickpeas, if using.

5. Squeeze with lemon juice and drizzle with balsamic vinegar, if desired.

> **MAKE-AHEAD TIP:** Make a big batch of quinoa ahead of time and have it ready for this and other meals for the week.

Per serving: Calories: 446; Total Fat: 21g; Saturated Fat: 5g; Cholesterol: 199mg; Sodium: 287mg; Carbohydrates: 49g; Fiber: 9g; Protein: 19g

Sesame Tofu and Brussels Sprouts Bowl

SERVES: 4 / **PREP TIME:** 10 minutes, plus 2 hours to press tofu (optional, see tip) / **COOK TIME:** 30 minutes
VEGETARIAN, NUT-FREE, DAIRY-FREE

Anytime you have a chance to cook something on a sheet pan, do it. Why? Because it makes for an easy cleanup. I love cooking, but the cleanup makes me less than happy at the end. So making a dish like this with impressive flavors and virtually no cleanup is a winner in my book. I make it over the weekend and then I have four meals done for the week. But be warned, this one is a bit spicy!

FOR THE MARINADE

4 garlic cloves, minced

1 tablespoon olive oil

1 tablespoon honey

¼ cup soy sauce

¼ cup Gochujang (page 258)

FOR THE BOWLS

16 ounces extra-firm tofu, pressed (see tip)

1 pound Brussels sprouts, halved

2 cups cooked white rice

1 tablespoon sesame seeds

TO MAKE THE MARINADE

Whisk together all of the ingredients for the marinade. Set aside.

TO MAKE THE BOWLS

1. Press the tofu for 15 minutes or up to 2 hours (see tip). Then cut the tofu into 1-inch cubes.

2. Preheat the oven to 400°F. Line a baking sheet with parchment paper.

3. Gently toss the tofu in marinade. Remove the tofu from the marinade (but keep the marinade for the Brussels sprouts in step 4) and place it on the baking sheet.

4. Toss the Brussels sprouts in the marinade, then remove them from the marinade and spread them out on the baking sheet with the tofu.

5. Bake for 20 minutes. Remove the baking sheet from the oven and gently flip the tofu and the Brussels sprouts. Return the baking sheet to the oven and roast until the tofu is golden brown, about 10 minutes more.

6. Toss in the sesame seeds with the tofu and Brussels sprouts.

7. In four large serving bowls, assemble the ingredients. For each bowl include ½ cup cooked rice, 4 ounces tofu, and 4 ounces Brussels sprouts.

SUBSTITUTION TIP: If you don't have gochujang, use a mild, hot, or chili sauce like Sriracha. Prefer it less spicy? Reduce the amount to 1 to 2 tablespoons of Gochujang (page 258) or Sriracha.

INGREDIENT TIP: To press the water out of the tofu, line a baking sheet with paper towels and place the block of tofu on the paper towels. Cover with another layer of paper towels. Place a cutting board over the top layer of paper towels and rest a weight (like a tea kettle) on top of the cutting board. Press the tofu for at least 15 minutes and up to 2 hours.

Per serving: Calories: 348; Total Fat: 10g; Saturated Fat: 1g; Cholesterol: 0mg; Sodium: 1213mg; Carbohydrates: 48g; Fiber: 6g; Protein: 20g

Grape Leaf Pilaf

SERVES: 4 / **PREP TIME:** 5 minutes / **COOK TIME:** 35 minutes
ONE-POT, QUICK-PREP, VEGETARIAN, NUT-FREE, DAIRY-FREE, GLUTEN-FREE

If you've ever had a dolma (aka stuffed grape leaf), then you know the joy it can bring. I love a stuffed grape leaf but decided I wanted to see what it would be like if I deconstructed it a bit and made it into a rice dish. The results were delicious and so satisfying. The lemon brightens the rice, and the grape leaf adds a hint of bitterness.

1 tablespoon olive oil

1 small yellow onion, diced

4 garlic cloves, diced

1 cup white rice, uncooked

2 cups vegetable broth or water

Juice and zest of 1 lemon

1 teaspoon salt

1 tablespoon fresh mint

1 tablespoon fresh dill

8 to 10 grape leaves, diced

1. In a medium saucepan, heat the oil over medium heat. Add the onion and garlic and sauté for 3 minutes, or until the onion begins to turn translucent.

2. Add the rice and toast it, stirring constantly, for 1 minute.

3. Pour in the broth and bring to a boil. Cover, then reduce the heat to low, and simmer for 20 minutes.

4. Remove from the heat and allow to sit for 10 minutes.

5. Fluff the rice with a fork, then stir in the lemon juice, zest, salt, mint, dill, and diced grape leaves.

INGREDIENT TIP: If you cannot find fresh grape leaves, you can buy them jarred and they work just as well. If you cannot find either, you can use chard instead.

Per serving: Calories: 227; Total Fat: 4g; Saturated Fat: 1g; Cholesterol: 0mg; Sodium: 1055mg; Carbohydrates: 43g; Fiber: 2g; Protein: 4g

Vegetable Risotto

SERVES: 6 / **PREP TIME:** 10 minutes / **COOK TIME:** 30 minutes
ONE-POT, QUICK-PREP, VEGETARIAN, NUT-FREE, GLUTEN-FREE

When I was in college, I was required to take a cooking class to learn how to cook, bake, and make substitutions. I got tasked with risotto and let me tell you I messed it up badly the first time I made it! The key to risotto is having enough liquid AND patience. I lacked the latter and ever since have realized patience is the key ingredient when making risotto. If you keep that in mind, you will be rewarded for it when the dish is finished.

2 tablespoons olive oil, divided

½ red onion, diced

3 garlic cloves

1 bunch asparagus, ends trimmed and chopped into thirds

1 red bell pepper, thinly sliced

1 cup arborio rice

4 cups vegetable broth

⅓ cup Parmesan cheese

Salt

Pepper

4 cups chopped kale

Lemon juice

1. In a large saucepan, heat 1 tablespoon of oil over medium heat. Add the onion and garlic and sauté for 3 minutes. Add the asparagus and bell pepper and stir. Cook for 3 to 5 minutes. Transfer the vegetables to a large bowl and set aside.

2. Return the pan to the heat, add the remaining tablespoon of oil and toast the rice, stirring constantly, for 1 minute.

3. Pour ½ cup of broth over the rice and stir frequently. As soon as the liquid is mostly absorbed, add another ½ cup of broth and stir until most of the liquid is absorbed. Repeat this process until all of broth is absorbed and the rice is creamy and tender.

4. Stir in the Parmesan cheese and season with salt and pepper.

5. Add the kale and let wilt. Turn off the heat and continue stirring.

6. Stir in the vegetables and a squeeze of fresh lemon juice.

> **SUBSTITUTION TIP:** If you can't find Arborio rice, look for another short grain like sushi rice or farro.

Per serving: Calories: 234; Total Fat: 7g; Saturated Fat: 2g; Cholesterol: 4mg; Sodium: 751mg; Carbohydrates: 37g; Fiber: 4g; Protein: 8g

Spaghetti Squash Primavera

SERVES: 6 / **PREP TIME:** 10 minutes / **COOK TIME:** 55 minutes
QUICK-PREP, VEGETARIAN, NUT-FREE, GLUTEN-FREE

Spaghetti squash is such a simple and healthy substitution for pasta. It is easy to make and is a nice vehicle for sauces like this primavera. Pasta is often used as a vehicle for sauces anyway, so why not throw in extra vegetables while we're at it? Speaking of primavera, it is just a fancy name for a sauce made from vegetables. Feel free to add any non-starchy vegetables you have on hand, like broccoli or snap peas, to this tasty and simple dish.

1 medium Spaghetti Squash (page 249)

1 tablespoon olive oil

1 small yellow onion, thinly sliced

2 stalks celery, diced

1 carrot, diced

3 garlic cloves, minced

1 bell pepper, sliced

1 yellow summer squash, chopped

1 (14.5-ounce) can diced tomatoes

Salt

Pepper

¼ cup grated Parmesan cheese

Fresh basil, chopped

1. Prepare the spaghetti squash according to the directions on page 249.

2. Meanwhile in a large skillet, heat the oil over medium heat. Add the onion, celery, and carrot and sauté for 3 to 4 minutes. Add the garlic and sauté for 1 minute more. Add the bell pepper, squash, and diced tomatoes. Season with salt and pepper. Simmer for 5 minutes.

3. When the spaghetti squash is done, shred it with a fork and add it to the skillet. Stir to coat the spaghetti squash with the sauce.

4. Top with the Parmesan and fresh basil.

> **INGREDIENT TIP:** If you can't find a spaghetti squash, feel free to use regular or gluten-free noodles, or try zucchini noodles.

Per serving: Calories: 89; Total Fat: 4g; Saturated Fat: 1g; Cholesterol: 3mg; Sodium: 223mg; Carbohydrates: 11g; Fiber: 3g; Protein: 4g

Five-Ingredient Veggie Lasagna

SERVES: 8 / **PREP TIME:** 20 minutes / **COOK TIME:** 50 minutes
5 INGREDIENTS OR LESS, VEGETARIAN, NUT-FREE, GLUTEN-FREE

Lasagna is one of those easy-to-make casseroles that can feed a family. This zucchini version, though it does not contain traditional pasta noodles, will do the same. It is packed with flavor and only has five ingredients to boot (minus the salt and pepper, of course). The zucchini holds the sauce and cheese and lets them do the talking while also helping you fill your plate with more vegetables.

3 zucchini, sliced in
   ½-inch rounds

½ teaspoon salt, plus more
   for salting zucchini

Cooking oil spray

15 ounces fresh
   ricotta cheese

1 large egg

¼ teaspoon pepper

2 cups pasta sauce or
   Homemade Marinara Sauce
   (page 266)

1½ cups mozzarella cheese,
   shredded

1. Lay zucchini on plate and lightly salt, allowing water to be drawn out for 10 minutes. Then pat with a paper towel and soak up any excessive moisture.

2. Preheat the oven to 375°F. Coat the inside of an 8-by-8-inch baking dish with cooking oil spray.

3. In a small bowl, whisk together the ricotta cheese, egg, salt, and pepper.

4. Put a ½ cup of pasta sauce in the bottom of the prepared baking dish. Spread it so it covers the bottom of the dish in an even layer. Top with ⅓ of the zucchini, then another ½ cup sauce. Then add ½ of the ricotta mixture, ½ cup mozzarella cheese, ⅓ of the zucchini, ½ cup sauce, the remaining ricotta, and ½ cup mozzarella cheese. Finish the lasagna with the remaining zucchini, ½ cup sauce, and the remaining mozzarella.

5. Cover with foil and cook for 30 minutes, remove cover, and cook for an additional 20 minutes or until the zucchini is fork-tender.

> **INGREDIENT TIP:** When choosing store-bought pasta sauce, look for those that have no added sugar.

Per serving: Calories: 198; Total Fat: 11g; Saturated Fat: 6g; Cholesterol: 59mg; Sodium: 648mg; Carbohydrates: 12g; Fiber: 2g; Protein: 12g

High Protein Pressure Cooker Mac & Cheese

SERVES: 4 / **PREP TIME:** 10 minutes / **COOK TIME:** 20 minutes
ONE-POT, 30 MINUTES OR LESS, QUICK-PREP, VEGETARIAN, NUT-FREE, GLUTEN-FREE

If you don't have a pressure cooker, you are missing out. Once you get over the initial learning curve, you will come to rely on it in your kitchen. It makes food in a fraction of the time that your slow cooker does, and everything you make with it comes out tender and flavorful. This mac and cheese is so easy to prepare and cook that it will it will become a go-to dinner when you have little time to spare.

1 tablespoon olive oil

1 small yellow onion, minced

3 garlic cloves, minced

1 bell pepper, chopped

8 ounces uncooked gluten-free pasta shells

2 cups vegetable broth

¼ teaspoon dry mustard

¼ teaspoon salt

¼ teaspoon pepper

¾ cup Cheddar cheese

¾ cup cottage cheese

Salt

Pepper

1. In a pressure cooker, use the sauté function and heat the oil in the pot along with the onion and sauté until it becomes translucent, about 3 to 4 minutes.

2. Add the garlic and bell pepper and sauté for 2 to 3 minutes more.

3. Turn off the sauté function, then add the pasta, broth, and spices.

4. Set the pressure cooker on manual (high). Close and cook for 5 minutes.

5. Quick release the vent, open the top, drain any excess liquid, and mix in the cheese and cottage cheese. Season with salt and pepper.

> **NOTE:** When venting your pressure cooker, use a kitchen towel to cover spout to limit splatter or heat ruining any of your kitchen cabinets.

Per serving: Calories: 381; Total Fat: 13g; Saturated Fat: 6g; Cholesterol: 30mg; Sodium: 916mg; Carbohydrates: 50g; Fiber: 3g; Protein: 17g

Butternut Squash Mac & Cheese

SERVES: 4 / **PREP TIME:** 15 minutes / **COOK TIME:** 30 minutes
VEGETARIAN, NUT-FREE

Mac and cheese is one of those foods that people think is unhealthy for them. Here's the secret: Make it with vegetables to increase the nutrient content. Then pair it with a salad and you are good to go.

1 small butternut squash, peeled, seeded, diced (about 2 cups)

½ teaspoon cinnamon

8 ounces uncooked pasta (a small size like shells or elbows)

1 cup milk

2 tablespoons unsalted butter

4 ounces goat cheese, crumbled

1 teaspoon garlic powder

½ teaspoon salt

¼ teaspoon pepper

1. Preheat the oven to 425°F. Line a baking sheet with parchment paper.

2. Place the butternut squash on the baking sheet and sprinkle with the cinnamon. Roast in the oven for 20 to 25 minutes, or until tender.

3. Meanwhile, in a large stockpot, boil 2 quarts of water over medium-high heat. Once the water reaches a boil, cook the pasta for 8 to 12 minutes, or according to package directions, until tender. Drain the pasta and set aside.

4. Return the stockpot to the stove and heat the milk and butter over low heat, whisking continuously until the butter has melted.

5. Add in the butternut squash to the milk and butter. Using an immersion blender, blend until smooth (alternatively, use a blender to blend—in batches, if necessary—then return to the pot).

6. Add the goat cheese and stir until it has melted.

7. Fold in the pasta and add the garlic powder, salt, and pepper.

> **SUBSTITUTION TIP:** If you don't have a butternut squash on hand, use sweet potatoes instead.

Per serving: Calories: 436; Total Fat: 17g; Saturated Fat: 11g; Cholesterol: 47mg; Sodium: 472mg; Carbohydrates: 57g; Fiber: 5g; Protein: 16g

Butternut Squash, Mushroom, and Goat Cheese Cauliflower Pizza

SERVES: 6 / **PREP TIME:** 10 minutes / **COOK TIME:** 25 minutes
QUICK-PREP, VEGETARIAN, NUT-FREE, GLUTEN-FREE

This veggie-packed pizza is sweet and savory all at once. The goat cheese ties the flavors together and adds some extra zing to it. I ate this as dinner one night, and it was such a nice change from the usual meat and potatoes. Feel free to add other toppings that you like or even use a store-bought pizza crust if you find it saves you time.

1 prepared Cauliflower Pizza Crust (page 267)

3 cups butternut squash, peeled, seeded, and chopped

2 garlic cloves, minced

½ teaspoon salt

¼ teaspoon pepper

1 tablespoon olive oil

1 tablespoon maple syrup

¼ cup liquid (broth, milk, or water)

8 ounces mushrooms, sliced

4 ounces goat cheese, crumbled

1 cup baby spinach

Pinch red pepper flakes

½ cup Crunchy Chickpeas (page 79) (optional)

1. Preheat the oven to 400°F. Line a baking sheet with parchment paper.

2. Place the butternut squash on the baking sheet and toss with the garlic, salt, and pepper. Spread the squash on the baking sheet in a single layer and bake for 15 to 20 minutes, or until tender.

3. Transfer the butternut squash to a blender or food processor. Add the oil, maple syrup, and liquid, and blend until smooth.

4. Place the cauliflower crust on the second baking sheet and spread the butternut squash on the crust like pizza sauce.

5. Top with the mushrooms, goat cheese, spinach, red pepper flakes, and chickpeas, if using.

6. Bake at 400°F for 5 minutes.

Per serving: Calories: 253; Total Fat: 13g; Saturated Fat: 7g; Cholesterol: 57mg; Sodium: 589mg; Carbohydrates: 22g; Fiber: 6g; Protein: 15g

Easy Homemade Falafel

SERVES: 8 (2 falafel per serving)

PREP TIME: 5 minutes, plus 10 minutes to chill / **COOK TIME:** 10 minutes

30-MINUTES OR LESS, VEGETARIAN, NUT-FREE, DAIRY-FREE

These falafel are easy to make as you rely on a food processor to do most of the work for you. A blender or an immersion blender would do the trick as well. These patties are very flavorful and even better when you pair with tzatziki or hummus. Enjoy them in a pita or over a salad.

¼ cup rolled oats

1 (15-ounce) can chickpeas, drained , rinsed, and patted dry

¼ cup fresh parsley

4 garlic cloves, minced

½ cup minced red onion

1 tablespoon sesame seeds

1 teaspoon cumin

½ teaspoon cayenne

½ teaspoon salt

½ teaspoon baking powder

1 large egg

1 tablespoon cornstarch (or more as needed for thickening)

¼ cup avocado oil for frying

1. To make oat flour, add rolled oats to food processor and pulse until oats form a flour.

2. Add the chickpeas, parsley, garlic, onion, sesame seeds, cumin, cayenne, salt, baking powder, egg, and cornstarch to the food processor and process until well-combined, about 30 seconds.

3. Form into 16 small patties. (If the dough is sticky, place it in the refrigerator for about 10 minutes, or until you can more easily form it into balls.)

4. In a large skillet, heat the avocado oil over medium heat.

5. Fry the falafel in batches for 2 to 3 minutes per side, working in batches as needed.

> **VARIATION TIP:** If you can find chickpea flour, use it in place of oat flour for a more authentic flavor.

Per serving (2 falafels): Calories: 159; Total Fat: 9g; Saturated Fat: 1g; Cholesterol: 23mg; Sodium: 159mg; Carbohydrates: 14g; Fiber: 3g; Protein: 5g

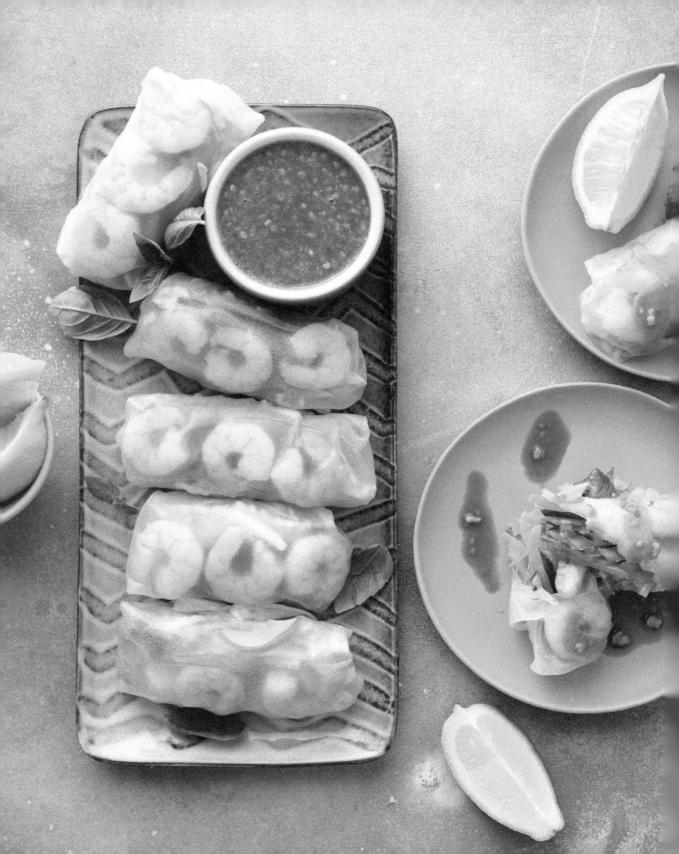

CHAPTER SEVEN

Seafood

148 Spring
Shrimp Rolls

150 Spicy
Shrimp Tacos

151 Shrimp
Pesto Pasta

152 Grilled Clams with
Lemon-Pepper
Ghee

153 Linguine
with Clams

154 Mussels Marinara

155 Scallop Risotto

156 Baked Crab Cakes
with Tartar Sauce

157 Tropical White
Fish Ceviche

158 Easy
Blackened Fish

159 Crispy Baked
Fish Sticks

160 Baked Fish
and Chips

161 Mediterranean
Fish in Parchment

162 Lemony Smoked
Salmon Roll-Ups
with Avocado

163 Deconstructed
Sushi Bowl

164 Honey-Lime
Salmon with
Watermelon Salsa

165 Sweet Potato
Salmon Cakes

167 Salmon
Tostada Salad

168 Maple-Glazed
Cedar Plank
Salmon

169 Easy Apple-
Tuna Salad

Spring Shrimp Rolls

SERVES: 8 / **PREP TIME:** 15 minutes

ONE-POT, 5 INGREDIENTS OR LESS, 30 MINUTES OR LESS, DAIRY-FREE

Spring rolls are a fun group activity. They are easy to make, so even the youngest of cooks can jump in on the fun. The best part about something like this is that you can personalize your spring roll with the ingredients that you like the most. When I make them, I like to add a little bit of everything, especially the avocado and shrimp, but use any combination of ingredients that suits you.

FOR THE PEANUT SAUCE

¾ cup peanut butter

⅓ cup soy sauce

⅓ cup water (plus more to thin)

3 tablespoons maple syrup

1 teaspoon sesame oil

1 tablespoon Sriracha

Juice of 2 limes

Pinch red pepper flakes

Pinch sesame seeds

FOR THE SPRING ROLLS

1 pound cooked shrimp (see tip), halved lengthwise

8 butter lettuce leaves, shredded

2 large carrots, julienned

2 avocados, diced

1 cucumber, thinly sliced

1 red bell pepper, thinly sliced

Fresh basil leaves

Warm water

16 rice paper wraps

TO MAKE THE PEANUT SAUCE

In a small bowl, whisk together all of the ingredients for the sauce and set aside.

TO MAKE THE SPRING ROLLS

1. Make sure that the shrimp, lettuce, carrots, avocados, cucumber, bell pepper, and basil leaves are all prepared, laid out, and easy to reach.

2. Fill a large shallow bowl with warm water. Dip the rice paper wraps into bowl one at a time and let sit for 5 to 10 seconds. Make sure the entire paper is moistened.

3. Remove and place on a clean, flat surface (a cutting board or a plate). Fill each wrap with the ingredients of your choice.

4. Fold the sides of the wrap toward the middle, then, starting at the bottom, roll away from your body until the filling is rolled up inside the spring roll. Repeat for each wrap.

5. Serve with the peanut sauce for dipping.

INGREDIENT TIP: To prepare and cook the shrimp yourself, bring a pot of water to boil over medium-high heat. While the water is heating, peel and devein the shrimp. Carefully place the shrimp in the boiling water and cook for 2 to 3 minutes, or until the shrimp are pink and opaque. Remove from the water and plunge into an ice water bath. Let cool in the ice water for 5 minutes. Drain and proceed with the recipe as directed.

Per serving: Calories: 371; Total Fat: 20g; Saturated Fat: 4g; Cholesterol: 110mg; Sodium: 843mg; Carbohydrates: 18g; Fiber: 6g; Protein: 19g

Spicy Shrimp Tacos

SERVES: 4 / **PREP TIME:** 5 minutes / **COOK TIME:** 5 minutes

30 MINUTES OR LESS, QUICK-PREP, NUT-FREE, DAIRY-FREE, GLUTEN-FREE

I find that people steer clear of shrimp and fish simply because they are scared to cook it. If you like fish and want to try to cook a simple fish dish at home, shrimp is a great place to start. Why? Because shrimp tells you when it's done! When the shrimp turn pink, and you can no longer see blue translucent colors, it's ready to eat. Ta-da!

1 pound shrimp, peeled and deveined

2 tablespoons avocado oil, divided

3 garlic cloves, minced

1 tablespoon Taco Seasoning (page 250)

Juice of ½ lime

8 hard taco shells

Avocado lettuce, red onion, and tomato, for topping (optional)

1. In a medium bowl, combine the shrimp, 1 tablespoon avocado oil, garlic, and Taco Seasoning. Toss to coat the shrimp with the oil and seasonings.

2. Heat the remaining oil in a large skillet over medium heat.

3. When the oil is hot, add the shrimp and cook for 3 to 4 minutes, flipping once.

4. The shrimp are done when they turn pink and opaque.

5. Squeeze the fresh lime juice over the shrimp. Fill the hard taco shells with the shrimp and your choice of toppings.

Per serving: Calories: 320; Total Fat: 15g; Saturated Fat: 2g; Cholesterol: 172mg; Sodium: 284mg; Carbohydrates: 19g; Fiber: 3g; Protein: 25g

Shrimp Pesto Pasta

SERVES: 4 / **PREP TIME:** 10 minutes / **COOK TIME:** 15 minutes
30 MINUTES OR LESS, QUICK-PREP

Cutting the amount of pasta in this recipe and replacing it with spiralized zucchini (or zucchini noodles) is a great way to lighten up the dish and an easy way to sneak in some extra vegetables. This is a quick dish that can be whipped up on a weeknight, in part because shrimp is one of the quickest-cooking proteins out there. I love keeping shrimp on hand in the freezer for a quick—and tasty—weeknight meal.

8 ounces spaghetti or linguine

1 pound medium/large shrimp, peeled and deveined (leave tail on)

1 cup Spinach-Walnut Pesto (page 265), divided

1 tablespoon olive oil

4 garlic cloves, minced

1 pint cherry tomatoes

1 zucchini, spiralized

Juice of ½ lemon

Grated Parmesan, for garnish

1. Bring a large pot of salted water to boil over high heat. Add the pasta and cook according to the package instructions. When the pasta is cooked, drain and set aside.

2. Meanwhile, in a small bowl, combine the shrimp with ¼ cup pesto. Cover and set aside.

3. In a large skillet, heat the oil over medium heat. Add the garlic and cook for 3 minutes, then add the cherry tomatoes and cook until bursting. Transfer the tomatoes and garlic to a medium bowl.

4. Return the skillet to the heat. Put the shrimp in the skillet and cook until pink, 2 to 3 minutes per side. Add the tomatoes back to the skillet.

5. Add the zucchini and the pasta to the skillet and mix well. Remove the skillet from the heat and mix the remaining ¾ cup pesto into the pasta.

6. Finish with a squeeze of lemon juice and sprinkling of grated Parmesan.

> **TIP:** If you don't have any zucchini, feel free to use 12 ounces of pasta in the recipe and cook as directed.

Per serving: Calories: 706; Total Fat: 41g; Saturated Fat: 6g; Cholesterol: 176mg; Sodium: 586mg; Carbohydrates: 81g; Fiber: 5g; Protein: 35g

Grilled Clams with Lemon-Pepper Ghee

SERVES: 8 / **PREP TIME:** 5 minutes / **COOK TIME:** 10 minutes
5 INGREDIENTS OR LESS, 30 MINUTES OR LESS, QUICK-PREP, DAIRY-FREE, NUT-FREE

If you are looking for a quick-and-easy recipe for your backyard barbecue or a spontaneous dinner with friends, use this clam recipe. It takes almost no time at all to cook. I make this dish to ward off hungry friends when I'm still preparing other dishes for a summer party, and it does the trick. The lemon-pepper ghee adds a nice finish, but feel free to serve the clams on their own.

½ cup Ghee
   (page 251), melted
Zest and juice of 1 lemon
¼ teaspoon pepper
2 pounds littleneck clams,
   scrubbed clean
Pinch sea salt

1. Preheat the grill to medium.

2. Meanwhile, in a small saucepan, warm the ghee, lemon zest, lemon juice, and pepper over low heat and whisk to combine. Leave over low heat until the clams are ready to eat.

3. Place the clams directly on the grill and cook for 8 to 10 minutes without turning. When the clams have opened, they can be removed from the grill and transferred to a medium bowl. Discard any clams that do not open.

4. Pour lemon-pepper ghee over the clams, sprinkle with salt, and serve.

> **INGREDIENT TIP:** When you buy clams and don't plan to use them immediately, make sure to store them in a breathable container (i.e., not a closed plastic bag) and throw away any clams that are not closed or do not close easily with a little help.

Per serving: Calories: 147; Total Fat: 14g; Saturated Fat: 10g; Cholesterol: 49mg; Sodium: 24mg; Carbohydrates: 2g; Fiber: 0g; Protein: 6g

Linguine with Clams

SERVES: 4 / **PREP TIME:** 5 minutes / **COOK TIME:** 25 minutes
ONE-POT, 30 MINUTES OR LESS, QUICK-PREP, NUT-FREE

I used to hate linguine with clams growing up and I'm not sure why. It's probably because many people have a preconceived notion that they don't like clams or fish. If you just give them a chance, you might also get past the notion and find a new easy dish to put on the menu during the week. This is a nice light dish, and, because the clams are canned, it can be made year-round. You can certainly use fresh clams and grill them (see Grilled Clams with Lemon-Pepper Ghee, page 152) then add them to this dish, but I prefer using canned so that I can skip the step of having to clean and cook them.

12 ounces linguine or spaghetti

½ cup dry white wine (or reserved pasta water)

2 tablespoons Ghee (page 251) or butter

2 shallots, minced

4 garlic cloves, minced

2 (6.5-ounce) cans chopped clams, drained and juice reserved

1 tablespoon cornstarch (optional)

¼ cup parsley, chopped

¼ cup grated Parmesan

Salt

Pepper

1. Bring a large pot of salted water to boil over high heat. Add the pasta and cook according to the package instructions. If you are using pasta water instead of wine, reserve ½ cup, then drain the pasta and set aside.

2. Using the same large pot (pasta removed), heat the ghee over medium heat until melted but not bubbling.

3. Add the shallots and cook for 2 minutes, then add the garlic and cook for 1 minute more.

4. Pour in the wine and stir, scraping up any brown bits from the sides and the bottom of the pot.

5. Whisk in the reserved clam juice and cornstarch and simmer for 5 minutes Add in the linguine, clams, and parsley to the pot and simmer for an additional 5 minutes.

6. Remove from the heat and add the grated Parmesan. Season with salt and pepper.

> **TIP:** Add some fresh vegetables to this dish, like sliced cherry tomatoes, to add some flavor and texture.

Per serving: Calories: 476; Total Fat: 11g; Saturated Fat: 6g; Cholesterol: 49mg; Sodium: 166mg; Carbohydrates: 67g; Fiber: 3g; Protein: 24g

Mussels Marinara

SERVES: 4 / **PREP TIME:** 5 minutes / **COOK TIME:** 10 minutes
ONE-POT, 5 INGREDIENTS OR LESS, 30 MINUTES OR LESS, QUICK-PREP, NUT-FREE

Mussels aren't just for the gym; they are also for the kitchen. Okay, that was a bad joke, but mussels are a quick and nutritious option in the kitchen. The zinc found in mussels helps build a healthy immune system, boosts metabolism, and helps repair tissues in the body, which are similar to the benefits of a good workout. Use these mussels and your other muscles and you'll be thankful you listened to my bad jokes.

4 cups Homemade
  Marinara Sauce
  (page 266)
2 pounds mussels,
  scrubbed clean (discard
  any that are open)
¼ cup grated Parmesan
¼ cup fresh parsley
Salt
Pepper
Baguette slices, toasted

1. In a large saucepan, heat the marinara sauce over medium heat until simmering.

2. When the sauce is simmering, add the mussels and cook until all of them open up, 3 to 5 minutes. Discard any that do not open.

3. Remove from the heat and transfer to a large serving bowl. Sprinkle with Parmesan cheese, parsley, salt, and pepper and serve with toasted baguette slices for dipping.

VARIATION TIP: If you have leftovers, remove the mussels from their shells and add to the marinara sauce. Discard the shells. Store leftovers without shells in a large airtight container for 3 to 4 days.

Per serving: Calories: 305; Total Fat: 9g; Saturated Fat: 2g; Cholesterol: 68mg; Sodium: 1075mg; Carbohydrates: 23g; Fiber: 4g; Protein: 34g

Scallop Risotto

SERVES: 4 / **PREP TIME:** 10 minutes / **COOK TIME:** 30 minutes
QUICK-PREP, NUT-FREE, GLUTEN-FREE

I love scallops and risotto but had never thought to put the two together. I'm glad I did because this recipe is super creamy and delicious. I find that this recipe is a good way to introduce you to cooking scallops. You can make the base risotto the night before and then cook the scallops right before eating so you can enjoy them fresh off the skillet.

3 tablespoons
    butter, divided

1 pound scallops

1 shallot, minced

3 garlic cloves, minced

1 cup arborio or short
    grain rice

⅓ cup dry white wine

4 cups vegetable broth

½ cup Parmesan
    cheese, grated

Juice of ½ lemon

¼ cup parsley, chopped

Salt

Pepper

1. In a medium skillet, heat 2 tablespoons of butter over medium heat. Add the scallops and cook for 3 minutes. Flip the scallops and cook for 1 minute more. Remove the scallops from the skillet, cover, and set aside.

2. In a large stockpot or Dutch oven, heat the remaining tablespoon of butter over medium heat, add the shallot and cook until translucent, 3 to 4 minutes.

3. Add the garlic and cook for an additional minute.

4. Add the rice and toast it, stirring continuously, for 1 minute. Pour in the white wine and stir, scraping up any brown bits stuck to the sides and the bottom of the pot.

5. Pour ½ cup of broth over the rice and stir frequently. As soon as the liquid is mostly absorbed, add another ½ cup of broth and stir until most of the liquid is absorbed. Repeat this process until all of broth is absorbed and the rice is creamy and tender.

6. Remove the risotto from the heat. Stir in the Parmesan, lemon, and parsley. Season with salt and pepper. Top with the scallops.

TIP: Make this dairy-free by using olive oil instead of butter.

Per serving: Calories: 429; Total Fat: 13g; Saturated Fat: 8g; Cholesterol: 70mg; Sodium: 1420mg; Carbohydrates: 44g; Fiber: 1g; Protein: 28g

Baked Crab Cakes with Tartar Sauce

SERVES: 4 / **PREP TIME:** 10 minutes / **COOK TIME:** 20 minutes
30 MINUTES OR LESS, QUICK-PREP, NUT-FREE, DAIRY-FREE, GLUTEN-FREE

I'm from Maryland so I couldn't leave out one of my favorite Maryland dishes: the crab cake. The problem with most crab cakes you find at generic restaurants is that they have far too much breading and not nearly enough crab. If I can't see and taste the crab in my crab cake, I'm not a happy camper.

FOR THE CRAB CAKES

1 pound lump crabmeat, picked clean of shells

½ cup crushed potato chips

1 green bell pepper, minced

3 garlic cloves, minced

1 large egg, beaten

2 tablespoons Homemade Mayo (page 254)

1 tablespoon Dijon mustard

1 tablespoon minced fresh parsley

1 teaspoon paprika or Old Bay Seasoning

½ teaspoon salt

¼ teaspoon pepper

FOR THE QUICK TARTAR SAUCE

½ cup Homemade Mayo (page 254)

1 tablespoon diced dill pickles

1 tablespoon lemon juice

½ teaspoon Dijon mustard

Salt

Pepper

TO MAKE THE CRAB CAKES

1. Preheat the oven to 400°F. Line a large baking sheet with parchment paper.

2. In a large bowl, add all of the ingredients for the crab cakes and mix by hand or with a large fork so the crab maintains its shape.

3. Form crab cake mixture into 8 large patties, squeezing it between your hands to bind the cake and let any excess liquid drain.

4. Place on the prepared baking sheet and bake in the oven for 20 minutes or until golden brown.

TO MAKE THE QUICK TARTAR SAUCE

While crab cakes are cooking, whisk together all of the ingredients for quick tartar sauce and refrigerate until the crab cakes are ready to eat.

Per serving: Calories: 488; Total Fat: 39g; Saturated Fat: 6g; Cholesterol: 106mg; Sodium: 1097mg; Carbohydrates: 18g; Fiber: 1g; Protein: 13g

Tropical White Fish Ceviche

SERVES: 6 / **PREP TIME:** 2 hours

NUT-FREE, DAIRY-FREE, GLUTEN-FREE

Ceviche is a great fish recipe because it smells fresh and fragrant, without the strong smell of a cooked fish dish. The citrus juices do all the work here, as they are what end up "cooking" the fish. This ceviche is great on its own or added to the top of a salad.

½ pound white fish (mahi-mahi, cod, tilapia, haddock, etc.), finely chopped

Juice of 3 to 4 limes

Juice of 1 orange

1 mango, diced

1 small bell pepper, diced

1 avocado, diced

1 jalapeño, seeded and diced

¼ cup thinly sliced red onion

2 tablespoons chopped cilantro

½ teaspoon salt

½ teaspoon pepper

1 sliced cucumber or tortilla chips, for serving

1. Place the white fish in a shallow bowl and cover with the lime juice and the orange juice.

2. Cover bowl and place in refrigerator for 1 to 2 hours, or until fish no longer looks raw when cut into.

3. Meanwhile, in a large bowl, combine the mango, bell pepper, avocado, jalapeño, red onion, cilantro, salt, and pepper. Stir gently, cover, and refrigerate.

4. After the fish has been in the citrus juice for 1 to 2 hours, add the fish to larger bowl of vegetables and season with additional salt and pepper, if desired.

5. Enjoy with cucumber slices or tortilla chips.

INGREDIENT TIP: The fish pieces are ready when they are no longer transparent. If you are not sure, let them sit in the citrus juice for 20 to 30 minutes longer. The smaller you slice the fish, the faster it will "cook."

Per serving: Calories: 128; Total Fat: 5g; Saturated Fat: 1g; Cholesterol: 21mg; Sodium: 227mg; Carbohydrates: 11g; Fiber: 3g; Protein: 10g

Easy Blackened Fish

SERVES: 4 / **PREP TIME:** 5 minutes / **COOK TIME:** 10 minutes

30 MINUTES OR LESS, QUICK-PREP, NUT-FREE, DAIRY-FREE, GLUTEN-FREE

I used to think blackened fish or chicken meant that it was burnt. Well, I was wrong, and I am so glad that I was. These blackened fish fillets are anything but burnt. The seasonings coat the white fish to make it a darker color but that's about it. Otherwise you get a nice flaky and tasty fish to pair with your favorite sides or to use in fish tacos.

2 teaspoons paprika

1 teaspoon
cayenne pepper

1 teaspoon dry mustard

1 teaspoon garlic powder

½ teaspoon cumin

½ teaspoon pepper

½ teaspoon salt

1½ pounds white fish,
patted dry and sliced
into 4 even-size fillets

2 tablespoons olive oil

1. In a small bowl, combine the paprika, cayenne, dry mustard, garlic powder, cumin, pepper, and salt. Mix until well combined.

2. Rub the spice mixture over the fish fillets.

3. In a large skillet, heat the oil over medium heat. Add the fish and cook for 3 to 4 minutes per side or until cooked through.

> **VARIATION TIP:** Make these for taco night and serve with tortillas, lettuce, tomatoes, and other toppings of your choice.

Per serving: Calories: 245; Total Fat: 9g; Saturated Fat: 1g; Cholesterol: 94mg; Sodium: 424mg; Carbohydrates: 1g; Fiber: <1g; Protein: 38g

Crispy Baked Fish Sticks

SERVES: 4 / **PREP TIME:** 10 minutes / **COOK TIME:** 20 minutes
30 MINUTES OR LESS, QUICK-PREP, GLUTEN-FREE

I'm not going to lie, I used to hate fish sticks as a kid. I would hope for mozzarella sticks and when I'd bite into a fish stick, I'd be severely disappointed. However, I made a promise to myself that I would eventually make a fish stick recipe that I would not only enjoy but look forward to. This fish stick recipe, while still not a mozzarella stick, will be on my rotation for years to come.

1 pound cod, flounder, or other white fish, cut into ½-inch sticks

½ teaspoon salt

¼ teaspoon pepper

½ cup tapioca flour

2 eggs, beaten

1 cup almond flour

¼ cup grated Parmesan cheese

1 teaspoon paprika

1 teaspoon garlic powder

½ teaspoon salt

¼ teaspoon black pepper

1. Preheat the oven to 425°F. Line a baking sheet with parchment paper.

2. Pat the fish dry with paper towels, then season with salt and pepper.

3. Put the tapioca flour on a plate and the beaten eggs into a small bowl.

4. In a large bowl, mix together the almond flour, Parmesan, paprika, garlic powder, salt, and pepper.

5. Dip the fish sticks first in tapioca flour, shaking any excess back onto the plate. Then dip the floured fish stick in egg, and, finally, roll it in the almond flour mixture and place on the baking sheet. Repeat this process for each fish stick.

6. Bake for 8 minutes. Turn the fish sticks over, then bake for an additional 8 minutes, or until the fish is cooked to an internal temperature of 145°F.

VARIATION TIP: Serve with your favorite ketchup, mustard, or barbecue sauce.

Per serving: Calories: 398; Total Fat: 19g; Saturated Fat: 3g; Cholesterol: 160mg; Sodium: 531mg; Carbohydrates: 20g; Fiber: 3g; Protein: 37g

Baked Fish and Chips

SERVES: 4 / **PREP TIME:** 10 minutes / **COOK TIME:** 30 minutes
QUICK-PREP, NUT-FREE

This is a very non-traditional spin on a very traditional dish. I find fish and chips to be far too greasy, so I often steer clear of them. This version is simple and straightforward and, most importantly, not greasy at all. The fish pairs well with malt vinegar, ketchup, or even barbecue sauce and is delicious served next to sweet potato fries (aka the "chips").

FOR THE CHIPS

2 large sweet potatoes, cut into wedges

1 tablespoon olive oil

Salt

Pepper

FOR THE FISH

½ cup flour

¼ teaspoon salt

¼ teaspoon pepper

1 large egg

¼ cup milk

1 cup old-fashioned oats

½ tablespoon garlic powder

¼ tablespoon paprika

1 teaspoon cayenne

1 pound cod or haddock, cut into 8 to 10 thin fillets

Ketchup (page 256)

Malt vinegar

TO MAKE THE CHIPS

1. Preheat the oven to 450°F. Line a baking sheet with aluminum foil.

2. In a large bowl, mix together the sweet potatoes, olive oil, salt, and pepper. Place the potatoes on the baking sheet in a single layer and bake for 20 minutes. When done, remove from the oven and set aside.

TO MAKE THE FISH

1. Line a second baking sheet with aluminum foil.

2. Take out three large bowls. In the first bowl, mix together the flour, salt, and pepper. In the second bowl, combine the egg and milk. In the third bowl, mix together the oats, garlic powder, paprika, and cayenne.

3. Dredge each fillet in the flour mixture, then dip into the egg mixture, and finally, coat with the oat mixture. Place each fillet on the baking sheet.

4. Bake for 4 to 5 minutes on each side, or until the internal temperature is 145°F.

5. Serve the fish and chips with ketchup and malt vinegar.

> **SUBSTITUTION TIP:** To make this recipe dairy-free, use a non-dairy milk alternative in place of the cow's milk.

Per serving: Calories: 389; Total Fat: 8g; Saturated Fat: 1g; Cholesterol: 111mg; Sodium: 280mg; Carbohydrates: 45g; Fiber: 6g; Protein: 34g

Mediterranean Fish in Parchment

SERVES: 4 / **PREP TIME:** 10 minutes / **COOK TIME:** 20 minutes
ONE-POT, 30 MINUTES OR LESS, QUICK-PREP, NUT-FREE, GLUTEN-FREE

A lot of people tell me that they hate cooking fish inside their house because of the smell. For some reason, the smell of this didn't waft through my house. Maybe it's the parchment or maybe it's the seasoning—either way it made for a tasty dish.

1 yellow onion, sliced

4 (6-ounce) cod fillets

1 pint cherry or grape tomatoes, halved

2 tablespoons capers

1 lemon, cut into 4 slices

2 tablespoons olive oil

4 garlic cloves, minced

¼ cup feta cheese, crumbled

1. Preheat the oven to 450°F and tear off four large parchment paper sheets.

2. Place ¼ of the onion on each sheet of parchment paper. Place a fish fillet on top of the onions on every sheet.

3. Top each fish fillet with ¼ of the tomatoes, ¼ of the capers, and 1 slice of lemon. Drizzle the olive oil over each fillet and sprinkle ¼ of the garlic and ¼ of the feta cheese on each fillet.

4. Fold the parchment paper to create a pouch and bake for 15 to 20 minutes or until fish flakes when tested with a fork. Let rest 5 minutes. Open the packet carefully to avoid a steam burn.

INGREDIENT TIP: If you don't have cod, use any white flaky fish in its place.

Per serving: Calories: 257: Total Fat: 11g: Saturated Fat: 2g: Cholesterol: 66mg: Sodium: 351mg: Carbohydrates: 10g: Fiber: 3g: Protein: 33g

Lemony Smoked Salmon Roll-Ups with Avocado

SERVES: 4 / PREP TIME: 10 minutes
5 INGREDIENTS OR LESS, 30 MINUTES OR LESS, QUICK-PREP, NUT-FREE, DAIRY-FREE, GLUTEN-FREE

These salmon roll-ups make for a light and tasty appetizer. It's like having a sushi roll without the hassle of having to get the sticky rice all over your hands. Make this as a snack for the family or use it as an appetizer at a party or gathering. And yes, you can eat the lemon slices, just make sure you slice them thin enough, so you are not getting too much rind in each bite.

4 ounces smoked salmon, cut into 8 slices

1 avocado, cut into 8 slices

8 thin slices cucumber

1 lemon, cut into 8 thin slices

Salt

Pepper

1. Wrap 1 slice of salmon around 1 slice each of avocado, cucumber, and lemon. Use a toothpick to hold the salmon roll together. Repeat to form 8 roll-ups.

2. Season with salt and pepper and enjoy!

MAKE-AHEAD TIP: Double or triple this recipe for a party. You can prepare them a few hours ahead and keep them in the refrigerator covered in plastic wrap until the party begins.

Per serving: Calories: 113; Total Fat: 8g; Saturated Fat: 1g; Cholesterol: 6mg; Sodium: 571mg; Carbohydrates: 7g; Fiber: 4g; Protein: 6g

Deconstructed Sushi Bowl

SERVES: 4 / PREP TIME: 10 minutes

30 MINUTES OR LESS, QUICK-PREP, DAIRY-FREE

I was introduced to sushi in college and have been addicted to it ever since. However, I don't get sushi all that often because I tend to make all of my meals for the week at home. This is a compromise dish that gives me the taste of sushi while also allowing me to eat and cook from home during the week. I like to make these bowls ahead of time and store them in four separate containers and small portable dressing containers so I can grab one on my way out the door for work and have a delicious lunch without the hassle.

FOR THE SUSHI

8 ounces smoked salmon

2 cups cooked white or brown rice

1 cup shelled edamame

2 carrots, cut into matchsticks

1 cucumber, chopped

1 avocado, sliced

2 sheets seaweed or nori paper, cut in half

FOR THE SAUCE

⅓ cup soy sauce

1 teaspoon Sriracha or Gochujang (page 258)

1 teaspoon sesame seeds

1 teaspoon sesame oil

½ teaspoon raw ginger, minced

TO MAKE THE SUSHI

Divide the ingredients evenly into four bowls or storage containers, folding the nori in half or shredding it and sprinkling it on top.

TO MAKE THE SAUCE

In a small bowl, whisk together the ingredients for the sauce. Dress each sushi bowl with the sauce if eating immediately. Otherwise, store, covered, in the refrigerator and dress each individual serving when ready to eat.

> **SUBSTITUTION TIP:** If you are comfortable eating raw fish, replace the smoked salmon with sushi-grade tuna or salmon.

Per serving: Calories: 343; Total Fat: 12g; Saturated Fat: 2g; Cholesterol: 13mg; Sodium: 2343mg; Carbohydrates: 38g; Fiber: 6g; Protein: 21g

Honey-Lime Salmon with Watermelon Salsa

SERVES: 4 / **PREP TIME:** 10 minutes / **COOK TIME:** 15 minutes
30 MINUTES OR LESS, QUICK-PREP, NUT-FREE, DAIRY-FREE, GLUTEN-FREE

Want a new salsa to add to your repertoire? This watermelon salsa is good on its own but even better over the salmon. The best part is you can treat your taste buds while also nourishing your body with the healthy omega-3 fats that salmon provides. Aside from all of that, you can get this delicious dish on the table in 30 minutes or less.

FOR THE SALMON

4 (6-ounce) salmon
   fillets, skin on

1 tablespoon olive oil

2 teaspoons honey

½ teaspoon salt

¼ teaspoon pepper

1 lime, cut into 4 slices

**FOR THE WATERMELON
   SALSA**

2 cups seedless
   watermelon, diced

¼ cup red onion, diced

1 jalapeño, seeded
   and diced

2 tablespoons chopped
   cilantro

½ teaspoon salt

¼ teaspoon pepper

Juice of 1 lime

TO MAKE THE SALMON

1. Preheat the oven to 400°F and tear off four large foil sheets.

2. Place each salmon fillet, skin-side down, onto a piece of foil.

3. Whisk together the oil, honey, salt, and pepper. Using a spoon, drizzle the honey mixture over the salmon and use the back of the spoon to spread it on each fillet evenly. Place a slice of lime on each fillet and close foil around salmon making a packet.

4. Bake the salmon packets on middle rack of the oven for 12 to 15 minutes or until fish easily flakes when tested with a fork. (Open the packets carefully to avoid a steam burn.)

TO MAKE THE WATERMELON SALSA

1. In a medium bowl, combine all of the ingredients for the watermelon salsa. Mix well.

2. When the salmon is done, open the packets carefully and scoop ¼ of salsa onto each fillet.

> **VARIATION TIP:** If you prefer to keep the smell of fish out of the house, cook these packets on the grill for a similar amount of time over medium high heat and check on them halfway through the cook time.

Per serving: Calories: 498; Total Fat: 22g; Saturated Fat: 3g; Cholesterol: 130mg; Sodium: 713mg; Carbohydrates: 12g; Fiber: 1g; Protein: 63g

Sweet Potato Salmon Cakes

SERVES: 4 / PREP TIME: 10 minutes / **COOK TIME:** 10 minutes
30 MINUTES OR LESS, QUICK-PREP, NUT-FREE, DAIRY-FREE, GLUTEN-FREE

I have been making these salmon cakes for a few years now. Canned salmon is a staple in my pantry because it keeps for a good amount of time and is really handy when I need to get dinner on the table fast. The sweet potato provides a nice sweet touch and makes the salmon cakes soft and delicious even when reheated. I like to serve mine with mustard over a salad.

2 (5-ounce) cans salmon packed in water, drained

1 small sweet potato, peeled, cooked, and mashed

1 large egg

2 garlic cloves, minced

2 green onions (greens and whites), minced

2 tablespoons flax meal, plus more to thicken as needed

1 tablespoon Dijon mustard

½ teaspoon paprika

½ teaspoon salt

¼ teaspoon pepper

Juice of 1 lemon

2 tablespoons avocado oil

1. In a medium bowl, mix together all of the ingredients except the avocado oil. Add more flax meal as needed to bind the mixture.

2. In a large skillet, heat the oil over medium heat until glistening.

3. Divide the salmon mixture into 8 equal portions and form them into patties. Place the patties in the skillet for 3 to 4 minutes per side or until golden brown on outside. Work in batches as needed.

TECHNIQUE TIP: A quick way to cook the sweet potato is to wrap it in a damp paper towel and microwave it for 5 to 7 minutes or until soft. After you remove it from the microwave, let it cool, then scoop out the flesh, and discard the skin.

Per serving: Calories: 225; Total Fat: 13g; Saturated Fat: 2g; Cholesterol: 78mg; Sodium: 446mg; Carbohydrates: 11g; Fiber: 2g; Protein: 14g

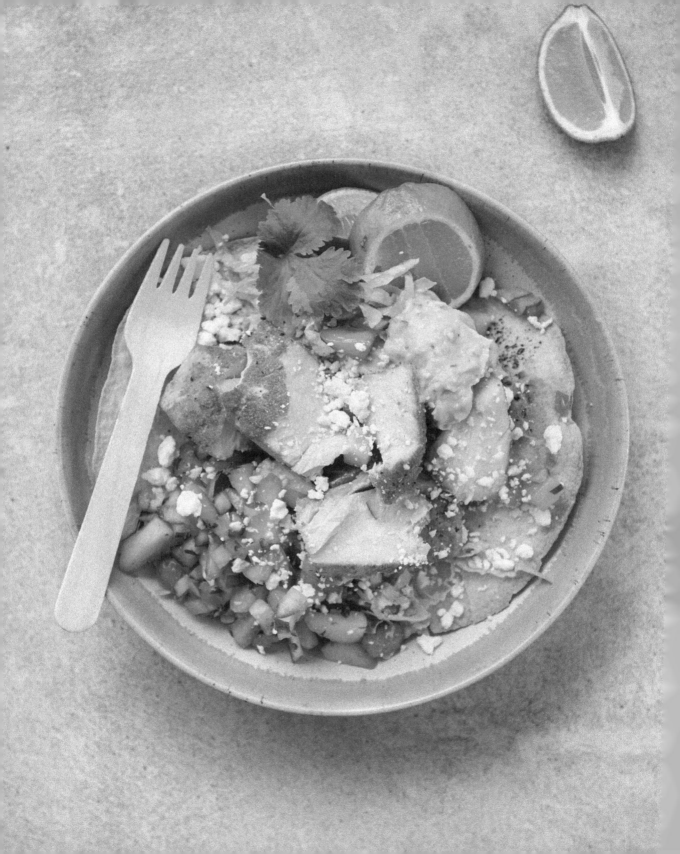

Salmon Tostada Salad

SERVES: 4 / **PREP TIME:** 10 minutes / **COOK TIME:** 10 minutes
30 MINUTES OR LESS, QUICK-PREP, NUT-FREE, GLUTEN-FREE

I once had a salmon tostada salad at a restaurant, and I've been dreaming about it ever since. I finally got the urge to make it on my own, and it made me feel fancy even though it's pretty simple and straightforward. It's like having taco night but adding more fruits and vegetables to the mix, which I will never complain about.

1 teaspoon paprika

½ teaspoon cayenne

½ teaspoon onion powder

½ teaspoon salt

¼ teaspoon cumin

¼ teaspoon ground black pepper

4 (6-ounce) salmon fillets, skin on

1 tablespoon olive oil

8 small corn tortillas

8 cups romaine lettuce, chopped

4 ounces feta or Cotija cheese, crumbled

½ cup Easy Guacamole (page 83)

1 cup Strawberry-Jalapeño Salsa (page 82)

1. Heat the grill to medium.

2. In a small bowl, mix together the paprika, cayenne, onion powder, salt, cumin, and pepper.

3. Rub the spice mixture evenly all over the fish fillets.

4. Place the fillets on the grill, skin-side down, and cook for 8 minutes, or until internal temperature reaches 145°F. (No turning necessary.)

5. Meanwhile, preheat the oven to 375°F. Rub the oil on both sides of each tortilla. Place the tortillas on a baking sheet or directly on the oven rack and bake for 5 minutes, or until crispy.

6. Assemble the four servings. In each bowl, place two corn tortillas, ¼ of the romaine lettuce, ¼ of the fish, ¼ of the cheese, ¼ of the guacamole, and ¼ of the salsa.

> **INGREDIENT TIP:** If you want to save some time, use corn tortilla chips instead of the baked corn tortillas.

Per serving: Calories: 704; Total Fat: 36g; Saturated Fat: 9g; Cholesterol: 155mg; Sodium: 1035mg; Carbohydrates: 26g; Fiber: 6g; Protein: 71g

Maple-Glazed Cedar Plank Salmon

SERVES: 4 / **PREP TIME:** 1 hour / **COOK TIME:** 20 minutes
30 MINUTES OR LESS, NUT-FREE, DAIRY-FREE

This is my husband's go-to method of making salmon. I was skeptical the first time he wanted to try it, but now I find myself requesting it often. This maple glaze combines beautifully with the cedar flavor. It does mean a little extra planning to use the cedar plank. We usually place the cedar in a water bath when we leave in the morning, and then it's ready to use when we get home for dinner.

1 to 2 cedar planks

¼ cup maple syrup

2 tablespoons lemon juice

1 tablespoon Dijon mustard

1 tablespoon soy sauce

½ teaspoon garlic powder

1 teaspoon paprika

4 (6-ounce) salmon fillets, cleaned and deboned

¼ teaspoon salt

¼ teaspoon pepper

Freshly squeezed lemon juice

1. Soak the cedar planks for at least 1 hour prior to grilling. Place the planks in a baking dish and cover with water. They will float, so weigh them down with something like a teapot or a heavy bowl to keep submerged.

2. In a large saucepan over medium heat, whisk together the maple syrup, lemon juice, mustard, soy sauce, garlic powder, and paprika and bring to a boil. Whisk constantly until the sauce thickens, 3 to 5 minutes. Remove the sauce from the heat and set aside.

3. When the cedar plank has fully soaked, heat the grill to medium-high.

4. Rub the salmon fillets with salt and pepper and place them skin-side down on the cedar plank.

5. Brush the salmon fillets with the maple glaze.

6. Place the cedar plank with the salmon on the grill and cook for 15 to 20 minutes or until internal temperature reaches 145°F.

Per serving: Calories: 481; Total Fat: 18g; Saturated Fat: 3g; Cholesterol: 130mg; Sodium: 594mg; Carbohydrates: 15g; Fiber: 0g; Protein: 62g

Easy Apple-Tuna Salad

SERVES: 4 / PREP TIME: 10 minutes

ONE-POT, 30 MINUTES OR LESS, QUICK-PREP, NUT-FREE, DAIRY-FREE, GLUTEN-FREE

It's easy to find excuses to not pack a lunch. This recipe is the opposite: It is an excuse for you *to* actually pack lunch. It takes less than 10 minutes to throw this all together, and you will have lunch all taken care of for a few days. Feel free to add or substitute the spices for others like paprika, cumin, or white pepper to change up the flavor and add an extra layer of depth.

2 (5-ounce) cans tuna in water, drained

½ cup Homemade Mayo (page 254)

1 tablespoon Dijon mustard

2 celery stalks, diced

1 apple, cored and diced

¼ cup dill pickles, minced

Salt

Pepper

Butter lettuce

1. Mix the tuna with the mayonnaise and mustard. Add the celery, apple, and pickles and mix well. Season with salt and pepper.

2. Serve in lettuce wraps or with cut up vegetables.

> **SUBSTITUTION TIP:** Swap out tuna for canned salmon for a different flavor but similar texture.

Per serving: Calories: 207: Total Fat: 15g: Saturated Fat: 2g: Cholesterol: 35mg: Sodium: 497mg: Carbohydrates: 5g: Fiber: 1g: Protein: 11g

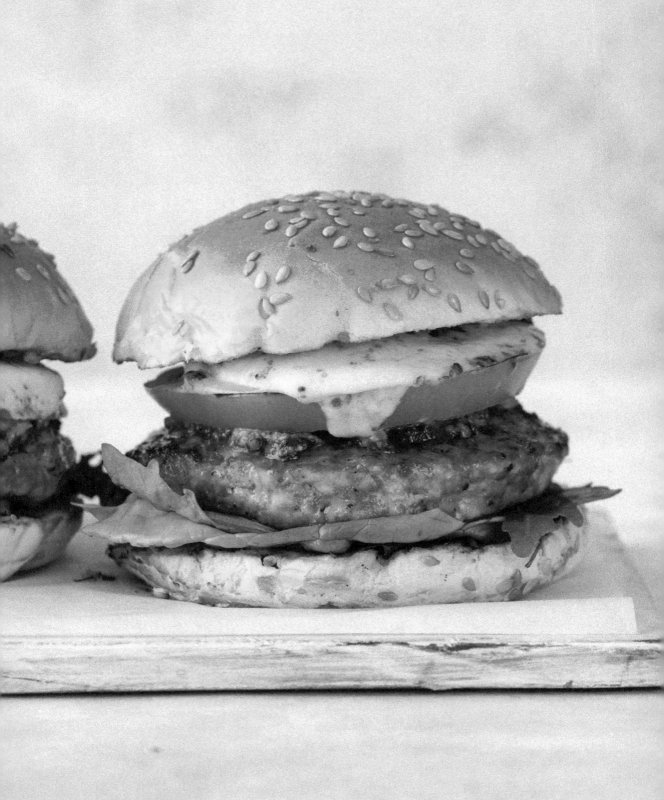

CHAPTER EIGHT

Chicken

172 Crispy Baked Wings

173 Lemon Greek Chicken Skewers

174 Grown-Up Chicken Tenders

175 Waldorf Chicken Salad

176 Spinach Artichoke Roll-Ups

177 Caprese Chicken Burgers

178 Egg Roll in a Bowl

179 Sheet Pan Sweet and Sour Chicken Rice Bowls

180 Paprika-Baked Chicken Thighs

181 BBQ Grilled Chicken

182 Pressure Cooker Butter Chicken

183 Sheet Pan Chicken Fajitas

184 Green Chicken Enchiladas

185 Skillet Peachy Chicken Picante

186 Chicken Marsala

187 Buffalo Chicken Cauliflower Pizza

189 Pressure Cooker Chicken Tikka Masala

190 Chicken Bruschetta Pasta

191 Pesto Chicken Alfredo with Spaghetti Squash

192 Chicken Parmesan over Zoodles

Crispy Baked Wings

SERVES: 4 / **PREP TIME:** 10 minutes / **COOK TIME:** 30 minutes
QUICK-PREP, NUT-FREE, DAIRY-FREE, GLUTEN-FREE

Wings are not my style when I go out to eat, as I'm not a fan of how they always seem to be soggy, greasy, and often fried. These wings are none of those things. They are crispy, lightly seasoned, and baked. Enjoy them tossed in your favorite barbecue sauce, or if you're like me, enjoy them as is out of the oven.

1 teaspoon garlic powder

1 teaspoon paprika

1 teaspoon chili powder

½ teaspoon salt

½ teaspoon ground black pepper

¼ teaspoon red pepper flakes (optional)

2 pounds chicken wings and drumsticks, separated

Sassy BBQ Sauce (page 257) (optional)

1. Preheat the oven to 400°F.

2. In a large bowl, mix together the garlic powder, paprika, chili powder, salt, pepper, and red pepper flakes, if using. Set aside.

3. Pat down the wings with a paper towel, squeeze out any excess juice and make the wings very dry (this step is key!).

4. Put the wings in the large bowl with spices and coat evenly, rubbing in the spices with your hands.

5. Place the wings on a greased cooling rack over a baking sheet in the oven and cook for 30 minutes or until internal temperature reaches 165°F.

6. Toss the wings in the sauce or enjoy as is.

> **VARIATION TIP:** If you prefer, you can make these on the grill. Heat the grill to medium high heat and turn chicken halfway through. They may take slightly less time to cook, so monitor closely.

Per serving: Calories: 431; Total Fat: 26g; Saturated Fat: 8g; Cholesterol: 108mg; Sodium: 490mg; Carbohydrates: 1g; Fiber: 1g; Protein: 47g

Lemon Greek Chicken Skewers

SERVES: 4 / **PREP TIME:** 15 minutes, plus 30 minutes to marinate / **COOK TIME:** 10 minutes
NUT-FREE, GLUTEN-FREE

Cooking chicken on skewers is a fun way to change things up. Even though the chicken is crispy on the outside, the yogurt does a great job of keeping the chicken from drying out. I recommend serving this dish over some turmeric rice so that it can sop up all the flavors of the marinade.

2 tablespoons olive oil

⅓ cup plain unsweetened Greek yogurt

Juice and zest of 1 large lemon

3 to 4 garlic cloves, minced

1 tablespoon oregano

¼ teaspoon salt

¼ teaspoon pepper

1½ pounds chicken breast, cubed

1 zucchini, sliced

1 small red onion, cut into a 1-inch dice

1 red bell pepper, cut into a 1-inch dice

1. In a large bowl, whisk together the olive oil, yogurt, lemon juice, lemon zest, garlic, oregano, salt, and pepper.

2. Pour half of the yogurt mixture into a freezer bag and add the cubed chicken. Seal the bag tightly and shake to coat evenly. Refrigerate for 30 minutes. Reserve the remaining marinade for basting.

3. Preheat the grill to medium heat.

4. Thread 5 or 6 skewers with the chicken, zucchini, red onion, and bell pepper. Discard the marinade you used for the raw chicken.

5. Place the skewers on grill, turning often and basting with the reserved marinade. Cook for 10 minutes, or until chicken is cooked to an internal temperature of 165°F.

VARIATION TIP: No grill? Bake in the oven for 20 minutes, turning once, and basting until the internal temperature reaches 165°F. Try serving with Grape Leaf Pilaf (page 138).

Per serving: Calories: 279; Total Fat: 12g; Saturated Fat: 3g; Cholesterol: 102mg; Sodium: 434mg; Carbohydrates: 10g; Fiber: 2g; Protein: 37g

Grown-Up Chicken Tenders

SERVES: 4 / **PREP TIME:** 15 minutes / **COOK TIME:** 20 minutes
NUT-FREE, GLUTEN-FREE

I am almost certain I ordered off the kids' menu until I was at least 16. I knew almost anywhere I went I could at least get some chicken fingers and French fries, which was all I wanted. The good news was we didn't often go out to eat as a family, because my mom cooked most meals from scratch—otherwise I might've turned into a chicken tender. However, every once in a while, I still wish I could get some chicken tenders off the kids' menu. This recipe is my grown-up dietitian approved version of a childhood favorite.

¼ cup cornstarch

2 eggs, beaten

1 cup grated
   Parmesan cheese

1 teaspoon garlic powder

1 teaspoon paprika

1 teaspoon oregano

1½ pounds chicken
   breast, cut into
   long strips

Ketchup (page 256)

Honey Mustard (page 255)

1. Preheat the oven to 425°F. Line a baking sheet with aluminum foil and place a greased cooling rack on top of it.

2. Take out three shallow dishes. In dish one, place the cornstarch. In dish two, place the eggs, and in dish three, combine the Parmesan cheese, garlic powder, paprika, and oregano.

3. Dredge each chicken strip in the cornstarch, then dip in the egg, then coat with the cheese and spice mixture. Place the coated chicken strip on the rack on the baking sheet. Repeat for each chicken strip.

4. Bake in the oven for 20 minutes or until the chicken is cooked through, or to an internal temperature of 165°F. Serve with ketchup and honey mustard.

VARIATION TIP: If you don't have a cooling rack, place the chicken on an aluminum foil–lined baking sheet and flip halfway through baking.

Per serving: Calories: 350; Total Fat: 14g; Saturated Fat: 6g; Cholesterol: 210mg; Sodium: 771mg; Carbohydrates: 9g; Fiber: 0g; Protein: 48g

Waldorf Chicken Salad

SERVES: 4 / **PREP TIME:** 10 minutes / **COOK TIME:** 20 minutes

30 MINUTES OR LESS, QUICK-PREP, GLUTEN-FREE

While this sounds like a fancy dish, it's actually incredibly easy to make and anything but fancy. This salad will provide some lunchtime variety, while also helping you get wholesome homemade food into the lunch bag, because it's quick and easy to make. Feel free to put it on a sandwich or toss it over greens.

1 pound chicken breast

½ cup plain unsweetened Greek yogurt

2 tablespoons Homemade Mayo (page 254)

2 celery stalks, sliced

1 pear, cored and sliced

1 cup red grapes, halved

¼ cup diced red onion

¼ cup chopped walnuts

Salt

Pepper

1. Put the chicken in a large stockpot and cover with water (or chicken stock). Bring to a boil over high heat. Once boiling, cover, reduce the heat to low, and simmer for 10 to 15 minutes, or until the chicken is cooked to an internal temperature of 165°F. Remove the chicken from the pot and allow to cool for 5 to 10 minutes.

2. Meanwhile, in a medium bowl, combine the yogurt, mayonnaise, celery, pear, grapes, onion, walnuts, salt, and pepper. Cover and refrigerate until the chicken is ready.

3. Dice the chicken and add it to the yogurt mixture.

> **SUBSTITUTION TIP:** Make this dish nut-free by swapping out the walnuts for pumpkin seeds or sunflower seeds.

Per serving: Calories: 276; Total Fat: 13g; Saturated Fat: 3g; Cholesterol: 75mg; Sodium: 249mg; Carbohydrates: 17g; Fiber: 3g; Protein: 26g

Spinach Artichoke Roll-Ups

SERVES: 8 / **PREP TIME:** 10 minutes / **COOK TIME:** 35 minutes

QUICK-PREP, NUT-FREE, GLUTEN-FREE

Sometimes chicken is boring, so using a roll-up recipe can keep you and your family interested and excited about dinner. I'll prepare these over the weekend and have them ready to go all week for lunch or dinner. It's a healthier and more substantive version of spinach artichoke dip.

Cooking oil spray

1 tablespoon olive oil

4 garlic cloves, minced

1 (14-ounce) can artichoke hearts, drained and chopped

8 cups baby spinach

2 ounces cream cheese

½ cup shredded Cheddar cheese

½ cup grated Parmesan cheese

1 teaspoon salt

½ teaspoon pepper

4 (4-ounce) chicken breasts

1. Preheat the oven to 400°F. Coat the inside of a 9-by-13-inch baking dish with cooking oil spray.

2. In a large skillet, heat the oil over medium heat. Add the garlic and cook for 3 minutes.

3. Add the artichokes and spinach and stir until spinach starts to wilt. Remove from the heat and stir in the cream cheese, Cheddar cheese, Parmesan, salt, and pepper. Set aside.

4. Butterfly the chicken breasts (don't cut all the way through) and open like a book. Place between 2 sheets of parchment paper and pound with a mallet (or rolling pin) until about ½- to ¼-inch thick.

5. Put ¼ of the spinach-artichoke mixture in each butterflied chicken breast and roll lengthwise. Place the rolled and stuffed chicken breast in the baking dish, seam-side down, and bake for 25 to 30 minutes, or until the chicken is cooked to internal temperature of 165°F.

6. Remove from the oven, and allow the chicken to cool for 5 minutes, then slice into pinwheels and serve over cauliflower rice or a salad.

TECHNIQUE TIP: Use toothpicks or kitchen twine to seal chicken together as some may fall apart when cooking.

Per serving: Calories: 182; Total Fat: 10g; Saturated Fat: 5g; Cholesterol: 51mg; Sodium: 636mg; Carbohydrates: 6g; Fiber: 5g; Protein: 19g

Caprese Chicken Burgers

SERVES: 4 / **PREP TIME:** 5 minutes / **COOK TIME:** 20 minutes
5 INGREDIENTS OR LESS, 30 MINUTES OR LESS, QUICK-PREP, GLUTEN-FREE

I like to get creative with burgers. This recipe is inspired by the fact that I love anything with Mediterranean flavors, but mostly because I love anything with fresh mozzarella cheese. For this recipe you are basically having a caprese salad on top of a burger; now that's something I can get behind.

¼ cup Spinach-Walnut Pesto (page 265), plus more for topping

1 pound ground chicken

1 tomato, sliced

4 (1-ounce) slices fresh mozzarella

4 hamburger buns

Lettuce, onions, and tomato, for topping (optional)

1. Heat the grill to medium-high.

2. Mix the pesto with the chicken and form 4 patties.

3. Grill the chicken patties for 8 minutes per side until cooked through and the internal temperature reaches 165°F.

4. During the last minute of cooking, top each patty with a bit more pesto, 1 slice of tomato, and 1 slice of mozzarella.

5. Meanwhile, spread pesto on the burger buns and when the burgers are done, place the buns on the grill for 2 to 3 minutes to toast and then place the burger on the bun.

> **SUBSTITUTION TIP:** Substitute chicken with beef or turkey if you prefer, but be mindful that cooking times will vary.

Per serving: Calories: 538; Total Fat: 29g; Saturated Fat: 8g; Cholesterol: 116mg; Sodium: 570mg; Carbohydrates: 43g; Fiber: 2g; Protein: 32g

Egg Roll in a Bowl

SERVES: 4 / **PREP TIME:** 10 minutes / **COOK TIME:** 15 minutes
ONE-POT, 30 MINUTES OR LESS, QUICK-PREP, DAIRY-FREE

This dish is easy to put together and would be an excellent make-ahead option for lunch or dinner for the week. I'm a fan of putting an egg on or in anything, because it gives a rich flavor and fills you up. The ground chicken can get sticky, so if you prefer to use ground turkey, pork, or beef, feel free to do so.

2 tablespoons sesame oil, divided

1 pound ground chicken

1 small sweet onion, diced

3 garlic cloves, minced

2 large carrots, diced

½ small head cabbage, shredded

2 large eggs, beaten

1 teaspoon freshly grated ginger

1 tablespoon rice vinegar

3 tablespoons soy sauce

1 to 2 teaspoons Sriracha (optional)

Sliced green onions (optional)

1. In a large skillet, heat 1 tablespoon of oil over medium heat. Add the chicken and cook until fully browned, about 8 minutes.

2. Add the remaining oil along with the onion, garlic, carrots, and cabbage and sauté for 3 to 4 minutes.

3. Make a well in the center of the skillet and pour in the eggs. Let the eggs sit for 20 to 30 seconds, then scramble and incorporate them into the rest of the mixture.

4. Add the ginger, rice vinegar, and soy sauce, and stir to combine.

5. Remove from the heat and top with Sriracha and green onions, if desired.

INGREDIENT TIP: You can either buy cabbage already shredded or use a food processor to make the shredding easier and more uniform.

Per serving: Calories: 350; Total Fat: 22g; Saturated Fat: 5g; Cholesterol: 188mg; Sodium: 844mg; Carbohydrates: 13g; Fiber: 3g; Protein: 27g

Sheet Pan Sweet and Sour Chicken Rice Bowls

SERVES: 4 / **PREP TIME:** 10 minutes / **COOK TIME:** 20 minutes
30 MINUTES OR LESS, QUICK-PREP, NUT-FREE, DAIRY-FREE

Sheet pan dinners are underrated in my opinion. If I can get everything to cook on one sheet pan, it means less mess in the kitchen for me to clean up when I'm done cooking. This dish pairs nicely over rice or cauliflower rice but can certainly be eaten on its own.

1½ to 2 pounds chicken breast, chopped

1 bell pepper, chopped

1 yellow onion, chopped

1 zucchini, chopped

1 (20-ounce) can pineapple chunks, drained and patted dry

1 tablespoon avocado oil

½ teaspoon garlic powder

¼ teaspoon ground ginger

1¼ cups Sweet-and-Sour Sauce (page 262)

3 cups cooked rice

1. Preheat the oven to 400°F. Line a baking sheet with parchment paper.

2. Place the chicken, bell pepper, onion, zucchini, and pineapple on the baking sheet. Drizzle the oil over the chicken, vegetables, and pineapple, and sprinkle with garlic powder and ginger. Stir to combine.

3. Spread the chicken, pineapple, and vegetables in a single layer on the baking sheet (use an extra baking sheet if you need more space).

4. Bake for 20 minutes, or until the chicken reaches an internal temperature of 165°F.

5. In a large bowl, toss the chicken, pineapple, and vegetables with the sweet-and-sour sauce and serve over rice.

MAKE-AHEAD TIP: If you're making the sweet-and-sour sauce ahead of time, use the juice from a can of pineapple and put the chunks themselves in a sealed container in the refrigerator until ready to use.

Per serving: Calories: 561: Total Fat: 8g; Saturated Fat: 1g; Cholesterol: 97mg; Sodium: 886mg; Carbohydrates: 89g; Fiber: 3g; Protein: 40g

Paprika-Baked Chicken Thighs

SERVES: 6 / **PREP TIME:** 5 minutes / **COOK TIME:** 45 minutes
QUICK-PREP, NUT-FREE, DAIRY-FREE, GLUTEN-FREE

Getting a healthy and delicious dinner on the table quickly is hard. However, when eating at home, not only can you feel proud of the meal you made, but you can control what goes into that meal. Don't let the time on this meal fool you; it takes 5 minutes to prepare and you can get plenty done in the kitchen and around the house while it is cooking.

Cooking oil spray

2 pounds boneless, skinless chicken thighs

¼ cup Ghee (page 251) or butter

5 to 6 garlic cloves, minced

2 tablespoons paprika

1 tablespoon oregano

½ teaspoon red pepper flakes

½ teaspoon dried parsley

¼ teaspoon salt

¼ teaspoon pepper

1. Preheat the oven to 425°F. Coat the inside of a 9-by-13-inch baking dish with cooking oil spray.

2. Pat the chicken thighs dry and place them in the baking dish.

3. In a small saucepan, heat the ghee and use a whisk to mix in the garlic, paprika, oregano, red pepper flakes, parsley, salt, and pepper. Pour the sauce over the chicken thighs.

4. Bake for 40 to 45 minutes or until the chicken reaches and internal temperature of 165°F.

> **SUBSTITUTION TIP:** If you prefer chicken breasts, you can use them in place of thighs, but note that the cooking time may need to be longer.

Per serving: Calories: 267; Total Fat: 19g; Saturated Fat: 9g; Cholesterol: 143mg; Sodium: 312mg; Carbohydrates: 3g; Fiber: 1g; Protein: 22g

BBQ Grilled Chicken

SERVES: 6 / **PREP TIME:** 5 minutes, plus 30 minutes to 2 hours / **COOK TIME:** 15 minutes
5 INGREDIENTS OR LESS, NUT-FREE, DAIRY-FREE, GLUTEN-FREE

Fun fact: You can grill year-round. I know most people leave the grilling to the summer months, but we like to use our grill rain or shine, sun or snow. The beauty of the grill is that you can do a bunch of meal prep all at once while leaving your kitchen pretty free for other meal items (or just to keep it clean). We use this recipe year-round for make-ahead dinners or lunches.

2 pounds chicken breast

1 cup Sassy BBQ Sauce (page 257), plus more for basting

1. Place the chicken and the barbecue sauce in a large freezer bag and seal tightly. Place the bag in the refrigerator and let the chicken marinate for at least 30 minutes or up to 2 hours.

2. Preheat the grill to medium-high heat.

3. Remove the chicken from the bag and discard the barbecue sauce left in the bag.

4. Grill the chicken for 7 minutes, then turn, and cook for 7 to 8 minutes more, or until the internal temperature reaches 165°F.

> **VARIATION TIP:** Replace the Sassy BBQ Sauce with any marinade you have on hand to change up the flavor and save on prep time.

Per serving: Calories: 169: Total Fat: 4g: Saturated Fat: 1g: Cholesterol: 87mg: Sodium: 476mg: Carbohydrates: 4g: Fiber: 1g: Protein: 31g

Pressure Cooker Butter Chicken

SERVES: 6 / **PREP TIME:** 5 minutes / **COOK TIME:** 30 minutes
ONE-POT, QUICK-PREP, NUT-FREE, GLUTEN-FREE

I call this recipe a "dump and run." Why? Because you can literally dump all the ingredients in and go for a run. Sorry, another bad joke. However, having a pressure cooker makes getting a delicious and nutritious meal on the table within the hour very easy. I like to serve this dish over rice, but it certainly holds up on its own and would also be good with pasta, couscous, or some bread to sop up all the goodness in the sauce.

1 tablespoon butter

3 garlic cloves, minced

1 yellow onion, diced

1 tablespoon grated ginger

6 ounces tomato paste

1 tablespoon garam masala

1 teaspoon paprika

½ teaspoon turmeric

½ teaspoon salt

¼ teaspoon pepper

¼ cup fresh parsley

1 (13.5-ounce) can full-fat coconut milk

½ cup full-fat plain unsweetened Greek yogurt

2 pounds chicken breast, chopped

1 tablespoon cornstarch

1. Put the butter, garlic, onion, ginger, tomato paste, garam masala, paprika, turmeric, salt, pepper, parsley, coconut milk, and yogurt into the pressure cooker and whisk.

2. Add the chicken, seal, and cook on manual (high) for 15 minutes.

3. Allow the pressure to naturally release for 10 minutes, then quick release until you are able to open.

4. Turn on the sauté function, whisk in the cornstarch, and cook for 3 to 5 minutes, or until the sauce thickens.

> **VARIATION TIP:** If you don't have a pressure cooker, you can use a slow cooker and cook on low for 6 to 8 hours or on high for 4 to 6 hours.

Per serving: Calories: 347; Total Fat: 18g; Saturated Fat: 3g; Cholesterol: 96mg; Sodium: 687mg; Carbohydrates: 11g; Fiber: 2g; Protein: 34g

Sheet Pan Chicken Fajitas

SERVES: 4 / **PREP TIME:** 5 minutes / **COOK TIME:** 30 minutes

5 INGREDIENTS OR LESS, QUICK-PREP, NUT-FREE, DAIRY-FREE, GLUTEN-FREE

Sheet pan chicken fajitas keep the mess out of the kitchen. Serve this up on a taco night or use it in a burrito bowl. I personally like to make a bowl filled with lettuce, rice, salsa, and beans, then top it with these chicken fajitas, a sprinkle of Cheddar cheese, and a few tablespoons of guacamole.

1½ to 2 pounds chicken breast, sliced

3 bell peppers (assorted colors), sliced

1 red onion, sliced

1 tablespoon avocado oil

1 tablespoon Taco Seasoning (page 250)

1. Preheat the oven to 400°F. Line a baking sheet with parchment paper.

2. In a large bowl, mix together all of the ingredients until evenly coated.

3. Spread the chicken mixture on the baking sheet in a single layer. Cook for 30 minutes or until the chicken is cooked through to an internal temperature of 165°F.

> **INGREDIENT TIP:** When slicing the chicken, make sure to cut even pieces so that they cook at an even rate, otherwise you may have pieces that dry out while others are not cooked through.

Per serving: Calories: 234; Total Fat: 7g; Saturated Fat: 1g; Cholesterol: 97mg; Sodium: 439mg; Carbohydrates: 8g; Fiber: 2g; Protein: 36g

Green Chicken Enchiladas

SERVES: 6 / **PREP TIME:** 15 minutes / **COOK TIME:** 25 minutes
NUT-FREE, GLUTEN-FREE

Chicken enchiladas are sometimes cumbersome to make, but once you get the hang of it, they become a go-to staple in any household. I like to make this recipe ahead of time as it holds up well for the week and makes a decent portion so you can sail smoothly through your week on tasty leftovers. Top with sour cream, olives, and extra salsa to liven it up after reheating.

Cooking oil spray

16 ounces mild salsa
  verde, divided

2 cups cooked,
  shredded chicken

1 green bell pepper, diced

1 small red onion, diced

12 corn tortillas

1 cup Cheddar cheese,
  shredded

1 tomato, diced

1 avocado, diced

1 jalapeño, diced

1. Preheat the oven to 400°F. Coat the inside of a 9-by-13-inch baking dish with cooking oil spray.

2. Reserve ¼ cup plus 2 tablespoons of salsa verde.

3. In a large bowl, mix together the chicken, bell pepper, onion, and the remaining salsa verde.

4. Spread the ¼ cup of reserved salsa verde evenly on the bottom of baking dish.

5. Wrap the tortillas in a damp paper towel and microwave for 30 seconds to soften.

6. Add about ⅛ of the chicken mixture down the center of the tortilla. Roll up the tortilla and place it seam-side down in baking dish. Repeat with all of the tortillas.

7. Top the rolled tortillas with the remaining 2 tablespoons of salsa verde, sprinkle with cheese, and cover the baking dish with foil. Bake for 20 minutes, then remove the foil and broil for 1 to 2 minutes.

8. Top with tomato, avocado, and jalapeño and enjoy!

SUBSTITUTION TIP: If you can't find salsa verde, use your favorite salsa.

Per serving: Calories: 574; Total Fat: 23g; Saturated Fat: 7g; Cholesterol: 118mg; Sodium: 922mg; Carbohydrates: 48g; Fiber: 9g; Protein: 36g

Skillet Peachy Chicken Picante

SERVES: 4 / **PREP TIME:** 10 minutes / **COOK TIME:** 45 minutes
ONE-POT, QUICK-PREP, NUT-FREE, DAIRY-FREE, GLUTEN-FREE

This dish is inspired by my husband. I asked him what meals reminded him of his child-hood and he recounted a chicken and peach dish that he loved and asked for frequently when he was growing up. The peaches add a sweet touch to this otherwise savory dish. Look for peaches that are on the riper side to bring out more flavor in this dish.

1 tablespoon Ghee (page 251) or butter

1 red onion, diced

3 garlic cloves, minced

1 jalapeño, seeded and diced

4 peaches, chopped

1 (14.5-ounce) can diced tomatoes

1 tablespoon honey

½ teaspoon salt

½ teaspoon pepper

¼ teaspoon red pepper flakes (optional)

1 pound chicken breast

1. Preheat the oven to 400°F.

2. In a large, oven-safe skillet, heat the ghee over medium heat. Add the onion and sauté for 3 to 5 minutes, or until soft-ened. Add the garlic, jalapeño, and peaches and sauté for 2 to 3 minutes more.

3. Add in the tomatoes, honey, salt, pepper, and red pepper flakes, if using. Simmer for 5 minutes. Add the chicken. Spoon the sauce over the chicken so it is completely coated with sauce. Place the skillet in the oven and cook for 30 minutes, or until internal temperature of the chicken reaches 165°F.

VARIATION TIP: If you do not have an oven-safe skillet, use a baking dish and transfer the chicken and sauce to the baking dish before placing in the oven.

Per serving: Calories: 228; Total Fat: 6g; Saturated Fat: 2g; Cholesterol: 73mg; Sodium: 698mg; Carbohydrates: 23g; Fiber: 3g; Protein: 25g

Chicken Marsala

SERVES: 4 / **PREP TIME:** 10 minutes / **COOK TIME:** 25 minutes
QUICK-PREP, NUT-FREE, DAIRY-FREE, GLUTEN-FREE

I used to despise mushrooms. I think mushrooms just tend to not be super kid-friendly even though they have a relatively mild flavor. However, I like to give foods a second chance, and if prepared well, I'll find a way to enjoy almost any food. This was one of the first dishes that brought mushrooms into my life for good. Pair this with some of your favorite pasta and maybe even enjoy a glass of wine to seal the deal.

1 to 1½ pounds
  chicken breasts

½ teaspoon salt

¼ teaspoon pepper

3 tablespoons
  cornstarch, divided

2 tablespoons butter

8 ounces white button
  mushrooms, sliced

¼ cup diced yellow onion

3 garlic cloves, minced

½ cup Marsala wine

½ cup chicken or
  beef broth

2 tablespoons
  fresh parsley

Salt

Pepper

1. Place the chicken, salt, pepper, and 2 tablespoons of the cornstarch in a large freezer bag and seal tightly. Shake the bag so that the cornstarch and spices coat the chicken.

2. In a large skillet, heat the butter over medium-high heat. Remove the chicken from the bag and shake off any extra cornstarch. Place the chicken in the skillet and brown for 2 to 3 minutes per side. Transfer the chicken to a plate and set aside.

3. Add the mushrooms to the skillet and sauté for 2 to 3 minutes, or until they start to soften. Add the onion and garlic and sauté for 1 to 2 minutes more.

4. Pour in the wine, broth, and remaining tablespoon of cornstarch. Stir, scraping up any brown bits from the sides and bottom of the skillet. Bring the liquid to a boil.

5. Reduce the heat to medium and return the chicken to the skillet. Cover and simmer for 15 minutes, or until the chicken is cooked through and the sauce has thickened. Garnish with the parsley and adjust the seasoning with the salt and pepper before serving.

Per serving: Calories: 253; Total Fat: 9g; Saturated Fat: 4g; Cholesterol: 81mg; Sodium: 598mg; Carbohydrates: 13g; Fiber: 1g; Protein: 25g

Buffalo Chicken Cauliflower Pizza

SERVES: 6 / **PREP TIME:** 5 minutes / **COOK TIME:** 5 minutes

30 MINUTES OR LESS, QUICK-PREP, NUT-FREE, GLUTEN-FREE

Buffalo chicken is a classic American flavor and always delicious on pizza. The cauliflower crust allows for a bit more vegetables to get on the table without compromising flavor. If you don't have any cooked chicken on hand, you can cook some quickly by boiling a chicken breast or two in water for 15 to 20 minutes.

1 Cauliflower Pizza Crust (page 267)

¼ cup Ghee (page 251) or butter

¼ cup hot sauce

½ teaspoon garlic powder

16 ounces cooked chicken, cubed

2 cups shredded mozzarella

½ red onion, sliced thin

2 cups arugula

2 green onions, sliced thin

½ cup blue cheese, crumbled

1. Preheat the oven to 400°F. Place the cauliflower crust on a parchment- or aluminum foil–lined baking sheet

2. In a large saucepan over medium heat, whisk together the ghee, hot sauce, and garlic powder. When melted and well combined, add in the cooked chicken, and stir to thoroughly coat the chicken with the sauce. Then remove from the heat.

3. Top the crust with the mozzarella cheese. Distribute the chicken, red onion, arugula, green onions, and blue cheese evenly over the pizza.

4. Bake for 5 minutes or until the cheese is melted.

> **VARIATION TIP:** Make this pizza your own by adding other toppings of your choice such as broccoli florets, mushrooms, green bell peppers, or chopped fresh tomatoes.

Per serving: Calories: 419; Total Fat: 26g; Saturated Fat: 17g; Cholesterol: 137mg; Sodium: 937mg; Carbohydrates: 13g; Fiber: 3g; Protein: 36g

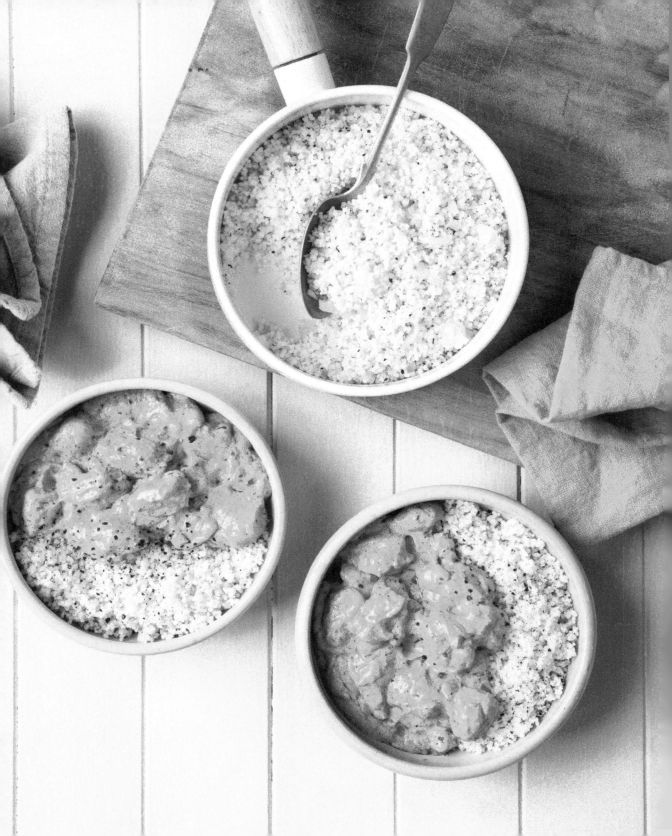

Pressure Cooker Chicken Tikka Masala

SERVES: 6 / **PREP TIME:** 5 minutes / **COOK TIME:** 15 minutes
ONE-POT, 30 MINUTES OR LESS, QUICK-PREP, NUT-FREE, DAIRY-FREE, GLUTEN-FREE

If you haven't gotten on board the pressure cooker train, it's time to do so. It's so satisfying to throw dinner in the pressure cooker knowing that you will get a delicious and tender meal in practically no time at all. You'll be shocked that something that cooks for such a short time can taste so good. The chicken in this dish practically melts in your mouth. Serve it over rice or eat it by itself—either way it's terrific.

1 yellow onion, diced

3 garlic cloves, minced

1 (14-ounce) can diced tomatoes

1 (13.5-ounce) can full-fat coconut milk

1 tablespoon garam masala

1 teaspoon turmeric

1 teaspoon grated fresh ginger

½ teaspoon salt

¼ teaspoon black pepper

2 to 3 pounds boneless, skinless chicken thighs

Lime juice and cilantro, for topping (optional)

1. Put the onion, garlic, diced tomatoes, coconut milk, garam masala, turmeric, ginger, salt, and pepper in a pressure cooker and use an immersion blender to blend.

2. Add the chicken, seal, and cook on manual (high) for 15 minutes.

3. Once finished, quick release until the pressure subsides.

4. Serve over rice and top with freshly squeezed lime juice and cilantro, if desired.

> **VARIATION TIP:** Use a slow cooker in place of a pressure cooker. Cook for 4 to 6 hours on high or 6 to 8 hours on low.

Per serving: Calories: 321; Total Fat: 21g; Saturated Fat: 3g; Cholesterol: 120mg; Sodium: 519mg; Carbohydrates: 5g; Fiber: 1g; Protein: 23g

Chicken Bruschetta Pasta

SERVES: 4 / **PREP TIME:** 10 minutes / **COOK TIME:** 20 minutes
30 MINUTES OR LESS, QUICK-PREP, NUT-FREE, DAIRY-FREE

If you've ever had bruschetta, you know it's a traditional Italian antipasto made of toasted bread rubbed with garlic and topped with fresh vegetables, most commonly fresh tomatoes and basil, with a hint of onion and balsamic. This recipe is a spin on bruschetta that allows you to make an entire meal of this classic appetizer.

FOR THE PASTA AND TOMATOES

8 ounces angel hair pasta

2 cups diced tomatoes

⅓ cup fresh basil, thinly sliced

¼ cup finely chopped red onion

3 garlic cloves, minced

1 tablespoon balsamic vinegar

1 tablespoon olive oil

¼ teaspoon salt

¼ teaspoon pepper

FOR THE CHICKEN

1½ pounds chicken breast, sliced

2 tablespoons olive oil, divided

½ teaspoon dried basil

½ teaspoon salt

¼ teaspoon pepper

Fresh basil leaves, Parmesan cheese, red pepper flakes, for topping (optional)

TO MAKE THE PASTA AND TOMATOES

1. Bring a large pot of salted water to boil over high heat. Add the pasta and cook according to the package instructions. When the pasta is cooked, drain and set aside.

2. Meanwhile, in a medium bowl, toss together the tomatoes, basil, onion, garlic, vinegar, oil, salt, and pepper. Set aside.

TO MAKE THE CHICKEN

1. In a medium bowl, combine the chicken with 1 tablespoon of the oil, basil, salt, and pepper.

2. In a large skillet, heat the remaining 1 tablespoon olive oil over medium heat. Add the chicken and sauté until cooked through and the internal temperature reaches 165°F.

3. Once the chicken is cooked, add tomato mixture to skillet with chicken and cook for an additional 3 minutes. Add the pasta to the skillet and fold the ingredients together gently using tongs.

4. Top with basil, Parmesan, and red pepper flakes, as desired.

Per serving: Calories: 485; Total Fat: 16g; Saturated Fat: 2g; Cholesterol: 97mg; Sodium: 716mg; Carbohydrates: 49g; Fiber: 3g; Protein: 43g

Pesto Chicken Alfredo with Spaghetti Squash

SERVES: 4 / **PREP TIME:** 5 minutes, plus 15 minutes to 2 hours to marinate / **COOK TIME:** 20 minutes
GLUTEN-FREE

I'm not a fan of jarred alfredo sauce because it tends to be too dense and overpowering. When making alfredo sauce at home—as with most food—you have far more control over the final flavor, and it doesn't end up being quite as dense. In this recipe, the alfredo is complemented by the pesto, which gives the dish an additional layer of flavor and texture.

1 pound chicken breast, cubed

¼ cup Spinach-Walnut Pesto (page 265)

⅓ cup Ghee (page 251) or butter

3 garlic cloves, minced

1 cup half-and-half

1 teaspoon oregano

1⅓ cups grated Parmesan

Salt

Pepper

1 cooked and shredded Spaghetti Squash (page 249)

1. Put the chicken and the pesto in a large freezer bag and seal tightly. Massage the pesto into the chicken through the bag so chicken is fully covered with the sauce. Refrigerate for 15 minutes or up to 2 hours.

2. Meanwhile in a medium saucepan, heat the ghee over medium heat. Add the garlic and cook for 2 minutes. Reduce the heat to low.

3. Whisk in the half-and-half and simmer for 2 minutes. Whisk in the oregano and Parmesan and season with salt and pepper.

4. In a large skillet over medium heat, cook the chicken (discard any excess pesto from the bag) until cooked through, or until it reaches an internal temperature of 165°F, about 10 minutes.

5. Pour the alfredo sauce over the chicken and simmer for 2 minutes. Remove from the heat and add the spaghetti squash, tossing gently to integrate the squash with the sauce. Season with additional salt and pepper, as desired.

> **SUBSTITUTION TIP:** You can substitute traditional spaghetti or linguine for the spaghetti squash, as desired.

Per serving: Calories: 602; Total Fat: 46g; Saturated Fat: 25g; Cholesterol: 160mg; Sodium: 943mg; Carbohydrates: 19g; Fiber: 2g; Protein: 40g

Chicken Parmesan over Zoodles

SERVES: 4 / **PREP TIME:** 15 minutes / **COOK TIME:** 30 minutes
NUT-FREE

I never knew that chicken parmesan was called chicken parmesan until I went to college. Growing up in an Italian family we didn't call it chicken parmesan; it was just our usual chicken meal. This rendition is just as delicious as what we would eat growing up in my honest Italian opinion.

2 large eggs

3 garlic cloves, minced

2 tablespoons
   fresh parsley

1½ to 2 pounds chicken
   breast, sliced in
   half horizontally to
   make cutlets

1½ cups bread crumbs

½ cup grated
   Parmesan cheese

1 teaspoon oregano

Salt

Pepper

⅓ cup oil, for frying

2 cups Homemade
   Marinara Sauce
   (page 266)

8 ounces fresh
   mozzarella, sliced

2 zucchinis, spiralized

1. Preheat the oven to 425°F. Line a baking sheet with parchment paper.

2. In a shallow dish, whisk the eggs with the garlic and parsley. Place the chicken in the dish, making sure that the chicken is coated with the egg mixture. Cover the dish with plastic wrap and refrigerate for 15 minutes.

3. Meanwhile in another shallow dish, combine the bread crumbs, Parmesan, oregano, salt, and pepper.

4. Remove the chicken from the refrigerator. Dredge the egg-coated chicken breast in the bread crumb mixture and set on a plate. Repeat for each cutlet.

5. In a large skillet, heat the oil until shimmering. Fry the chicken for 4 to 5 minutes per side.

6. Place the chicken cutlets on the baking sheet and top each one with ¼ cup marinara sauce and a slice of mozzarella and bake for 15 to 20 minutes, or until cooked through or until the chicken reaches an internal temperature of 165°F.

7. Serve over zucchini noodles with extra sauce as desired.

Per serving: Calories: 719; Total Fat: 41g; Saturated Fat: 14g; Cholesterol: 240mg; Sodium: 904mg; Carbohydrates: 30g; Fiber: 4g; Protein: 58g

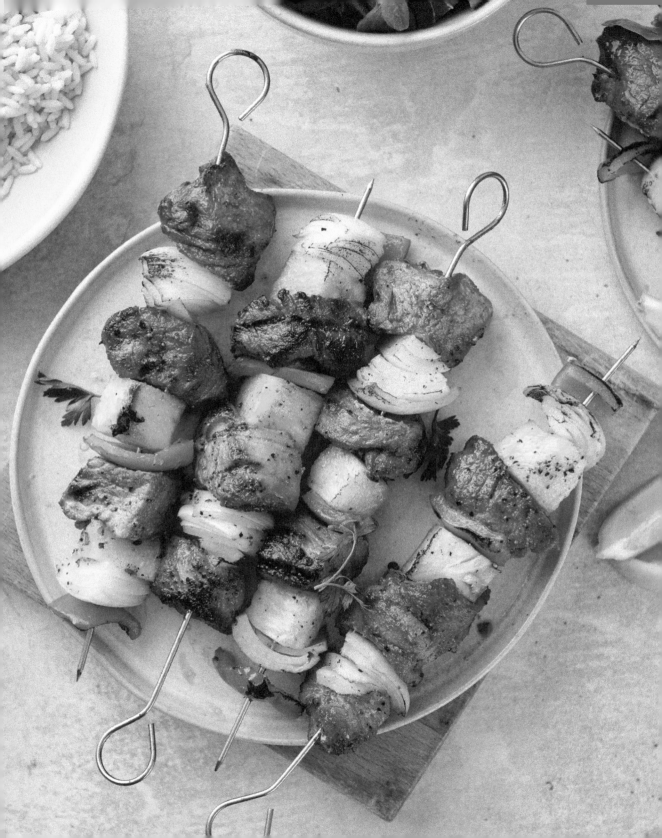

CHAPTER NINE

Pork

196 Asian Lettuce Wraps with Hoisin Sauce

197 Hawaiian Pork Kebabs

198 Crispy Baked Bacon

199 Loaded Baked Potatoes

200 Dairy-Free Bacon Mac & "Cheese"

201 Grilled Sausage, Peppers, and Onions

202 Chorizo Stuffed Sweet Potatoes

203 Spinach-Sausage-Pumpkin Pasta Bake

204 Carnitas

206 BBQ Pulled Pork

207 Piggy Nachos

208 BBQ Ribs

209 Pork Fried Cauliflower Rice

210 Pork Bibimbap

211 Pork Ramen Noodle Bowls

212 Honey Mustard Pork Chops

213 Pork Chops with Apples and Onions

215 Stuffed Pork Tenderloin

216 Pork and White Bean Stew

217 Pesto, Prosciutto, and Roasted Red Pepper Cauliflower Pizza

Asian Lettuce Wraps with Hoisin Sauce

SERVES: 4 / **PREP TIME:** 10 minutes / **COOK TIME:** 15 minutes
ONE-POT, 30 MINUTES OR LESS, QUICK-PREP, DAIRY-FREE

The inspiration for this recipe came from a meal I once had at a chain restaurant. I love the idea of using lettuce as a vehicle for a meal. It's basically just a way to get your food from your plate to your mouth without using a fork, which can be a nice change of pace.

FOR THE HOISIN SAUCE

¼ cup soy sauce

2 tablespoons
   peanut butter

1 tablespoon maple syrup

2 teaspoons apple
   cider vinegar

2 teaspoons sesame oil

1 teaspoon Sriracha

1 garlic clove, minced

Salt

Pepper

FOR THE WRAPS

2 teaspoons sesame oil

1 teaspoon minced
   fresh ginger

3 garlic cloves, minced

1 pound ground pork

1 large carrot, cut into
   matchsticks

4 green onions (greens
   and whites), chopped

4 large lettuce leaves
   (romaine, butter, or
   iceberg)

¼ cup chopped unsalted
   roasted peanuts

TO MAKE THE HOISIN SAUCE

Whisk together all of the ingredients for the hoisin sauce. Set aside.

TO MAKE THE WRAPS

1. In a large skillet, heat the oil over medium heat. Add the ginger and garlic and cook for 2 minutes.

2. Add the pork and cook until it is no longer pink, 5 to 6 minutes.

3. Add the carrot and green onion and cook for 2 to 3 minutes more, or until the vegetables have softened.

4. Stir in the hoisin sauce and continue to cook until sauce thickens, 3 to 4 minutes. Remove from the heat.

5. Divide the pork into 8 lettuce wraps and top with chopped peanuts.

Per serving (2 wraps): Calories: 465; Total Fat: 36g; Saturated Fat: 11g; Cholesterol: 82mg; Sodium: 1032mg; Carbohydrates: 12g; Fiber: 2g; Protein: 24g

Hawaiian Pork Kebabs

SERVES: 6 / **PREP TIME:** 20 minutes, plus 20 minutes to 2 hours to marinate / **COOK TIME:** 15 minutes
NUT-FREE, DAIRY-FREE

I love a good Hawaiian pizza; I'm not going to lie. That's where the inspiration for these kebabs came from. I love the combination of ham and pineapple and wondered what they would taste like on the grill. Whoever thought up the pork and pineapple duo is a genius and should get to enjoy this recipe, free of charge. I like to eat these kebabs over a salad with a little bit of rice, but I won't blame you if you eat them right off the skewer.

⅓ cup soy sauce

1 tablespoon honey

½ teaspoon paprika

½ teaspoon garlic powder

½ teaspoon onion powder

¼ teaspoon cumin

¼ teaspoon salt

¼ teaspoon pepper

2 pounds boneless pork
   loin, chopped

Cooking oil spray

2 bell peppers, chopped

1 pineapple, cored
   and chopped

1 yellow onion, chopped

1. In a large freezer bag or baking dish, combine the soy sauce, honey, paprika, garlic powder, onion powder, cumin, salt, and pepper. Mix well.

2. Add the pork and coat evenly with the sauce. Marinate for 20 minutes or up to 2 hours.

3. Preheat the grill to medium and spray with cooking oil spray.

4. Remove the pork from the marinade. Discard the marinade.

5. Assemble the kebabs. Divide the pork, peppers, pineapple, and onion evenly among 6 skewers.

6. Grill the kebabs for 12 to 15 minutes or until the internal temperature reaches 145°F.

> **VARIATION TIP:** If you don't have a grill, roast the kebabs in the oven on a baking sheet at 400°F for 15 to 20 minutes, turning once. Cook until the pork has cooked through.

Per serving: Calories: 293; Total Fat: 11g; Saturated Fat: 4g; Cholesterol: 73mg; Sodium: 1424mg; Carbohydrates: 20g; Fiber: 2g; Protein: 30g

Crispy Baked Bacon

SERVES: 2 / **PREP TIME:** 5 minutes / **COOK TIME:** 15 minutes
ONE-POT, 5 INGREDIENTS OR LESS, 30 MINUTES OR LESS, QUICK-PREP, NUT-FREE, DAIRY-FREE, GLUTEN-FREE

This is the only way I make bacon. It is the easiest and most delicious way I've found. Not to mention, it is so much nicer to cook bacon without having to stand 2 feet away to avoid getting splattered with the bacon grease. Once you cook bacon this way, you'll never go back.

4 bacon slices

1. Preheat the oven to 400°F. Line a baking sheet with parchment paper.

2. Arrange the bacon on the baking sheet in a single layer. Bake for 15 minutes or until crisped to your liking.

> **INGREDIENT TIP:** Make sure you watch the bacon! Every oven is different, and bacon can go from not cooked to burnt in no time.

Per serving: Calories: 87: Total Fat: 6g: Saturated Fat: 2g: Cholesterol: 20mg: Sodium: 325mg: Carbohydrates: 0g: Fiber: 0g: Protein: 7g

Loaded Baked Potatoes

SERVES: 4 / **PREP TIME:** 10 minutes / **COOK TIME:** 1 hour, plus 5 minutes to cool
ONE-POT, QUICK-PREP, NUT-FREE, GLUTEN-FREE

I only like a baked potato if it is crispy on the outside and creamy on the inside. If it's anything less, I'm out. I also love loading it with as many toppings as possible to make it a rich and decadent experience. Feel free to add your own favorite toppings to make this recipe your own, or maybe even switch up the type of potato to see what flavors and textures other potatoes have to offer.

4 medium russet potatoes

2 teaspoons olive oil

1 teaspoon sea salt

1 tablespoon Ghee (page 251) or butter

2 teaspoons garlic powder

6 slices cooked bacon, crumbled

1 cup, plus ¼ cup shredded Cheddar cheese

½ cup plain unsweetened Greek yogurt

½ cup sliced green onions

Salt

Pepper

1. Preheat the oven to 400°F. Line a baking sheet with parchment paper.

2. Pierce each potato with a fork or knife 8 to 10 times.

3. Rub each potato with olive oil and sprinkle with sea salt. Place the potatoes on the baking sheet and bake for 50 to 60 minutes or until fork-tender. Cool for 5 minutes.

4. Slice the potatoes in half lengthwise. Scoop out most of the insides (leaving a little inside) and put it into a large bowl. Repeat with each potato, putting all of the potatoes in the same bowl. Leave the potato skins on the baking sheet (do not discard).

5. Add to the potatoes the butter, garlic powder, bacon, 1 cup of shredded Cheddar cheese, yogurt, and green onions. Season with salt and pepper and mix until creamy.

6. Scoop the filling back into each potato half. Top each potato half with 2 tablespoons of shredded Cheddar and broil for 1 to 2 minutes.

> **INGREDIENT TIP:** To speed up the cooking time, microwave the potatoes for a few minutes before putting them in the oven.

Per serving: Calories: 400; Total Fat: 23g; Saturated Fat: 13g; Cholesterol: 61mg; Sodium: 1069mg; Carbohydrates: 31g; Fiber: 3g; Protein: 17g

Dairy-Free Bacon Mac & "Cheese"

SERVES: 8 / **PREP TIME:** 10 minutes / **COOK TIME:** 30 minutes
QUICK-PREP, NUT-FREE, DAIRY-FREE, GLUTEN-FREE

I have a lot of people in my life who have a sensitivity or intolerance to dairy. I have always wondered how I could make them a dairy-free mac and "cheese," and this one does the trick. The combination of the creaminess from the sweet potato and the "cheesy" flavor of the nutritional yeast helps make this almost taste like you're eating the real deal.

16 ounces gluten-free pasta

4 bacon slices, chopped into 1-inch pieces

4 garlic cloves, minced

1 yellow onion, chopped

1 sweet potato, chopped

1 small head cauliflower, chopped

2 cups chicken or vegetable broth

¼ cup nutritional yeast

½ teaspoon salt

¼ teaspoon pepper

1. Bring a large pot of salted water to boil over high heat. Add the pasta and cook according to the package instructions. When the pasta has cooked, drain and set aside.

2. In a medium saucepan, cook the bacon over medium heat until crispy. Using a slotted spoon, remove the bacon from the pan and place on a paper towel–lined plate. Reserve 2 tablespoons of the bacon grease in the pan.

3. Put the garlic and onion into the pan and sauté for 2 minutes. Add the sweet potato, cauliflower, and broth, and bring to a boil. Reduce the heat to low, cover, and simmer for 15 minutes, or until the sweet potato is fork-tender.

4. Using an immersion blender set on high, blend the vegetables until smooth. Stir in the nutritional yeast, salt, and pepper.

5. Pour the sauce over the cooked pasta and stir to coat evenly.

INGREDIENT TIP: If you can tolerate some dairy, use grated Parmesan cheese in place of nutritional yeast.

Per serving: Calories: 272; Total Fat: 2g; Saturated Fat: 1g; Cholesterol: 6mg; Sodium: 483mg; Carbohydrates: 55g; Fiber: 6g; Protein: 9g

Grilled Sausage, Peppers, and Onions

SERVES: 4 / **PREP TIME:** 5 minutes / **COOK TIME:** 15 minutes

5 INGREDIENTS OR LESS, 30 MINUTES OR LESS, QUICK-PREP, NUT-FREE, DAIRY-FREE, GLUTEN-FREE

Is there anything that screams summer more than grilled sausage, peppers, and onions? I would argue not, but that's just me. Feel free to use whatever pork sausage you prefer. I like supporting my local butcher and buying freshly made sausages to grill up on a nice summer evening. Pair this with a side salad or load it onto a sandwich roll.

2 yellow onions, sliced in rings

2 bell peppers, sliced in rings

1 teaspoon olive oil

1 teaspoon paprika

½ teaspoon salt

¼ teaspoon pepper

1 pound pork sausage links

1. Preheat the grill to medium heat.

2. In a large bowl, toss the onions, peppers, oil, paprika, salt, and pepper.

3. Place the vegetables in aluminum foil and fold the foil to make into a closed packet.

4. Place the sausage and the foil packet directly on the grill and grill for 15 minutes or until the vegetables are softened and the sausage is cooked to an internal temperature of 160°F.

> **VARIATION TIP:** No time to grill? Roast the sausages and vegetables on a baking sheet in the oven at 400°F for 15 to 20 minutes or until the sausage is cooked through.

Per serving: Calories: 423; Total Fat: 35g; Saturated Fat: 11g; Cholesterol: 81mg; Sodium: 1080mg; Carbohydrates: 10g; Fiber: 2g; Protein: 17g

Chorizo Stuffed Sweet Potatoes

SERVES: 4 / **PREP TIME:** 10 minutes / **COOK TIME:** 1 hour 10 minutes
QUICK-PREP, NUT-FREE, GLUTEN-FREE

The sweetness of the sweet potato paired with the saltiness of the chorizo is a winning combo in this dish. The sweet potatoes also do an excellent job of soaking up all the excess juices from the chorizo mixture, so don't worry about licking your plate clean.

4 medium sweet potatoes, scrubbed clean

2 tablespoons olive oil, divided

½ teaspoon salt

¼ teaspoon pepper

1 bell pepper, chopped

1 yellow onion, chopped

1 pound ground chorizo

1 ounce crumbled Cotija cheese

¼ cup cilantro

1. Preheat the oven to 400°F. Line a baking sheet with parchment paper.

2. Pierce the potatoes with a fork 5 to 10 times each.

3. Using 1 tablespoon of the olive oil, rub a bit of oil on each potato and sprinkle with salt and pepper. Place the potatoes on the baking sheet and bake for 45 to 60 minutes or until fork-tender.

4. Meanwhile, in a large skillet, heat the remaining tablespoon of oil over medium heat.

5. Add the bell pepper and onion and cook until the onion is softened.

6. Add the chorizo, stirring and breaking it up into small pieces as you cook. Sauté until cooked through, about 10 minutes.

7. Cut the potatoes in half lengthwise. Then, using a slotted spoon, remove a generous spoonful of chorizo filling from the skillet and place it on top of each potato half. Top with the cheese and cilantro. If you prefer your cheese melted, place the filled potatoes under the broiler for 2 to 3 minutes.

Per serving: Calories: 583; Total Fat: 37g; Saturated Fat: 12g; Cholesterol: 70mg; Sodium: 1216mg; Carbohydrates: 40g; Fiber: 5g; Protein: 21g

Spinach-Sausage-Pumpkin Pasta Bake

SERVES: 6 / **PREP TIME:** 10 minutes / **COOK TIME:** 30 minutes
QUICK-PREP, NUT-FREE

This dish idea was presented to me by a friend. I had never had this combination before. It was something she loved growing up and wondered if I could recreate it. I'm not sure if I did her childhood dish any justice, but I sure enjoyed the results. It's a spin on baked ziti with a fall harvest feel. Make this ahead of time, but don't be surprised if it's all gone after one night.

12 ounces ziti or penne pasta

Cooking oil spray

1 pound ground mild or medium Italian sausage

5 ounces baby spinach

1 (15-ounce) can pumpkin purée

1 teaspoon salt

¼ teaspoon pepper

1 cup mozzarella cheese, shredded

¼ cup Parmesan cheese, grated

1. Bring a large pot of salted water to boil over high heat. Add the pasta and cook according to the package instructions. When the pasta has cooked, drain and set aside.

2. Preheat the oven to 400°F. Coat the inside of a 9-by-13-inch baking dish with cooking oil spray.

3. In a large skillet, crumble the sausage and stir, breaking it up as it browns. Sauté until cooked through, 8 to 10 minutes.

4. Add the spinach and cook until wilted. Add pumpkin, salt, and pepper and stir to combine.

5. Remove from heat. Stir in the cooked pasta and cheese.

6. Transfer to the baking dish and bake for 15 to 20 minutes, or until the cheese is bubbling.

> **SUBSTITUTION TIP:** Make this dish gluten-free by substituting in gluten-free pasta for the wheat pasta.

Per serving: Calories: 534; Total Fat: 24g; Saturated Fat: 9g; Cholesterol: 71mg; Sodium: 1243mg; Carbohydrates: 50g; Fiber: 5g; Protein: 28g

Carnitas

SERVES: 12 / **PREP TIME:** 10 minutes / **COOK TIME:** 8 hours
ONE-POT, QUICK-PREP, NUT-FREE, GLUTEN-FREE

I love any meal that can be made in one pot. These carnitas are easy to make as you just toss everything into the slow cooker, set it, and forget it. The addition of the lime aioli and pickled onions are nice to have, but if you are short on time or motivation, you can leave them out of the picture and just enjoy the carnitas over a salad, in tacos, or on their own.

FOR THE CARNITAS

3 to 4 pounds boneless
   pork shoulder

1½ teaspoons oregano

1½ teaspoons cumin

1½ teaspoons paprika

1 teaspoon salt

½ teaspoon pepper

1 orange

2 limes

4 garlic cloves,
   roughly chopped

1 cup broth

1 tablespoon olive oil
   (optional)

16 corn tortillas

Cotija cheese, crumbled

FOR THE LIME AIOLI

½ cup Homemade Mayo
   (page 254)

Zest and juice of 1 lime

Salt

Pepper

FOR THE ONIONS

¾ cup vinegar

1 tablespoon honey

½ tablespoon salt

1 small red onion,
   thinly sliced

TO MAKE THE CARNITAS

1. Pat the pork with paper towels to dry and cut into 2-inch chunks.

2. In a small bowl, mix together the oregano, cumin, paprika, salt, and pepper. Rub the spice mixture on the pork and then place the pork in a slow cooker.

3. Slice the orange and the limes in half, squeeze the juice into slow cooker, then put the orange and limes halves into slow cooker. Add the garlic. Pour in the broth over everything. Cover and cook on low for 8 hours or on high for 6 hours.

4. Transfer the cooked pork to a cutting board. Using two forks, shred the pork.

5. Optional step: In a large skillet, heat the oil over medium-high heat. Add the pork and cook for 3 to 5 minutes, or until the pork is a bit crispy. Season with salt and pepper, as desired.

6. Serve on warmed corn tortillas and top with lime aioli, pickled onions, and Cotija cheese.

TO MAKE THE LIME AIOLI

In a small bowl, mix together all of the ingredients for lime aioli. Cover and refrigerate.

TO MAKE THE ONIONS

1. In a small saucepan over medium heat, simmer the vinegar, honey, and salt until the honey has dissolved.

2. Place the onion in a small glass jar and pour the vinegar mixture over it, let sit at room temperature for 1 to 2 hours, then cover and refrigerate.

> **VARIATION TIP:** If you have a pressure cooker, make the carnitas in the pressure cooker on manual (high) and reduce time to 1 hour of cooking.

Per serving (2 with ⅛ of the meat + 1 tablespoon aioli + ⅛ of the onions): Calories: 423; Total Fat: 28g; Saturated Fat: 8g; Cholesterol: 81mg; Sodium: 675mg; Carbohydrates: 21g; Fiber: 3g; Protein: 21g

BBQ Pulled Pork

SERVES: 10 to 12 (about 5-6 cups) / **PREP TIME:** 10 minutes / **COOK TIME:** 1 hour 30 minutes

ONE-POT, 5 INGREDIENTS OR LESS, QUICK-PREP, NUT-FREE, DAIRY-FREE

Pulled pork is an easy protein to make ahead and enjoy for the entire week—or to make and feed a lot of people at a party. I make it and freeze any that I don't use, because it reheats well. This goes nicely with a slaw, on a sandwich, or a combination of both.

3 to 4 pounds boneless pork shoulder, cut into 5 to 6 equal-size chunks

Salt

Pepper

2 tablespoons olive oil

1 cup Sassy BBQ sauce (page 257)

1. Season the pork with salt and pepper.

2. In a pressure cooker, on the sauté function, heat the oil. In batches, brown the pork on all sides, 1 to 2 minutes per side. Remove the pork from the pressure cooker and set aside.

3. Turn the pressure cooker off and pour in the barbecue sauce.

4. Put the pork back into the pressure cooker. Seal and set on manual (high) for 1 hour.

5. When done, naturally release the pressure for 15 to 20 minutes.

6. Transfer the pork to a cutting board. Using two forks, shred the pork.

7. Thicken the barbecue sauce by turning pressure cooker to sauté and simmer for 5 minutes until the volume is reduced and the sauce is thickened.

8. Toss the pulled pork in the reduced sauce and serve.

> **VARIATION TIP:** If you don't have a pressure cooker, you can use a slow cooker and cook the pork on low for 6 to 8 hours or high for 4 to 6 hours.

Per serving: Calories: 362; Total Fat: 28g; Saturated Fat: 9g; Cholesterol: 90mg; Sodium: 220mg; Carbohydrates: 2g; Fiber: 0g; Protein: 23g

Piggy Nachos

SERVES: 6 / **PREP TIME:** 5 minutes / **COOK TIME:** 10 minutes

ONE-POT, 30 MINUTES OR LESS, QUICK-PREP, NUT-FREE, GLUTEN-FREE

I love nachos; they are easy to put together and filling. Make sure you load up your nachos with more vegetables than cheese so that you are filling up on plenty of fiber as well as vitamins and minerals. Nachos are a good kitchen clean-out meal. Add anything in your refrigerator or pantry that sounds good in the moment. Nachos are incredibly filling and also work well as an appetizer or a snack to satisfy hungry guests prior to dinner.

10 ounces corn tortilla chips

2 cups cooked BBQ Pulled Pork (page 206)

1 tomato, chopped

1 jalapeño, seeded and diced

1 small red onion, chopped

½ cup Cheddar cheese, shredded

Sassy BBQ Sauce (page 257), to drizzle (optional)

Green onions, sliced, for topping

Avocado, sliced, for topping

1. Preheat the oven to 400°F. Line a baking sheet with parchment paper.

2. Layer the chips on the baking sheet and top with the pork, tomato, jalapeño, and red onion. Sprinkle the cheese liberally over the top. Drizzle with barbecue sauce, if desired.

3. Bake for 10 minutes, or until the cheese is melted.

4. Top with the green onions and avocado.

> **VARIATION TIP:** Change up the tortilla chips with sweet potato chips or other vegetable chips to change the flavor of the dish.

Per serving: Calories: 551; Total Fat: 34g; Saturated Fat: 9g; Cholesterol: 76mg; Sodium: 419mg; Carbohydrates: 35g; Fiber: 4g; Protein: 23g

BBQ Ribs

SERVES: 6 / **PREP TIME:** 5 minutes / **COOK TIME:** 3 hours 5 minutes

ONE-POT, QUICK-PREP, DAIRY-FREE, NUT-FREE

Ribs are a real test of patience. They are quite easy to prepare, but you must be patient if you want the meat to get so tender that it practically falls off the bone like at your favorite barbecue joint. The longer you can let the ribs sit in the oven, the better. If you have time, I'd also suggest letting the ribs sit with the rub in the refrigerator for a few hours before cooking—or even overnight—to let the flavors sink in.

Cooking oil spray

2 tablespoons
coconut sugar

1 tablespoon chili powder

1 tablespoon paprika

1 tablespoon
onion powder

1 teaspoon salt

2 racks pork ribs
(2½ to 3 pounds
per rack)

1 cup Sassy BBQ sauce
(page 257)

1. Preheat the oven to 325°F. Line a large 9-by-13-inch baking dish with foil and coat the foil with cooking oil spray.

2. In a small bowl, mix together the coconut sugar, chili powder, paprika, onion powder, and salt.

3. Remove the white membrane from back side of ribs, then rub the spice mixture evenly over ribs. Place the seasoned ribs in the baking dish.

4. Cover and seal tightly with foil. Bake for 2 to 3 hours or until tender and meat starts to pull away from the bones.

5. Remove from the oven, discard the juices, and toss the ribs in the barbecue sauce.

6. Turn the oven to broil. Place the ribs under the broiler for 5 minutes, or until they are golden and crispy.

INGREDIENT TIP: Feel free to use your favorite barbecue sauce or omit it all together and enjoy the ribs as is.

Per serving: Calories: 757; Total Fat: 41g; Saturated Fat: 8g; Cholesterol: 219mg; Sodium: 857mg; Carbohydrates: 10g; Fiber: 2g; Protein: 79g

Pork Fried Cauliflower Rice

SERVES: 4 / **PREP TIME:** 10 minutes / **COOK TIME:** 20 minutes
ONE-POT, 30 MINUTES OR LESS, QUICK-PREP, DAIRY-FREE

Fried rice can have a bad reputation mostly because it is often drowning in soy sauce and the portions are always gigantic. This recipe reduces the soy sauce but has a rich flavor AND you can feel good eating it because cauliflower rice is not nearly as dense as rice. Certainly, if you prefer, you can swap out the cauliflower rice for regular white or brown rice; just make sure you cook it before adding it to this dish.

2 tablespoons sesame oil, divided

2 large eggs, beaten

3 garlic cloves, minced

1 small red onion, minced

1 carrot, diced

1 pound ground pork

½ teaspoon salt

¼ teaspoon black pepper

½ cup frozen peas

1 medium head cauliflower, riced

¼ cup soy sauce

1 to 2 teaspoons Sriracha (optional)

3 green onions, thinly sliced for topping

1. In a large skillet, heat 1 tablespoon of sesame oil over medium heat. Add the eggs and let them sit for 20 to 30 seconds before scrambling. Stir the eggs and fully scramble and cook through. Remove from the skillet and set aside.

2. Put the remaining oil in skillet, then add the garlic, onion, and carrot, and sauté until the onion softens, about 3 minutes.

3. Add the pork, salt, and pepper to the skillet, and sauté until no pink is showing, about 8 minutes.

4. Stir in the peas and cauliflower rice, and sauté until the cauliflower is slightly softened, 3 to 5 minutes.

5. Mix in the soy sauce and Sriracha, if using.

6. Fold in the eggs and sprinkle with green onions.

INGREDIENT TIP: If you don't like spicy food, leave out the Sriracha, but if you're like me and love sweating while eating, make sure to include it, as it gives this dish a nice extra layer of flavor.

Per serving: Calories: 471; Total Fat: 34g; Saturated Fat: 11g; Cholesterol: 175mg; Sodium: 1363mg; Carbohydrates: 16g; Fiber: 6g; Protein: 28g

Pork Bibimbap

SERVES: 4 / PREP TIME: 10 minutes / COOK TIME: 15 minutes
ONE-POT, 30 MINUTES OR LESS, QUICK-PREP, NUT-FREE, DAIRY-FREE

Bibimbap is the word for Korean rice mixed with meat and assorted vegetables. I love the word, but I love the food even more. Make sure to finish this dish off by adding in some of your favorite kimchi; just be warned, some kimchi is very spicy.

1 tablespoon sesame oil

1 pound ground pork

¼ teaspoon salt

Pinch pepper

1 red bell pepper, cut in thin strips

2 carrots, cut into matchsticks

8 ounces mushrooms, sliced

2 tablespoons soy sauce

2 tablespoons Gochujang (page 258)

3 cups cooked white rice

1 cucumber, cut into matchsticks

4 eggs, fried or cooked to liking

Kimchi, sesame seeds, and spinach, for topping (optional)

1. In a large skillet, heat the oil over medium heat. Add the pork, salt, and pepper and cook until there is no pink showing, about 8 minutes. Transfer the pork to a medium bowl.

2. Put the bell pepper, carrots, and mushrooms in the skillet and cook for 3 to 4 minutes. Sprinkle with salt and pepper.

3. Add the soy sauce and gochujang, and stir to cover all of the vegetables. Remove from the heat.

4. Assemble the bibimbap in four bowls. In each bowl place ¾ cup rice, ¼ of the cooked vegetables, ¼ of the cucumber, ¼ of pork, and top with 1 egg. Add extra soy sauce and gochujang, as desired. Add extra toppings to your liking.

> **VARIATION TIP:** You can use any type of ground meat or vegetables with this dish. Experiment and make it your own!

Per serving: Calories: 610; Total Fat: 33g; Saturated Fat: 11g; Cholesterol: 268mg; Sodium: 888mg; Carbohydrates: 45g; Fiber: 3g; Protein: 32g

Pork Ramen Noodle Bowls

SERVES: 4 / **PREP TIME:** 10 minutes / **COOK TIME:** 20 minutes

30 MINUTES OR LESS, QUICK-PREP, NUT-FREE, DAIRY-FREE

Ramen noodles remind me of college when we would grab a quick option for dinner or snacks. However, ramen has made a comeback, just make sure you toss out that mystery salt packet that comes in every package. By dressing up your ramen and adding protein and vegetables to it, you end up making yourself a grown-up ramen meal that is filling and healthy. I'd call that a win-win.

4 (3-ounce) packages ramen noodles, seasoning packets discarded

1 tablespoon avocado oil

1 yellow onion, sliced thin

1 red bell pepper, sliced thin

4 garlic cloves, minced

1 pound ground pork

1 teaspoon paprika

½ teaspoon salt

¼ teaspoon ginger

¼ teaspoon black pepper

8 ounces mushrooms, sliced

3 cups baby spinach

¼ cup soy sauce

1 to 2 teaspoons Sriracha (optional)

2 green onions, sliced, for topping

Salt

Pepper

1. Bring a large pot of water to a boil. Add the ramen noodles, cook for 3 to 4 minutes. Drain, rinse with cold water, and set aside.

2. In a large skillet, heat the oil over medium heat. Add the onion and sauté for 3 minutes.

3. Add the bell pepper and garlic, and sauté for 1 minute more.

4. Add the pork, paprika, salt, ginger, and pepper, and cook until no longer pink, 5 to 6 minutes.

5. Add mushrooms and spinach to the pork and cook for 2 to 3 minutes, or until the mushrooms and soft and the spinach is wilted.

6. Add the ramen noodles to pork and stir in the soy sauce and Sriracha. Top with green onions. Season with salt and pepper, as needed.

> **INGREDIENT TIP:** Use gluten-free ramen noodles to make this dish gluten-free.

Per serving: Calories: 769; Total Fat: 44g; Saturated Fat: 17g; Cholesterol: 82mg; Sodium: 1588mg; Carbohydrates: 63g; Fiber: 3g; Protein: 32g

Honey Mustard Pork Chops

SERVES: 2 / **PREP TIME:** 5 minutes, plus 20 minutes to marinate / **COOK TIME:** 10 minutes
5 INGREDIENTS OR LESS, NUT-FREE, DAIRY-FREE, GLUTEN-FREE

Sometimes the best meals are those that have minimal ingredients and require minimal effort. This is one of those dishes. You can marinate these pork chops for longer than 20 minutes—you could even put them in the refrigerator to marinate the night before so they are ready to cook when you get home from work.

2 boneless pork chops
¼ teaspoon salt
¼ teaspoon black pepper
¼ cup Honey Mustard (page 255)
1 teaspoon avocado oil

1. Place the pork chops on a large platter. Season the pork chops on both sides with salt and pepper.

2. With a brush or the back of a spoon, spread the honey mustard on the pork chops. Cover the chops with plastic wrap and allow to marinate for 20 minutes in the refrigerator.

3. In a large skillet, heat the oil over medium heat. Place the pork chops in the skillet and cook for 4 to 5 minutes on each side, or until internal temperature reaches 145°F.

4. Serve with extra honey mustard for dipping.

> **INGREDIENT TIP:** If you don't have time to make your own honey mustard, grab some from the store, just make sure there is no high-fructose corn syrup on the ingredient label.

Per serving: Calories: 202; Total Fat: 9g; Saturated Fat: 2g; Cholesterol: 56mg; Sodium: 1094mg; Carbohydrates: 6g; Fiber: 0g; Protein: 21g

Pork Chops with Apples and Onions

SERVES: 4 / **PREP TIME:** 10 minutes / **COOK TIME:** 35 minutes
ONE-POT, QUICK-PREP, NUT-FREE, DAIRY-FREE, GLUTEN-FREE

Have you ever had so many apples you didn't know what to do with them? Maybe that's just an upstate New York problem, but it seems like we constantly have an overload of apples in our house. This dish is easy to make and makes the house smell like fall. If you don't have any apple cider, you can use apple juice or even broth instead to make it a more savory dish.

1 tablespoon olive oil

4 boneless pork chops

1 teaspoon salt

1 teaspoon cinnamon

¼ teaspoon black pepper

3 apples, cored and sliced

1 sweet onion, sliced

½ cup broth

½ cup apple cider

1 tablespoon
   Dijon mustard

Salt

Pepper

1. Preheat the oven to 400°F.

2. In a large skillet, heat the oil over medium-high heat.

3. Season the pork chops with the salt, cinnamon, and pepper, then add them to the skillet and cook for 4 to 5 minutes per side. Transfer the pork chops to a platter and set aside.

4. Add the apples and the onion to the skillet (add extra oil if needed) and sauté until softened, 3 to 4 minutes.

5. Pour in the broth and apple cider. Stir in the mustard and simmer for 5 minutes, or until the liquid is reduced by half.

6. Return the pork chops and any juices that have collected on the plate back to the skillet. Place the skillet in the oven. Cook for 15 minutes or until the pork is cooked through.
Add salt and pepper as desired.

VARIATION TIP: If you don't have an oven-safe skillet, transfer all of the ingredients to a baking dish prior to putting in the oven to cook.

Per serving: Calories: 256; Total Fat: 9g; Saturated Fat: 3g; Cholesterol: 56mg; Sodium: 1400mg; Carbohydrates: 21g; Fiber: 3g; Protein: 22g

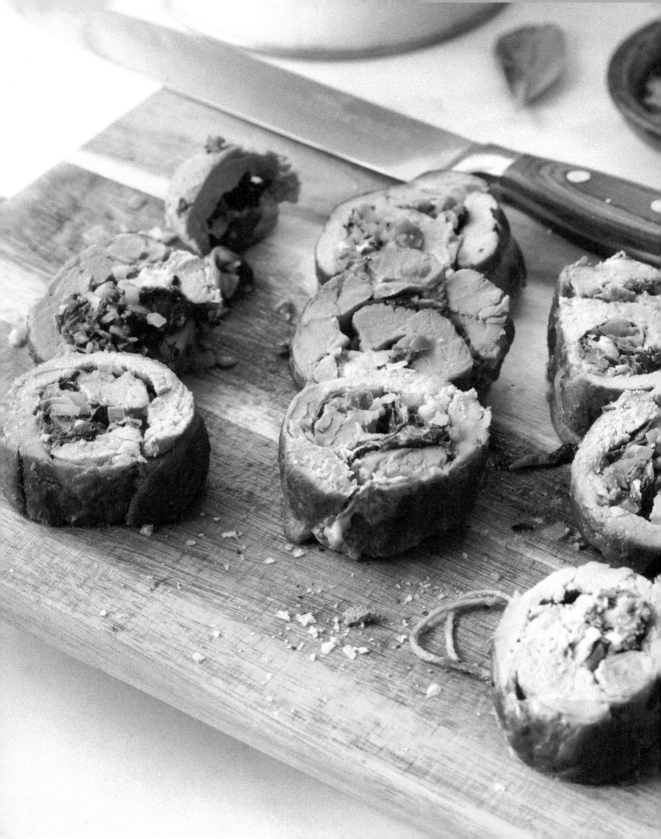

Stuffed Pork Tenderloin

SERVES: 8 / **PREP TIME:** 15 minutes / **COOK TIME:** 50 minutes

NUT-FREE, GLUTEN-FREE

A pork tenderloin can be intimidating to cook, but if done correctly, can make for an enjoyable meal. I find that tenderizing the meat by pounding it down makes it easier to cook and eat. If you're not a fan of goat cheese, feel free to substitute a different soft cheese or omit the cheese altogether.

¼ cup sun-dried tomatoes

2 pounds pork tenderloin, trimmed

Salt

Pepper

2 tablespoons olive oil, divided

4 garlic cloves, minced

2 shallots, diced

4 ounces goat cheese

5 ounces baby spinach

1. Preheat the oven to 400°F.

2. Place the sun-dried tomatoes in a bowl. Boil water in a kettle and pour the hot water over tomatoes and allow to sit for 10 minutes or until ready to use. Drain and chop before using.

3. Prepare the pork tenderloin by trimming off any excess fat, then cut a slit down the center of tenderloin so it opens like a book (do not cut completely through). Open it up and place it between two sheets of parchment paper or plastic wrap. Pound the pork with meat mallet until it is ½-inch thick.

4. Season each side of the pork generously with salt and pepper. Set aside.

5. In a large cast iron or oven-safe skillet, heat the oil over medium heat. Add the garlic and shallots and sauté for 3 to 5 minutes.

6. Add the goat cheese, spinach, and sun-dried tomatoes and sauté until the spinach is wilted. Remove from the heat and season with salt and pepper.

7. Spread filling over the middle of the pork tenderloin, then roll it up and wrap with kitchen twine in 3 or 4 places.

8. Using the same large skillet, heat the remaining tablespoon of oil over medium heat. When hot, add the pork and brown on all sides.

9. Transfer the skillet to the oven and cook for 40 minutes or until the internal temperature reaches 145°F.

Per serving: Calories: 218; Total Fat: 10g; Saturated Fat: 4g; Cholesterol: 56mg; Sodium: 228mg; Carbohydrates: 5g; Fiber: 1g; Protein: 28g

Pork and White Bean Stew

SERVES: 4 / PREP TIME: 10 minutes / **COOK TIME:** 45 minutes
ONE-POT, QUICK-PREP, NUT-FREE, DAIRY-FREE, GLUTEN-FREE

As I've been known to say, "There's nothing better than bacon," and that holds true for this recipe. Bacon is one of those foods that universally brings joy to the plate. It is so flavorful and can be a part of a healthy diet as long as used in moderation. When looking for bacon, try to find a center cut and if possible, from a pasture-raised pig. Quality is key when buying bacon, so don't skimp on it!

6 bacon slices, chopped

1 yellow onion, minced

4 garlic cloves, minced

2 celery stalks, minced

1 pound pork tenderloin, trimmed of fat and cubed

½ cup dry white wine

1 (15-ounce) can cannellini beans, drained and rinsed

4 cups chicken or Easy Broth (page 253)

2 teaspoons paprika

½ teaspoon salt

¼ teaspoon pepper

4 cups chopped kale

1. Heat a large stockpot or Dutch oven over medium heat. Place the bacon in the pot and cook until crispy.

2. Using a slotted spoon, remove the bacon and place it on a paper towel–lined plate. Reserve 2 tablespoons of bacon grease in the pot and return it to the heat.

3. Add the onion and cook for 2 to 3 minutes, then add the garlic and celery and cook until softened, 2 to 3 minutes more.

4. Add the pork and cook, stirring occasionally, until the pork is browned on all sides.

5. Pour in the white wine, stirring to scrape up any brown bits on the sides or the bottom of the pot.

6. Add the bacon, beans, broth, paprika, salt, pepper, and kale. Stir and bring to a simmer.

7. Turn heat to low and simmer for 30 minutes or until the pork is cooked to an internal temp of 145°F.

> **INGREDIENT TIP:** You can use any lean cut of pork including pork chops or ham steak in place of the pork tenderloin in this recipe.

Per serving: Calories: 370; Total Fat: 8g; Saturated Fat: 3g; Cholesterol: 65mg; Sodium: 1625mg; Carbohydrates: 32g; Fiber: 9g; Protein: 40g

Pesto, Prosciutto, and Roasted Red Pepper Cauliflower Pizza

SERVES: 6 / **PREP TIME:** 5 minutes / **COOK TIME:** 5 minutes
30 MINUTES OR LESS, QUICK-PREP, GLUTEN-FREE

There is nothing that pizza can't fix. It makes for an easy meal and frankly, makes you feel like you're a kid all over again. The cauliflower pizza crust is a staple, and once you make it, you'll realize how easy it is and how you feel healthy while eating a pizza. It's a weird but satisfying experience.

1 Cauliflower Pizza Crust (page 267)

½ cup Spinach-Walnut Pesto (page 265)

1 cup shredded mozzarella

2 ounces prosciutto

⅔ cup chopped roasted red peppers

1 cup arugula

1. Preheat the oven to 400°F. Line a baking sheet with parchment paper.

2. Place the cauliflower crust on the baking sheet.

3. Spread the pesto on the cauliflower crust and top with the mozzarella, prosciutto, roasted red peppers, and arugula.

4. Bake for 5 minutes or until the cheese is melted and the crust is slightly golden.

> **INGREDIENT TIP:** Use a pre-made crust from the freezer aisle if you prefer to make this without making your own crust. Cook the crust per package instructions.

Per serving: Calories: 295; Total Fat: 21g; Saturated Fat: 7g; Cholesterol: 61mg; Sodium: 847mg; Carbohydrates: 20g; Fiber: 3g; Protein: 17g

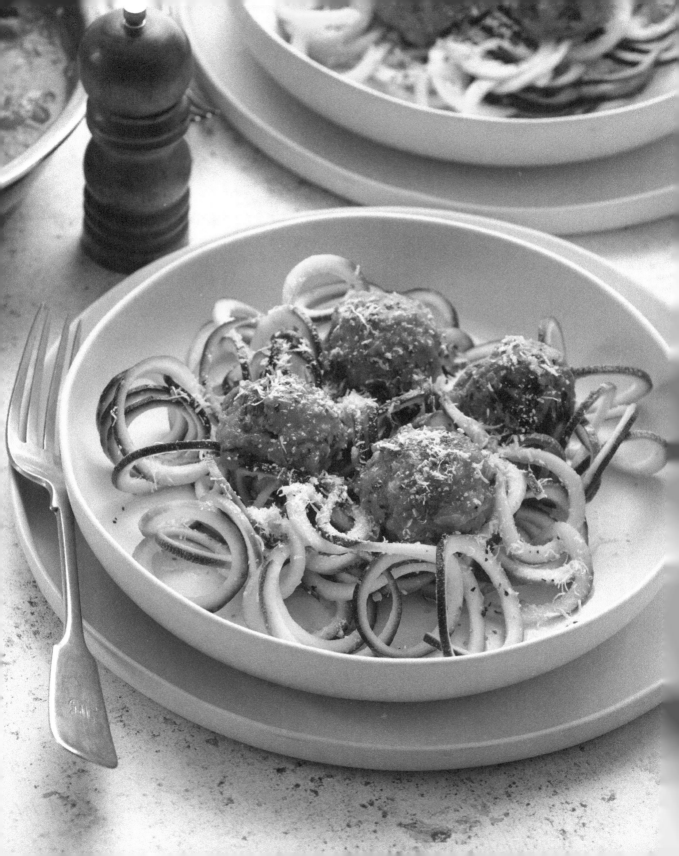

CHAPTER TEN

Beef and Lamb

220 Beef Tacos
in Lettuce

221 Bacon-Wrapped
Meatloaf Muffins

222 Taco
Cauliflower Pizza

223 Burger Bowls

224 Barbacoa
Beef Bowls

225 Pressure Cooker
French Dip
Sandwiches

227 Apple, Brie, and
Caramelized
Onion Burger

228 Steak and Pepper
Roll-Ups

229 Mongolian Beef
and Broccoli

230 One-Skillet
Pepper Steak

231 Skillet Garlic-
Herb Steak

232 Chili-Stuffed
Peppers

233 Spinach
Meatballs and
Zucchini Noodles

234 Spaghetti Squash
Bolognese

235 One-Pot
Taco Pasta

236 Sweet Potato and
Butternut Squash
Shepherd's Pie

238 Lamb
Kofta Kebabs

239 Lamb Gyros

240 Feta Lamb Burgers

241 Pressure Cooker
Lamb Meatballs

243 Greek Lamb Bowls
with Turmeric
Cauliflower
Rice and
Cucumber Salsa

245 Lamb
Lollipops with
Chimichurri Sauce

Beef Tacos in Lettuce

SERVES: 4 / **PREP TIME:** 5 minutes / **COOK TIME:** 20 minutes
ONE-POT, 30 MINUTES OR LESS, QUICK-PREP, NUT-FREE, DAIRY-FREE, GLUTEN-FREE

Taco Tuesday should be Tacos Every Day because tacos are delicious, but, more importantly, they are fantastically easy to make. For some recipes, the simpler the better, and that is true in this case. I love to make these into a taco bowl by using lettuce as the base, topping with the beef mixture, salsa, avocado, and of course a bit of Cheddar cheese.

1 tablespoon olive oil

1 pound lean ground beef

1 tablespoon
tomato paste

1 tablespoon Taco
Seasoning (page 250)

¼ teaspoon black pepper

1 yellow onion, chopped

3 small bell
peppers, chopped

Lettuce, for serving

1. In a large skillet, heat the oil over medium heat, add the ground beef, and cook until light brown, 5 to 7 minutes.

2. Add the tomato paste, taco seasoning, and pepper. Reduce the heat to low and add the onion and bell peppers, and cook for 5 to 10 minutes until flavors are well combined.

3. Serve over lettuce wraps with your favorite toppings.

> **SUBSTITUTION TIP:** If you aren't a fan of lettuce, substitute tortillas for the lettuce wraps.

Per serving: Calories: 231; Total Fat: 12g; Saturated Fat: 3g; Cholesterol: 65mg; Sodium: 271mg; Carbohydrates: 7g; Fiber: 2g; Protein: 24g

Bacon-Wrapped Meatloaf Muffins

MAKES: 12 muffins / **PREP TIME:** 15 minutes / **COOK TIME:** 35 minutes
NUT-FREE, GLUTEN-FREE

Bacon makes everything better. Wrapping these meatballs in bacon allows the meat to hold on to its moisture and gives the meatballs such a depth of flavor, you'll be tempted to have more. If you are looking for a more filling meal, try these with Ketchup (page 256) and Mashed Parmesan Cauliflower (page 91).

Cooking oil spray
1 pound ground beef
1 large egg
1 tablespoon tomato paste
1 small yellow onion, diced
3 garlic cloves, minced
¼ cup fresh parsley, diced
2 tablespoons grated Parmesan cheese
1 teaspoon paprika
½ teaspoon salt
¼ teaspoon pepper
12 bacon slices

1. Preheat the oven to 400°F. Coat the muffin cups of a 12-cup muffin tin with cooking oil spray.

2. Mix all of the ingredients except the bacon in a large bowl. Add additional Parmesan cheese as needed to thicken.

3. Form the meat mixture into 12 meatballs, then wrap each meatball with a piece of bacon either around the outside or like you are wrapping a bow on a present.

4. Place one meatball into each muffin cup, press down, so the meatball fills the cup, and bake for 30 minutes, or until the bacon is cooked through.

5. Turn the oven to broil and finish the meatballs under the broiler for 3 to 5 minutes to brown the top of each muffin.

Per muffin: Calories: 115; Total Fat: 6g; Saturated Fat: 2g; Cholesterol: 48mg; Sodium: 316mg; Carbohydrates: 1g; Fiber: 0g; Protein: 12g

Taco Cauliflower Pizza

SERVES: 6 / **PREP TIME:** 5 minutes / **COOK TIME:** 15 minutes
30 MINUTES OR LESS, QUICK-PREP, NUT-FREE, GLUTEN-FREE

Tacos on pizza? That's a thing? It is now. If you haven't had tacos on pizza, then you are most certainly missing out. Run, don't walk, to your nearest grocery store and pick up the items to make this meal so you can treat yourself, and if you feel like sharing, you can treat others around you as well.

1 Cauliflower Pizza Crust (page 267)

½ pound lean ground beef

1 tablespoon Taco Seasoning (page 250)

½ cup canned black beans, drained and rinsed

½ cup tomato sauce

2 cups shredded Cheddar cheese

1 bell pepper, chopped

1 tomato, chopped

Avocados, green onions, jalapeños, olives, plain unsweetened Greek yogurt, or sour cream, for topping (optional)

1. Preheat the oven to 400°F. Line a baking sheet with parchment paper.

2. Place the cauliflower crust on the baking sheet.

3. In a large skillet over medium heat, cook the ground beef and taco seasoning until the beef is browned and no pink is showing.

4. Stir in the beans.

5. Top the crust with the tomato sauce and sprinkle with Cheddar cheese.

6. Spread the meat and bean mixture evenly over the pizza, and top with the bell pepper and tomato.

7. Bake for 5 minutes or until the cheese is melted. Add toppings as desired.

> **SUBSTITUTION TIP:** If you don't have any taco seasoning, feel free to use spices of your choice including paprika, cumin, salt, and pepper.

Per serving: Calories: 342; Total Fat: 20g; Saturated Fat: 12g; Cholesterol: 97mg; Sodium: 768mg; Carbohydrates: 15g; Fiber: 4g; Protein: 26g

Burger Bowls

SERVES: 4 / **PREP TIME:** 10 minutes / **COOK TIME:** 15 minutes

ONE-POT, 30 MINUTES OR LESS, QUICK-PREP, NUT-FREE, GLUTEN-FREE

I love burgers, as evidenced by all of the burger recipes in this cookbook. However, one day I thought of making my burger into a bowl so that I could just throw everything together and not have to worry about the presentation. Feel free to add your favorite toppings and sauces to this burger bowl and get inspired by the other burger recipes in this book to put your own spin it.

1 tablespoon avocado oil

1 pound lean ground beef

2 tablespoons Ketchup (page 256), plus more for serving

1 tablespoon yellow mustard, plus more for serving

1 teaspoon garlic powder

1 teaspoon onion powder

Paprika

1 small red onion, sliced thin

8 ounces mushrooms, sliced thin

1 head butter lettuce, shredded

1 to 2 tomatoes, chopped

½ cup dill or Quick Pickles (page 259)

1 avocado, sliced

½ cup Cheddar cheese, shredded

Air-Fryer Sweet Potato Tots (page 94)

1. In a large skillet over medium heat, heat the oil until glistening.

2. Add the ground beef and cook until no pink is showing. Mix in the ketchup, mustard, garlic powder, onion powder, and paprika. Stir to combine, then transfer the beef mixture to a medium bowl.

3. Return the skillet to the heat and add extra oil if the pan is dry. Sauté the onion and mushrooms until softened, 3 to 5 minutes.

4. Assemble four burger bowls. Divide the lettuce, meat, onion, mushrooms, tomatoes, pickles, avocado, cheese, and sweet potato tots evenly among the bowls.

5. Drizzle with extra ketchup and mustard, as desired.

> **VARIATION TIP:** If you prefer, you can form the meat into four burger patties and grill them up, 5 minutes per side over medium heat.

Per serving: Calories: 451; Total Fat: 23g; Saturated Fat: 7g; Cholesterol: 77mg; Sodium: 519mg; Carbohydrates: 31g; Fiber: 8g; Protein: 32g

Barbacoa Beef Bowls

SERVES: 6 / **PREP TIME:** 10 minutes / **COOK TIME:** 8 hours
ONE-POT, QUICK-PREP, NUT-FREE, GLUTEN-FREE

Burrito bowls are a crowd favorite and these barbacoa bowls are no different. The nice part is you can put the barbacoa in before you leave in the morning, and then you have dinner ready for you when you get home. I personally love the sauce and add extra to my bowl. I like it so much that I keep a jar of it in the refrigerator to use with other dishes.

FOR THE BARBACOA BEEF

2 chipotle peppers in adobo sauce

2 tablespoons tomato paste

4 garlic cloves

½ cup yellow onion, roughly chopped

Juice of 2 limes

2 tablespoons apple cider vinegar

1 tablespoon oregano

2 teaspoons ground cumin

2 teaspoons smoked paprika

1 teaspoon salt

½ teaspoon ground black pepper

½ cup Easy Broth (page 253) or water

2 pounds beef shoulder roast, cut in 2-inch slabs

FOR THE BOWLS

4 cups cauliflower, riced

1 (15-ounce) can black beans, drained and rinsed

1 to 2 avocados, chopped

4 ounces Cotija cheese, crumbled

1 pint cherry tomatoes, halved

1. In a slow cooker, add all of the ingredients for the barbacoa except the beef, then use an immersion blender and blend on high until smooth (or, alternatively, use a blender).

2. Add the beef to the slow cooker. Cover and cook for 4 to 6 hours on high or for 6 to 8 hours on low.

3. When the beef is cooked, transfer it to a cutting board. Using two forks, shred the beef. (Do not discard the sauce in the slow cooker!)

4. Assemble the bowls. In each bowl, place an equal portion of the cauliflower rice, beans, avocado, cheese, tomatoes, beef, and barbacoa sauce from the slow cooker.

INGREDIENT TIP: If there is leftover barbacoa sauce, save it and use it either as a sauce for your bowls or use over eggs or in another recipe. Freeze any leftovers after 1 week.

Per serving: Calories: 509; Total Fat: 22g; Saturated Fat: 8g; Cholesterol: 107mg; Sodium: 1256mg; Carbohydrates: 25g; Fiber: 8g; Protein: 50g

Pressure Cooker
French Dip Sandwiches

SERVES: 8 / **PREP TIME:** 10 minutes / **COOK TIME:** 2 hours 10 minutes
QUICK-PREP, NUT-FREE

I had a French dip sandwich at a restaurant on a whim because I asked the waitress what her favorite dish on the menu was. I was not disappointed. I went home eager to try making it myself. Since I had no idea where to start, I figured I'd try my pressure cooker since it is great for making meat very tender, which that sandwich had been. The pressure cooker allows you to do minimal work and enjoy maximum rewards. Top this sandwich with cheese or add some vegetables and make me proud.

3 pounds beef rump roast, fat trimmed

1 teaspoon salt

½ teaspoon pepper

2 tablespoons olive oil

2 medium yellow onions, sliced

1 cup dry red wine

2 cups beef broth

8 rolls

8 slices Swiss cheese

1. Cut the beef into large chunks, season with salt and pepper, and let it sit on a platter for a few minutes.

2. Turn a pressure cooker to sauté and pour in the oil.

3. When the oil is hot, place the meat in the pressure cooker and sear on all sides until the meat is golden brown on the outside, 3 to 4 minutes.

4. Remove the meat from the pressure cooker and place it on a clean platter.

5. Put the onions in the pressure cooker and sauté for 3 to 5 minutes or until they start to turn translucent. Add the wine and stir, scraping up any brown bits on the sides or the bottom of the pressure cooker. Simmer for 1 to 2 minutes.

6. Pour in the beef broth and return the beef and any juice that has collected on the platter back into the slow cooker.

7. Cancel the sauté function, close the top, and seal it (making sure the vent is closed) and turn on manual (high) for 90 minutes.

8. After 90 minutes, allow the pressure cooker to naturally release pressure for 20 to 25 minutes.

CONTINUED

9. After that, open the vent and finish depressurizing manually. Remove the lid.

10. Transfer the beef to a cutting board. Using two forks, shred the beef.

11. Reserve the onions and liquid for dipping.

12. Evenly distribute the beef among the 8 rolls, top with the cheese, and place the sandwiches on a baking sheet. Turn on the broiler and put the sandwiches under the broiler for 2 to 3 minutes until the cheese is melted.

13. Serve the sandwiches with a small bowl of the reserved broth for dipping.

> **VARIATION TIP:** If you don't have a pressure cooker, brown the beef with oil in a skillet on the stovetop and then place all ingredients (except the cheese and rolls) in a slow cooker and cook on low for 6 to 8 hours.

Per serving: Calories: 577; Total Fat: 27g; Saturated Fat: 11g; Cholesterol: 95mg; Sodium: 1054mg; Carbohydrates: 34g; Fiber: 1g; Protein: 42g

Apple, Brie, and Caramelized Onion Burger

SERVES: 4 / **PREP TIME:** 5 minutes / **COOK TIME:** 30 minutes
QUICK-PREP, NUT-FREE, GLUTEN-FREE

One of my favorite things to do while traveling is to find the best burger in town. I find a burger can tell me a lot about the city or town that I'm in. I forget what town I was in when I had Brie on a burger, but I remember thinking what a great idea it was. Brie provides a mild yet buttery taste that makes this burger (and any burger, for that matter) irresistible. I have included a few burger recipes in this cookbook to help you get a feel for my style and to enjoy some delicious burgers, of course. This one might be my favorite one. Shhh! Don't tell the others!

1 tablespoon olive oil

2 onions, peeled and sliced

¼ teaspoon salt, plus more for seasoning

¼ teaspoon pepper, plus more for seasoning

1 pound lean ground beef

1 apple, cored and sliced

4 ounces Brie, sliced

4 hamburger buns

1. In a large skillet, heat the oil over medium heat.

2. Add the onions and cook for 20 minutes until caramelized, stirring frequently. Stir in the salt and pepper.

3. Form the beef into four patties and season with salt and pepper.

4. Grill the patties for about 5 minutes per side.

5. During the last minute of grilling, place the apple slices and Brie slices on top of each patty and continue grilling until the Brie is slightly melted.

6. Place the patties on the burger buns and enjoy!

> **VARIATION TIP:** Mix this up by using sliced pears or goat cheese in place of apples and Brie.

Per serving: Calories: 510; Total Fat: 21g; Saturated Fat: 8g; Cholesterol: 93mg; Sodium: 686mg; Carbohydrates: 44g; Fiber: 3g; Protein: 35g

Steak and Pepper Roll-Ups

SERVES: 4 / **PREP TIME:** 15 minutes, plus 20 minutes to marinate / **COOK TIME:** 10 minutes
NUT-FREE, DAIRY-FREE

This recipe was a quite a nice surprise. It is almost like steak sushi. The combination of spices and vegetables was/is just right, and I am always sad when it's all gone. Make sure when you buy the meat that it is extra thin so that it doesn't take a long time to cook and is thin enough to soak up the marinade in a timely manner.

⅓ cup soy sauce

1 tablespoon honey

1 teaspoon minced
fresh ginger

2 garlic cloves, minced

1 teaspoon sesame seeds

½ teaspoon salt

½ teaspoon pepper

1 pound flank steak, thinly
sliced into 16 strips

1 bell pepper, sliced

1 zucchini, sliced in
matchsticks

1 green onion, sliced into
2-inch strips

2 teaspoons olive oil

1. Preheat the grill to medium.

2. In a medium bowl, mix together the soy sauce, honey, ginger, garlic, sesame seeds, ¼ teaspoon of salt, and pepper. Add the meat to the sauce, stir, and let marinate for 15 to 20 minutes.

3. Meanwhile, in a medium bowl, toss the bell pepper, zucchini, and green onions in the olive oil and ¼ teaspoon each of the salt and pepper. Grill the vegetables for 4 to 5 minutes, turning to grill all sides evenly. Transfer the vegetables to a platter and let cool.

4. Turn the grill up to medium-high.

5. Remove the steak from the marinade and discard the marinade. Wrap each strip of beef around a small portion of vegetables and secure with a toothpick. Repeat until all of the beef and vegetables are used.

6. Grill on high for 4 to 5 minutes or until cooked through.

> **SUBSTITUTION TIP:** If you can't find thin beef, use some lean cut of beef, place between two sheets parchment paper or plastic wrap, and use a meat mallet to pound meat into thin pieces.

Per serving (4 roll-ups): Calories: 245; Total Fat: 11g; Saturated Fat: 4g; Cholesterol: 57mg; Sodium: 1565mg; Carbohydrates: 11g; Fiber: 1g; Protein: 25g

Mongolian Beef and Broccoli

SERVES: 4 / **PREP TIME:** 10 minutes / **COOK TIME:** 15 minutes
ONE-POT, 30 MINUTES OR LESS, QUICK-PREP, NUT-FREE, DAIRY-FREE

Mongolian beef may be one of my favorite meals. I love the umami flavor that this dish has, and I'm not going to lie, I'm a big broccoli fan. I used to hate broccoli growing up but now I try to have it weekly, if I can. Pair this with rice, and you'll be so glad you did because it will soak up all the marinade so none of it will go to waste.

1½ pounds flank steak, sliced into 3-by-½-inch strips

¼ cup cornstarch

2 tablespoons olive oil

3 garlic cloves, minced

1 teaspoon grated fresh ginger

1 head broccoli, cut into florets

4 green onions (green and white parts), chopped

¾ cup soy sauce

¼ cup maple syrup

¼ cup water

Zest and juice of 1 orange

Red pepper flakes (optional)

Green onion, sliced thin (optional)

Cooked rice

1. On a large plate, coat the steak with the cornstarch. Tap off any extra cornstarch and set aside.

2. In a large skillet, heat the oil over medium heat. Sauté the garlic and ginger for 2 minutes, then add the steak to skillet until browned on both sides. Transfer the steak to a plate and set aside.

3. Add extra oil to the skillet, if necessary. Put the broccoli, green onions, soy sauce, maple syrup, water, orange zest, and orange juice into the skillet. Bring to a simmer and cook for 5 to 10 minutes or until the sauce has reduced by half.

4. Return the steak and any juices that have collected on the plate back to the skillet and cook for 2 to 3 minutes.

5. Garnish with the red pepper flakes and the sliced green onion if desired. Serve over rice.

> **VARIATION TIP:** You can omit the cornstarch and just brown the beef without it. But note, it may not hold on to the marinade as much.

Per serving: Calories: 486; Total Fat: 20g; Saturated Fat: 7g; Cholesterol: 85mg; Sodium: 2863mg; Carbohydrates: 36g; Fiber: 6g; Protein: 42g

One-Skillet Pepper Steak

SERVES: 4 / **PREP TIME:** 15 minutes, plus 20 minutes to marinate / **COOK TIME:** 15 minutes
ONE-POT, NUT-FREE, DAIRY-FREE

Having a one-skillet meal is always welcome. I'm not a fan of having to do a lot of dishes, so this is ideal—and delicious, too! While this recipe is full of flavor, you could always add more vegetables to the mix, like broccoli and snap peas; just use what you have available.

¼ cup soy sauce

¼ cup water

2 teaspoons maple syrup

1 tablespoon cornstarch

½ teaspoon black pepper

1 pound flank steak, cut into ¼- to ½-inch slices

2 tablespoons avocado oil, divided

2 bell peppers, sliced into strips

1 yellow onion, sliced into strips

3 garlic cloves, minced

1-inch piece of fresh ginger, peeled and minced

Red pepper flakes (optional)

Cooked rice

1. In a small baking dish or large freezer bag, combine the soy sauce, water, maple syrup, cornstarch, and pepper. Add the steak and coat well with the sauce. Let marinate in the refrigerator for 20 minutes (or longer, if possible).

2. In a large skillet over medium heat, heat 1 tablespoon of the oil until glistening.

3. Add the peppers and onion, and stir until the vegetables have softened, about 8 minutes. Transfer the vegetables to a medium bowl and set aside.

4. Heat the remaining tablespoon of oil in the skillet. Add the garlic and ginger and sauté for one minute.

5. Remove the steak from the marinade (discard extra marinade) and cook until browned on each side, about 2 minutes per side.

6. Return the peppers and onions to the skillet and toss to combine.

7. Top with red pepper flakes, if using, and serve over rice.

> **TECHNIQUE TIP:** Cook the peppers and onions while the steak marinates to save time.

Per serving: Calories: 307; Total Fat: 15g; Saturated Fat: 5g; Cholesterol: 57mg; Sodium: 983mg; Carbohydrates: 17g; Fiber: 2g; Protein: 25g

Skillet Garlic-Herb Steak

SERVES: 4 / PREP TIME: 5 minutes / COOK TIME: 10 minutes, plus 5 minutes to rest
ONE-POT, 5 INGREDIENTS OR LESS, 30 MINUTES OR LESS, QUICK-PREP, NUT-FREE, DAIRY-FREE, GLUTEN-FREE

Steak is one of those foods that most people save for a special occasion. However, this skillet steak takes no time at all to make and should definitely not be left for only special occasions. Eat this steak with potatoes, some Mashed Parmesan Cauliflower (page 91), or place it on top of a salad. I prefer to slice it up after I cook it so that I can heat up any left-overs in desired portions.

2 (8-ounce) New York strip or rib-eye steaks, trimmed of excess fat

1 teaspoon salt

½ teaspoon pepper

1 teaspoon thyme

1 teaspoon rosemary

1 tablespoon butter or Ghee (page 251)

4 garlic cloves, minced

1. Season both sides of steak with salt, pepper, thyme, and rosemary. Set aside.

2. In a large skillet, heat the butter over medium–high heat. Add the garlic and sauté for 1 minute.

3. Add the steaks and sear 3 minutes per side. Reduce the heat to medium and cook, turning frequently until internal temp reads 130°F.

4. Remove from the heat and let rest for 5 minutes before slicing.

> **MAKE-AHEAD TIP:** For more flavorful steaks, season them with the salt, pepper, thyme, and rosemary, then cover and refrigerate overnight.

Per serving: Calories: 245; Total Fat: 10g; Saturated Fat: 5g; Cholesterol: 74mg; Sodium: 654mg; Carbohydrates: 2g; Fiber: 0g; Protein: 35g

Chili-Stuffed Peppers

SERVES: 6 / **PREP TIME:** 10 minutes / **COOK TIME:** 30 minutes
QUICK-PREP, NUT-FREE, GLUTEN-FREE

One of my biggest complaints over any stuffed pepper recipe is that there is always too much filling and not enough pepper. I made sure in this recipe that there were equal amounts of both. If for some reason you should have too much filling, save some to eat it by itself for a later meal.

Cooking oil spray

1 tablespoon oil

1 yellow onion, diced

4 garlic cloves, minced

6 bell peppers, tops removed and cores removed and discarded

1 pound lean ground beef

1 (14.5-ounce) can diced tomatoes

1 tablespoon chili powder

1 tablespoon cumin

2 teaspoons salt

1 teaspoon paprika

1 tablespoon tomato paste

1 cup shredded Cheddar cheese

1 cup plain unsweetened Greek yogurt mixed with juice of 1 lime, for topping (optional)

1. Preheat the oven to 400°F. Coat the inside of a baking dish with cooking oil spray.

2. In a large skillet, heat the oil over medium heat. Add the onion and sauté for 2 minutes, then add the garlic and chopped pepper tops, and sauté 1 minute more.

3. Add the beef and sauté until no pink is showing, 5 to 7 minutes.

4. Stir in the tomatoes, spices, and tomato paste.

5. Fill each pepper with the beef mixture and top with cheese.

6. Place the stuffed peppers in the baking dish and roast for 30 minutes or until the peppers are soft and the cheese is melted. Top with the lime Greek yogurt, if desired.

> **SUBSTITUTION TIP:** You can use any type of ground meat in this recipe. Feel free to change it up based on what flavor you are craving or what's on sale.

Per serving: Calories: 298; Total Fat: 14g; Saturated Fat: 6g; Cholesterol: 60mg; Sodium: 1163mg; Carbohydrates: 21g; Fiber: 5g; Protein: 22g

Spinach Meatballs and Zucchini Noodles

SERVES: 4 / **PREP TIME:** 10 minutes / **COOK TIME:** 30 minutes
QUICK-PREP, NUT-FREE, GLUTEN-FREE

Hiding some vegetables or greens in a dish can be a great way to get even the pickiest of eaters to eat something healthy. I love to stuff my meatballs full of good ingredients so that I can feel good that both myself and others are eating a well-balanced meal.

FOR THE MEATBALLS

Cooking oil spray

1 pound lean ground beef

2 cups spinach, chopped

½ cup diced onion

3 garlic cloves, minced

1 large egg

1 teaspoon oregano

¼ teaspoon pepper

¼ teaspoon salt

FOR THE NOODLES

1 tablespoon olive oil

3 garlic cloves, minced

2 zucchini, spiralized

2 tablespoons grated
   Parmesan cheese

Salt

Pepper

2 cups Homemade
   Marinara Sauce
   (page 266)

TO MAKE THE MEATBALLS

1. Preheat the oven to 400°F. Coat the surface of a roasting pan with cooking oil spray.

2. In a large bowl, combine all of the meatball ingredients. Mix well.

3. Form 16 golf ball–size meatballs and place them on the roasting pan. Roast for 30 minutes.

TO MAKE THE NOODLES

1. In a large skillet, heat the oil over medium heat. Add the garlic and sauté for 3 minutes.

2. Add the zucchini and sauté for 3 to 5 minutes until softened. Remove from the heat and season with the Parmesan cheese, salt, and pepper.

3. In a large saucepan, heat the marinara sauce over medium heat.

4. When the meatballs are done cooking, gently add them to the marinara sauce, then pour the sauce and the meatballs over the zucchini noodles.

Per serving: Calories: 304; Total Fat: 15g; Saturated Fat: 4g; Cholesterol: 113mg; Sodium: 457mg; Carbohydrates: 15g; Fiber: 4g; Protein: 30g

Spaghetti Squash Bolognese

SERVES: 4 to 6 / **PREP TIME:** 10 minutes / **COOK TIME:** 1 hour 5 minutes
QUICK-PREP, NUT-FREE, GLUTEN-FREE

This recipe is one of my go-to meals. I have a list of about 10 meals that I use as my fallback recipes. These are recipes that I can make whenever I'm in a pinch time-wise or if I'm lacking inspiration in the kitchen, or when I'm craving a tried-and-true meal. I can get this on the table without having to wonder how it will turn out. I recommend finding a few recipes that you like and don't take much time, then start your go-to recipe list today—perhaps you could begin with this very recipe.

1 Spaghetti Squash (page 249)

1 tablespoon olive oil

1 small yellow onion, diced

4 garlic cloves, minced

1 bell pepper, diced

2 celery stalks, diced

1 pound ground beef

1 (28-ounce) can crushed tomatoes

2 tablespoons tomato paste

1 teaspoon oregano

¼ cup grated Parmesan

Salt

Pepper

Red pepper flakes (optional)

1. Prepare the spaghetti squash according to the directions on page 249.

2. Meanwhile, in a large skillet, heat the oil over medium heat. Add the onion and cook for 2 to 3 minutes, or until the onion starts to turn translucent.

3. Add the garlic, bell pepper, and celery, and cook for an additional 2 to 3 minutes.

4. Add the ground beef and cook and stir, breaking apart, until the beef is browned, and no pink is showing.

5. Add the tomatoes, tomato paste, and oregano, and simmer for 8 to 10 minutes, or until the beef is cooked through.

6. Add the spaghetti squash, Parmesan, salt, pepper, and red pepper flakes, if using.

> **MAKE-AHEAD TIP:** Make the spaghetti squash ahead of time and then make the bolognese when ready to eat.

Per serving: Calories: 351; Total Fat: 14g; Saturated Fat: 5g; Cholesterol: 70mg; Sodium: 606mg; Carbohydrates: 27g; Fiber: 7g; Protein: 31g

One-Pot Taco Pasta

SERVES: 6 / **PREP TIME:** 10 minutes / **COOK TIME:** 20 minutes
ONE-POT, 30 MINUTES OR LESS, QUICK-PREP, NUT-FREE

Did someone say tacos? I'm pretty sure we have some form of tacos almost every week in my house. This one-pot pasta was new to us though. I was looking for a way to have all the flavors of tacos without the mess and with a way to create a meal that we could eat throughout the week. This one-pot pasta was a crowd pleaser and made me especially happy because there were very few dishes to clean up.

1 tablespoon olive oil

1 small red onion, diced

3 garlic cloves, minced

1 pound lean ground beef

1 tablespoon Taco Seasoning (page 250)

2 tablespoons tomato paste

1 bell pepper, diced

1 (15-ounce) can black beans, drained and rinsed

1 (14.5-ounce) can diced tomatoes

3 cups chicken broth

8 ounces elbow macaroni

1 cup shredded Cheddar cheese

Juice of 1 lime

2 tablespoons cilantro, chopped

1 jalapeño, seeded and diced

Avocado, cheese, jalapeños, lime wedges, sour cream, for topping (optional)

1. In a large stockpot or Dutch oven, heat the oil over medium heat. Add the onion and garlic and sauté for 2 minutes, or until the onion starts to soften.

2. Add the ground beef and cook until brown, 5 to 7 minutes.

3. Stir in the taco seasoning, tomato paste, and bell pepper.

4. Add the black beans, diced tomatoes, and broth and bring to a slow boil.

5. Add the macaroni and cook for 8 to 10 minutes or until the pasta is done.

6. Stir in the cheese and top with the lime juice, cilantro, and diced jalapeño. Serve with the toppings of your choice.

> **SUBSTITUTION TIP:** Make this a gluten-free dish by replacing the traditional macaroni with a gluten-free version.

Per serving: Calories: 444; Total Fat: 15g; Saturated Fat: 7g; Cholesterol: 62mg; Sodium: 952mg; Carbohydrates: 48g; Fiber: 6g; Protein: 30g

Sweet Potato and Butternut Squash Shepherd's Pie

SERVES: 6 / **PREP TIME:** 10 minutes / **COOK TIME:** 50 minutes to 1 hour
QUICK-PREP, NUT-FREE, GLUTEN-FREE

I always veered away from shepherd's pie because I thought it was a big tasteless meat pie. I was wrong. The combination of spices plus the butternut squash and sweet potato create a flavorful and slightly sweet and savory experience. This dish reheats well so make it ahead of time and have leftovers for the week.

FOR THE SWEET POTATO AND BUTTERNUT SQUASH TOPPING

1 sweet potato, peeled and chopped

1 (1½-pound) butternut squash, peeled, seeded, and cut into chunks

1 tablespoon olive oil

2 tablespoons butter, melted

¼ cup grated Parmesan cheese

FOR THE BEEF FILLING

1 tablespoon olive oil

1 yellow onion, minced

3 garlic cloves, minced

1 bell pepper, diced

3 carrots, diced

1 pound ground beef

8 ounces white button mushrooms, sliced

1 (14.5-ounce) can diced tomatoes

1 cup Easy Broth (page 253)

1 teaspoon rosemary

1 teaspoon thyme

1 teaspoon salt

½ teaspoon pepper

TO MAKE THE SWEET POTATO AND BUTTERNUT SQUASH TOPPING

1. Preheat the oven to 400°F. Line a baking sheet with parchment paper.

2. In a large bowl, toss the sweet potato and butternut squash with the oil. Spread the potatoes and squash on the baking sheet and bake for 30 minutes or until fork-tender.

3. Transfer the potatoes and squash to a blender. Add the butter and Parmesan cheese and blend until smooth. Set aside.

1. In a large oven-safe skillet, heat the oil over medium heat. Add the onion and cook for 2 to 3 minutes, then add the garlic, bell pepper, and carrots, and cook for 1 minute more.

2. Add the beef and cook until browned, about 5 minutes.

3. Add the mushrooms, tomatoes, broth, rosemary, thyme, salt, and pepper, and stir. Simmer for 5 minutes to thicken. Remove from the heat.

4. Top the meat mixture with the butternut squash and sweet potato. Put the skillet in the oven. Cook the shepherd's pie, uncovered, for 15 to 20 minutes.

> **INGREDIENT TIP:** If you have a large enough butternut squash (over 2 pounds), feel free to omit the sweet potato. Alternatively, if you wish to just use sweet potatoes, use 3 or 4 total.

Per serving: Calories: 327; Total Fat: 15g; Saturated Fat: 6g; Cholesterol: 57mg; Sodium: 911mg; Carbohydrates: 29g; Fiber: 7g; Protein: 21g

Lamb Kofta Kebabs

SERVES: 4 / **PREP TIME:** 15 minutes, plus 15 minutes to chill / **COOK TIME:** 10 minutes
NUT-FREE, GLUTEN-FREE

When seasoned appropriately, lamb may be one of my favorite proteins. These kebabs are seasoned with an interesting combination of seasonings, ones that I do not normally pair with meat, but it works. This is great served with Turmeric Rice (page 93). If you want to keep this dairy-free, the kebabs taste great without the dipping sauce and could be paired with some Ketchup (page 256) or even some hummus if you would like an alternative sauce to pair it with.

FOR THE LAMB KOFTA

1 pound ground lamb

1 small onion, chopped

3 garlic cloves, chopped

2 tablespoons fresh mint, finely chopped

1 teaspoon cumin

1 teaspoon salt

½ teaspoon cinnamon

¼ teaspoon turmeric

¼ teaspoon black pepper

FOR THE MINT YOGURT

½ cup plain unsweetened Greek yogurt

¼ cup feta, crumbled

2 tablespoons mint, finely chopped

1 tablespoon lemon

Salt

Pepper

TO MAKE THE LAMB KOFTA

1. Mix all of the ingredients for lamb kofta in a blender or food processor until there are no big chunks of onion.

2. Form into 4 equal balls and flatten to create long ovals. Place the lamb ovals on a dish and refrigerate, covered, for at least 15 minutes.

3. Preheat a grill to medium high.

4. Remove the lamb from the refrigerator and thread it onto skewers lengthwise (about 2 per skewer). Grill for 5 to 6 minutes, then flip over and grill for an additional 5 minutes or until the lamb is cooked through.

TO MAKE THE MINT YOGURT

In a small bowl, whisk together all of the ingredients for mint yogurt. Serve alongside the lamb.

Per serving: Calories: 391; Total Fat: 31g; Saturated Fat: 14g; Cholesterol: 97mg; Sodium: 774mg; Carbohydrates: 5g; Fiber: 1g; Protein: 22g

Lamb Gyros

SERVES: 4 / **PREP TIME:** 5 minutes / **COOK TIME:** 45 minutes
QUICK-PREP, NUT-FREE, GLUTEN-FREE

This might be one of my favorite recipes from this cookbook. I don't like to play favorites, but I was pleasantly surprised by these and was unable to save any for leftovers. You can eat these on their own or serve them in a pita topped with the tomatoes and tzatziki. I was wary to have to bake these twice, but I highly recommend taking the extra step as it helps to crisp them up and make them perfect for a sandwich or pita.

1 pound ground lamb

4 bacon slices, chopped

3 garlic cloves, chopped

1 teaspoon oregano

1 teaspoon onion powder

1 teaspoon salt, plus more for seasoning

½ teaspoon pepper, plus more for seasoning

2 tomatoes, diced

1 cucumber, diced

1 small red onion, diced

Juice of 1 lime

Pita

Tzatziki (page 261)

1. Preheat the oven to 325°F. Line a baking sheet with parchment paper.

2. Place the lamb, bacon, garlic, oregano, onion powder, 1 teaspoon salt, and ½ teaspoon pepper in a food processor and process until well combined.

3. Form the lamb mixture into a long flat loaf, place on the baking sheet and bake until the internal temperature reaches 155°F, 30 to 35 minutes. Remove from the oven, transfer to cutting board, and let cool for 5 minutes. Reserve the baking sheet.

4. Meanwhile, in a medium bowl, toss together the tomatoes, cucumber, onion, and lime. Season with salt and pepper.

5. Turn the oven to broil. Slice the lamb loaf into thin slices. Place the slices on the baking sheet. Return the baking sheet to the oven and broil for 2 to 4 minutes.

6. Serve with pita, the tomato mixture, and tzatziki.

Per serving: Calories: 402; Total Fat: 30g; Saturated Fat: 13g; Cholesterol: 93mg; Sodium: 819mg; Carbohydrates: 8g; Fiber: 2g; Protein: 24g

Feta Lamb Burgers

SERVES: 4 / **PREP TIME:** 15 minutes / **COOK TIME:** 10 minutes
30 MINUTES OR LESS, QUICK-PREP, NUT-FREE, GLUTEN-FREE

As I've mentioned before, I'm a fan of trying new burgers, as there are so many ways you can make them your own. The tomato paste really helps to bind these burgers together and keep them moist. If you need these to be dairy-free, you could leave out the feta cheese and then just use it as a topping for those that want the cheese flavor.

⅓ cup sun-dried tomatoes

Cooking oil spray

1 pound ground lamb

⅓ cup feta cheese, crumbled

1 tablespoon tomato paste

½ teaspoon cumin

½ teaspoon salt

¼ teaspoon pepper

1. In a medium bowl, cover sun-dried tomatoes with boiling water and let soak for 10 to 15 minutes or until softened. Drain and dice.

2. Preheat the grill to medium. Lightly coat the grill with cooking oil spray.

3. Combine all of the ingredients and form 4 evenly shaped patties.

4. Grill until the internal temperature reaches 145°F, about 5 minutes per side.

VARIATION TIP: If you don't have ground lamb, feel free to use any type of ground meat for these burgers.

Per serving: Calories: 369; Total Fat: 29g; Saturated Fat: 13g; Cholesterol: 94mg; Sodium: 622mg; Carbohydrates: 4g; Fiber: 1g; Protein: 21g

Pressure Cooker Lamb Meatballs

SERVES: 4 / **PREP TIME:** 10 minutes / **COOK TIME:** 15 minutes
30 MINUTES OR LESS, QUICK-PREP, NUT-FREE

I'm a sucker for meatballs because they are incredibly easy to eat, and they freeze well. The freezing usually only happens if I make extra or if I have a lot of other food to get through during the week. Otherwise, I eat these up in no time. Pair these meatballs with a marinara sauce or with tzatziki, warmed pita bread, and hummus.

1 pound ground lamb

3 ounces feta, crumbled

Juice and zest of 1 lemon

¼ cup fresh parsley, chopped

¼ cup minced onion

1 large egg

2 tablespoons plain bread crumbs

1 cup Easy Broth (page 253)

¼ teaspoon salt

¼ teaspoon black pepper

¼ cup kalamata olives, diced

1 tablespoon tomato paste

1. In a large bowl, mix all of the ingredients together until well combined.

2. Form the mixture into 12 to 16 ping-pong ball–size meatballs.

3. Place a trivet in pressure cooker and place meatballs on top of the trivet. (It's okay if the meatballs have to be stacked on top of each other.)

4. Seal the pressure cooker.

5. Cook on manual (high) for 7 minutes. Allow the pressure cooker to naturally release for 5 minutes when done, then quick release the remaining pressure.

6. Serve over greens or in a pita.

> **VARIATION TIP:** Make these in the oven by placing the meatballs on a greased roasting pan and baking at 400°F for 15 to 20 minutes, or until the lamb is cooked through.

Per serving: Calories: 442; Total Fat: 34g; Saturated Fat: 15g; Cholesterol: 148mg; Sodium: 670mg; Carbohydrates: 8g; Fiber: 1g; Protein: 24g

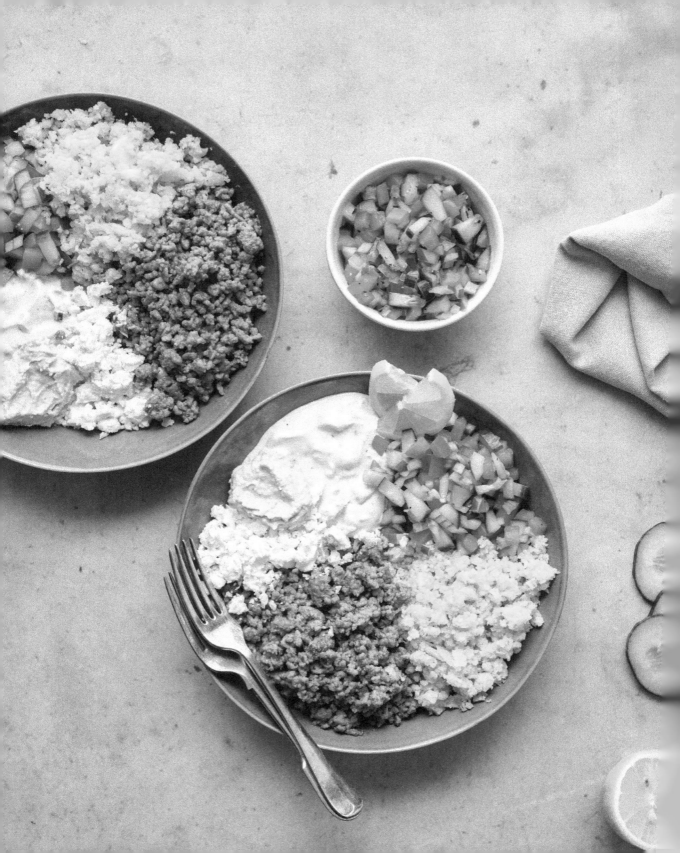

Greek Lamb Bowls with Turmeric Cauliflower Rice and Cucumber Salsa

SERVES: 4 / **PREP TIME:** 10 minutes / **COOK TIME:** 15 minutes
30 MINUTES OR LESS, QUICK-PREP, NUT-FREE, GLUTEN-FREE

I will eat most of my meals in a bowl as it allows me to experience all the flavors combined together. I also love that it's easier to prepare, because you can just throw everything in a bowl or in covered containers in the refrigerator and you're ready to go. If you don't have lamb, don't worry. This recipe works well with other ground meats, like chicken and turkey, in case you need a change or need to use what you have on hand. I make this recipe fairly often as I can't resist the easy preparation.

FOR THE CUCUMBER SALSA

1 small red
  onion, chopped

1 cucumber, chopped

1 red bell
  pepper, chopped

Juice of 1 lemon

1 teaspoon apple
  cider vinegar

Salt

Pepper

**FOR THE TURMERIC
  CAULIFLOWER RICE**

1 tablespoon olive oil

1 head cauliflower, stem
  removed and riced

½ teaspoon turmeric

Salt

Pepper

FOR THE LAMB BOWLS

1 teaspoon salt

1 teaspoon oregano

½ teaspoon black pepper

½ teaspoon garlic powder

¼ teaspoon turmeric

1 pound ground lamb

1 tablespoon
  tomato paste

½ cup hummus of choice

½ cup feta cheese,
  crumbled

Tzatziki (page 261)

CONTINUED

TO MAKE THE CUCUMBER SALSA

In a large bowl, mix all of the ingredients together, cover, and set aside.

TO MAKE THE TURMERIC CAULIFLOWER RICE

1. In a large skillet, heat the olive oil over medium heat. Add the cauliflower and cook for 5 minutes, or until the cauliflower is cooked down and tender.

2. Season with the turmeric, salt, and pepper. Remove from the heat and set aside.

TO MAKE THE LAMB BOWLS

1. In a small bowl, mix together the salt, oregano, pepper, garlic powder, and turmeric.

2. In a larger skillet over medium heat, combine the lamb and the spice mixture and cook, stirring occasionally, until the lamb is no longer pink.

3. Mix the tomato paste into the lamb. Remove from the heat.

4. Divide the cauliflower rice, lamb mixture, hummus, cucumber salsa, and feta evenly among four bowls. Top each bowl with 2 tablespoons of tzatziki.

SUBSTITUTION TIP: Make this dairy-free by omitting feta cheese and tzatziki.

Per serving: Calories: 610; Total Fat: 43g; Saturated Fat: 19g; Cholesterol: 119mg; Sodium: 1232mg; Carbohydrates: 28g; Fiber: 8g; Protein: 32g

Lamb Lollipops with Chimichurri Sauce

SERVES: 4 / **PREP TIME:** 15 minutes / **COOK TIME:** 10 minutes
30 MINUTES OR LESS, NUT-FREE, DAIRY-FREE, GLUTEN-FREE

We had lamb lollipops for the first time at a restaurant when we were celebrating our anniversary. We don't normally pick lamb, but for one reason or another we thought the lamb lollipops looked interesting. They were delicious! I decided to try my hand at them, and it was definitely worth it. The chimichurri sauce is not necessary, but it adds an extra level of flavor that ties this dish together. Serve over rice or as an appetizer.

FOR THE CHIMICHURRI SAUCE

1 cup cilantro

⅔ cup fresh parsley

⅓ cup fresh mint

1 tablespoon dried oregano

4 garlic cloves

½ cup olive oil

¼ cup lemon juice

1 teaspoon salt

FOR THE LAMB

1 pound (about 8) lamb rib chops

½ teaspoon salt

½ teaspoon pepper

¼ cup olive oil

4 garlic cloves, minced

TO MAKE THE CHIMICHURRI SAUCE

Put all of the ingredients for the chimichurri sauce in a blender and blend on high until smooth. Set aside.

TO MAKE THE LAMB

1. Season the lamb chops with the salt and pepper. Let sit for 15 minutes.

2. In a large skillet, heat the oil over medium heat. Add the garlic and sauté for 1 minute.

3. Add the lamb chops and cook for 3 minutes per side, or until both sides are browned and the lamb is cooked to an internal temperature of 145°F.

4. Serve with chimichurri sauce spooned over the top of each rib chop.

> **INGREDIENT TIP:** If you have extra herbs after using them for this recipe, dice them and place them in an ice cube tray, fill with water, cover, and freeze until ready to use.

Per serving: Calories: 581; Total Fat: 51g; Saturated Fat: 9g; Cholesterol: 75mg; Sodium: 959mg; Carbohydrates: 6g; Fiber: 2g; Protein: 24g

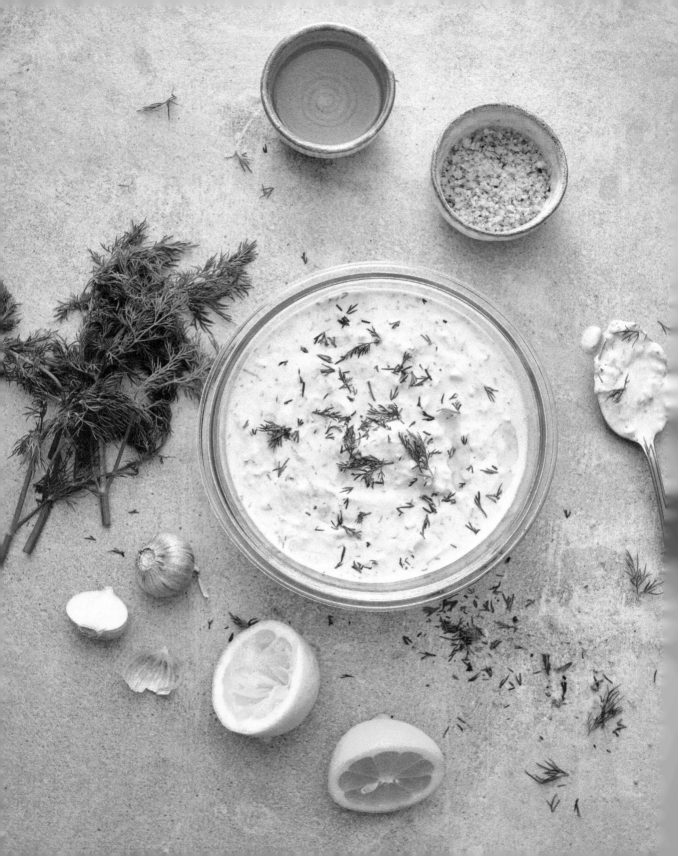

CHAPTER ELEVEN

Staples and Sauces

248 Poached Eggs

249 Spaghetti Squash

250 Taco Seasoning

251 Ghee

252 Almond Butter

253 Easy Broth

254 Homemade Mayo

255 Honey Mustard

256 Ketchup

257 Sassy BBQ Sauce

258 Gochujang

259 Quick Pickles

260 Maple Vinaigrette

261 Tzatziki

262 Sweet-and-Sour Sauce

263 Enchilada Sauce

265 Spinach-Walnut Pesto

266 Homemade Marinara Sauce

267 Cauliflower Pizza Crust

Tzatziki, Page 261

Poached Eggs

SERVES: 1 / **PREP TIME:** 5 minutes / **COOK TIME:** 5 minutes
ONE-POT, 5 INGREDIENTS OR LESS, 30 MINUTES OR LESS, QUICK-PREP, VEGETARIAN, NUT-FREE, DAIRY-FREE, GLUTEN-FREE

I love eggs and poached eggs are my absolute favorite way to eat them. I will warn you: Poached eggs take practice. So, try your hand at these, but if they don't turn out perfectly the first time, chalk it up to a learning experience, and try, try again. Once you get the hang of it, you'll be putting poached eggs on everything.

6 cups water

Pinch salt

1 teaspoon vinegar

2 large eggs

1. Fill a medium saucepan with the water.

2. Add the salt and the vinegar and bring the water to a boil over high heat.

3. Crack each egg in its own small bowl or ramekin, and set aside.

4. When the water reaches a boil, turn down the heat until it comes to a slow and steady simmer.

5. Using a spoon or spatula, swirl the water in a circle to create a vortex and slide the egg(s) into water.

6. Cook for 4 minutes and then remove the eggs with a slotted spoon and place on a paper towel–lined plate to blot.

7. If you prefer your yolks on the runnier side, cook for 3 minutes. If you prefer them hard, cook for 5 to 6 minutes.

Per serving: Calories: 144; Total Fat: 10g; Saturated Fat: 3g; Cholesterol: 372mg; Sodium: 297mg; Carbohydrates: 1g; Fiber: 0g; Protein: 13g

Spaghetti Squash

MAKES: 1 spaghetti squash / **PREP TIME:** 5 minutes / **COOK TIME:** 45 minutes

OME-POT, 5 INGREDIENTS OR LESS, QUICK-PREP, VEGETARIAN, NUT-FREE, DAIRY-FREE, GLUTEN-FREE

I had no idea what a spaghetti squash was until a few years ago. Once I discovered it though, I was hooked. You can eat it as is or use it in place of pasta. I personally love cooking it for the week and then having it as a side dish ready to go for whatever we have on hand like meatballs, chicken, or fish.

1 (2- to 3-pound)
  spaghetti squash

1. Preheat the oven to 400°F. Line a baking sheet with foil.

2. Cut the spaghetti squash in half lengthwise and scoop out the seeds.

3. Place the spaghetti squash cut-sides down and bake for 45 minutes or until the skin is easy to push in and when tested with a fork, the strands pull out easily.

> **INGREDIENT TIP:** Microwave the spaghetti squash for 1 to 2 minutes prior to cutting. It will make it easier to slice through.

Per recipe (~ 2.5 cups for a 2-pound squash): Calories: 105; Total Fat: 1g; Saturated Fat: 0g; Cholesterol: 0mg; Sodium: 70mg; Carbohydrates: 25g; Fiber: 5g; Protein: 3g

Taco Seasoning

MAKES: ⅔ cup / **PREP TIME:** 5 minutes

30 MINUTES OR LESS, QUICK-PREP, VEGETARIAN, NUT-FREE, DAIRY-FREE, GLUTEN-FREE

Making taco seasoning at home can be a game changer to your cooking. Not only is it lower in sodium than store-bought taco seasonings, I also think it's far tastier. Don't believe me? Try it for yourself.

¼ cup chili powder

1 tablespoon paprika

1 tablespoon cumin

1 tablespoon salt

1 teaspoon garlic powder

1 teaspoon onion powder

1 teaspoon oregano

½ teaspoon ground
  black pepper

Combine all of the ingredients in a glass container, cover/seal, and shake to combine. Store in your pantry at room temperature until ready to use.

MAKE-AHEAD TIP: Make-ahead a week or two in advanced and store in an airtight container so you can use in recipes like Vegetarian Black Bean Enchiladas (page 131) and Spicy Shrimp Tacos (page 150).

Per serving (1 tablespoon): Calories: 8; Total Fat: 0g; Saturated Fat: 0g; Cholesterol: 0mg; Sodium: 666mg; Carbohydrates: 1g; Fiber: 0g; Protein: 0g

Ghee

MAKES: 3 cups / **PREP TIME:** 5 minutes / **COOK TIME:** 40 minutes

ONE-POT, 5 INGREDIENTS OR LESS, VEGETARIAN, QUICK-PREP, NUT-FREE, GLUTEN-FREE

My husband is lactose intolerant, so we try to make everything at home as dairy-free as possible. Ghee helps to retain the flavor of butter in the dishes that we cook without causing him any stomach woes. It's easy to make, and you can make it while you are doing other things in the kitchen. It can be stored at room temperature until ready to use.

2 pounds unsalted butter, cut into even chunks

1. In a large saucepan, melt the butter over medium heat and bring to a slow boil.

2. Reduce the heat and simmer for 15 minutes.

3. Using a spoon, remove the white solids and continue to simmer for another 15 minutes. Brown solids will form on the bottom of the pan. Continue to skim white solids off the top.

4. Remove the ghee from the heat and allow to cool for 5 minutes.

5. Line a fine mesh strainer with cheesecloth and strain the ghee into a medium bowl to remove the remaining milk solids.

6. Store in an airtight container in a dark cool place in the kitchen or pantry for up to 1 month or in the refrigerator for up to 3 months.

> **VARIATION TIP:** If you don't have a cheesecloth, use a coffee filter in a fine mesh strainer.

Per serving (1 tablespoon): Calories: 136; Total Fat: 15g; Saturated Fat: 10g; Cholesterol: 41mg; Sodium: 2mg; Carbohydrates: 0g; Fiber: 0g; Protein: 0g

Almond Butter

MAKES: 2 cups / **PREP TIME:** 5 minutes

ONE-POT, 5 INGREDIENTS OR LESS, 30 MINUTES OR LESS, QUICK-PREP, VEGETARIAN, DAIRY-FREE, GLUTEN-FREE

This is one of those items that you can certainly go out and buy, but how satisfying is it to make something on your own? Making almond butter is simple and, in my opinion, is tastier than the varieties found in stores. I used it in a few recipes in this book, too, so that you won't be left just eating it from the jar, not that that would be a bad thing.

16 ounces raw almonds

1. Place the almonds in a food processor and process until creamy. It will be necessary to pulse a few times and scrape down the sides every few minutes. Be patient!

2. Store in an airtight container in the refrigerator for up to 1 week.

> **VARIATION TIP:** Add ½ teaspoon vanilla and ¼ teaspoon cinnamon to make a cinnamon-vanilla almond butter.

Per serving (2 tablespoons): Calories: 163; Total Fat: 14g; Saturated Fat: 1g; Cholesterol: 0mg; Sodium: 0mg; Carbohydrates: 6g; Fiber: 3g; Protein: 6g

Easy Broth

MAKES: 12 cups / **PREP TIME:** 5 minutes / **COOK TIME:** 8+ hours

ONE-POT, 5 INGREDIENTS OR LESS, QUICK-PREP, NUT-FREE, DAIRY-FREE, GLUTEN-FREE

Broth is one of the easiest things you can make in your kitchen, and it allows you to use all of your food—even the parts you may usually throw away. It's nice to have broth on hand for the countless recipes in this book that use it as a base. By changing up the bones and the vegetables, you can make a different flavor every time. My favorite is beef stock with onions, celery, and carrots.

2 to 4 pounds bones
(e.g., beef, chicken,
pork, oxtail, etc.)

3 to 4 quarts water
(depending on size of
your slow cooker)

2 tablespoons apple
cider vinegar

5 to 6 garlic
cloves, smashed

2 to 3 cups assorted
vegetables, including
scraps and ends
(optional)

½ teaspoon salt

1. Place all of the ingredients in a slow cooker. Cover and cook on low for a least 8 hours or up to 24 hours.

2. Strain the broth through a fine-mesh strainer. Cool and store in glass jars. Refrigerate for up to 1 week or freeze until ready to use.

> **INGREDIENT TIP:** When cooking, save your vegetable ends and scraps, freeze them, and then toss them in your slow cooker when making broth.

Per serving (1 cup): Calories: 19; Total Fat: 0g; Saturated Fat: 0g; Cholesterol: 0mg; Sodium: 141mg; Carbohydrates: 4g; Fiber: 2g; Protein: 1g

Homemade Mayo

MAKES: 1½ cups / **PREP TIME:** 15 minutes

ONE-POT, 30 MINUTES OR LESS, VEGETARIAN, NUT-FREE, DAIRY-FREE, GLUTEN-FREE

I am not usually a fan of anything mayonnaise-based; it just has never been one of my favorite condiments. However, making my own mayonnaise has changed the game for me. This homemade mayonnaise is creamy and flavorful without any extra additives. Be patient with this one to ensure that the oil emulsifies properly. I also recommend splurging on some nice avocado oil as its mild flavor is perfect for this recipe.

1 large egg

1 tablespoon Dijon mustard

1 tablespoon apple cider vinegar

¼ teaspoon salt, plus more as desired

¾ cup avocado oil

Pinch garlic powder

1 teaspoon lemon juice

1. Put the egg in a 2-cup liquid measuring cup or bowl. Using an immersion blender, blend on high for 20 seconds (should be frothy).

2. Add the mustard, vinegar, and salt, and blend for another 20 seconds.

3. Then, while still blending, add the oil drop by drop until it begins to emulsify (turn whitish and look creamy).

4. Then, add the rest of the oil in a fine stream while still blending until all of the oil is used up.

5. If not creamy or thick enough, add an extra ¼ cup of oil in a slow and steady stream.

6. Mix in additional salt as needed and the garlic powder and lemon juice. Store in an airtight container in the refrigerator for up to 2 weeks.

> **VARIATION TIP:** If you don't have an immersion blender, you can make this in a regular blender—just make sure you go slow.

Per serving (2 tablespoons): Calories: 137; Total Fat: 14g; Saturated Fat: 2g; Cholesterol: 15mg; Sodium: 84mg; Carbohydrates: 0g; Fiber: 0g; Protein: 0g

Honey Mustard

MAKES: 1½ cups / **PREP TIME:** 5 minutes

ONE-POT, 30 MINUTES OR LESS, QUICK-PREP, VEGETARIAN, NUT-FREE, DAIRY-FREE, GLUTEN-FREE

Honey mustard used to be my favorite condiment for pairing with chicken fingers and curly fries at the pool when I was little. A lot has changed with my diet since then. I can't tell you the last time I had chicken fingers and curly fries (not that I'm opposed!). However, one thing hasn't changed, I still love honey mustard. Once you realize how easy it is to make for yourself, you may never need to buy it again.

¼ cup Dijon mustard

2 tablespoons
   yellow mustard

2 tablespoons Homemade
   Mayo (page 254)

¼ cup honey

¼ teaspoon salt

¼ teaspoon cayenne

¼ teaspoon garlic powder

In a medium bowl, mix together all of the ingredients. Serve immediately or store in an airtight container in the refrigerator for up to a week.

> **INGREDIENT TIP:** Use local honey to change up the flavor of your honey mustard.

Per serving (¼ cup): Calories: 79; Total Fat: 3g; Saturated Fat: 0g; Cholesterol: 3mg; Sodium: 407mg; Carbohydrates: 12g; Fiber: 0g; Protein: 0g

Ketchup

MAKES: 2½ cups / **PREP TIME:** 10 minutes

ONE-POT, 30 MINUTES OR LESS, QUICK-PREP, VEGETARIAN, NUT-FREE, DAIRY-FREE, GLUTEN-FREE

Ketchup is a family staple for many. The problem with ketchup is that it's usually loaded with sugar, and sometimes even high-fructose corn syrup. When you make ketchup yourself, you get to enjoy the tomato flavor and control how much sugar gets added. It might take some getting used to, but I think over time you'll find homemade ketchup to be quite enjoyable.

12 ounces tomato paste

¼ cup coconut sugar

¾ cup water

½ cup apple cider vinegar

1 teaspoon onion powder

1 teaspoon garlic powder

Pinch red pepper flakes

½ teaspoon salt

Pinch pepper

1. In a large bowl, combine all of the ingredients together and whisk until smooth.

2. Refrigerate overnight. Then check the consistency and add water, if necessary, to reach desired consistency. Store in an airtight jar in the refrigerator for up to 2 weeks.

Per serving (¼ cup): Calories: 79; Total Fat: 0g; Saturated Fat: 0g; Cholesterol: 0mg; Sodium: 642mg; Carbohydrates: 19g; Fiber: 3g; Protein: 3g

Sassy BBQ Sauce

MAKES: 4 cups / **PREP TIME:** 5 minutes / **COOK TIME:** 25 minutes

ONE-POT, 30 MINUTES OR LESS, QUICK-PREP, VEGETARIAN, NUT-FREE, DAIRY-FREE

This barbecue sauce gets its name from my nickname "The Sassy Dietitian." I decided one day that I wanted to try my hand at a homemade barbecue sauce because when I looked at the labels for all the barbecue sauces on the shelves, their ingredient lists were all full of sugar and fillers. It took me a few times to get this recipe right. The final result is a great-tasting barbecue sauce made of real foods.

1 tablespoon avocado oil

4 garlic cloves, minced

1 (14.5-ounce) can diced tomatoes

1 (6-ounce) can tomato paste

2 tablespoons soy sauce

2 tablespoons Dijon mustard

2 tablespoons maple syrup

1 tablespoon apple cider vinegar

1 teaspoon garlic powder

1 teaspoon onion powder

1 teaspoon chili powder

½ teaspoon salt

½ teaspoon pepper

1. In a large saucepan, heat the oil over medium heat.

2. Add the garlic cloves and sauté for 3 to 4 minutes until slightly golden.

3. Add all of the remaining ingredients and mix well. Bring the barbecue sauce to a simmer.

4. Using an immersion blender, blend the ingredients until smooth. Add water to thin, as needed.

5. Lower the heat and simmer on low for 20 minutes, stirring occasionally.

6. Store in a sealed airtight container in the refrigerator for up to 2 weeks.

> **VARIATION TIP:** If you don't have an immersion blender, at step 3 put all of the ingredients into a blender or food processor and blend on high until smooth. Add water to thin, as needed.

Per serving (½ cup): Calories: 68; Total Fat: 2g; Saturated Fat: 0g; Cholesterol: 0mg; Sodium: 708mg; Carbohydrates: 11g; Fiber: 2g; Protein: 2g

Gochujang

MAKES: 1¼ cups / **PREP TIME:** 5 minutes

ONE-POT, 5 INGREDIENTS OR LESS, 30 MINUTES OR LESS, QUICK-PREP, VEGETARIAN, DAIRY-FREE

I love a good Asian dish, however, without the right seasoning it can fall flat. This Gochujang—otherwise known as red chile paste—is simple to make and very flavorful. If you aren't a huge fan of spice, you may want to reduce the amount of red pepper flakes.

½ cup miso paste

⅓ cup maple syrup

⅓ cup soy sauce

4 garlic cloves, minced

¼ cup red pepper flakes

Pinch salt

1. Put all of the ingredients into a blender and blend well. Add water as needed to thin.

2. Store in and airtight container in the refrigerator for up to one week.

Per serving (¼ cup): Calories: 75; Total Fat: 0g; Saturated Fat: 0g; Cholesterol: 0mg; Sodium: 1045mg; Carbohydrates: 17g; Fiber: 0g; Protein: 1g

Quick Pickles

MAKES: 2 cups / **PREP TIME:** 15 minutes

ONE-POT, 30 MINUTES OR LESS, QUICK-PREP, VEGETARIAN, NUT-FREE, DAIRY-FREE, GLUTEN-FREE

My friends and I had a pickling party one year and I've been hooked on pickling food ever since. It takes relatively little time and is a great way to use up vegetables that might otherwise go bad in the refrigerator. Make sure you have salt and vinegar on hand, and you will be ready to pickle anything!

1 cucumber, sliced

4 garlic cloves, smashed

1 teaspoon whole black peppercorns

½ teaspoon dried dill

½ cup vinegar

1 tablespoon sugar

1 teaspoon salt

1. In a medium bowl, mix the cucumber, garlic, black peppercorns, and dill. Set aside.

2. In a small saucepan, heat the vinegar, sugar, and salt over medium heat until the sugar and salt are dissolved.

3. Pour the liquid over the cucumbers and stir to coat.

4. Allow to cool, then serve or pour into jars, adding extra vinegar to cover, if necessary.

5. Store in a sealed glass jars in the refrigerator up to 2 months.

> **VARIATION TIP:** You can make this recipe with other vegetables including carrots, beets, onions, or radishes.

Per serving (½ cup): Calories: 28; Total Fat: 0g; Saturated Fat: 0g; Cholesterol: 0mg; Sodium: 584mg; Carbohydrates: 7g; Fiber: 1g; Protein: 1g

Maple Vinaigrette

MAKES: ½ cup / **PREP TIME:** 5 minutes

ONE-POT, 5 INGREDIENTS OR LESS, 30 MINUTES OR LESS, QUICK-PREP, VEGETARIAN, NUT-FREE, DAIRY-FREE, GLUTEN-FREE

Dressings are easy to make, but people often end up buying them anyway because it seems more convenient. This maple vinaigrette is a nice addition to any salad, and you can make it ahead of time and add it as you wish. I keep it on hand in the refrigerator as a go-to for everyday salads.

¼ cup extra-virgin olive oil

¼ cup maple syrup

1 tablespoon Dijon mustard

½ tablespoon apple cider vinegar

Juice of 1 lemon

Pinch salt

Pinch pepper

1. Whisk together all of the ingredients and refrigerate until ready to use.

2. Prior to each use, very briefly warm the dressing in the microwave and shake well before serving, since the maple syrup and the oil will congeal in the refrigerator.

3. Store in an airtight container for up to 1 week.

Per serving (2 tablespoons): Calories: 177; Total Fat: 13g; Saturated Fat: 2g; Cholesterol: 0mg; Sodium: 130mg; Carbohydrates: 14g; Fiber: 0g; Protein: 0g

Tzatziki

SERVES: 4 / **PREP TIME:** 15 minutes
ONE-POT, 5 INGREDIENTS OR LESS, 30 MINUTES OR LESS, VEGETARIAN, NUT-FREE, GLUTEN-FREE

Tzatziki is not only fun to say but it's also fun to eat. I sometimes sneak a few bites with a spoon when I'm done making it. Otherwise, I enjoy tzatziki with a slew of recipes in this book, including the Greek Lamb Bowls (page 243) and Lamb Gyros (page 239). You can certainly add other spices to it to make it your own, like dill, crushed red pepper, and garlic powder, but I'll leave that decision up to you.

1 cucumber, finely grated

Pinch salt, plus more for seasoning

7 ounces full-fat plain unsweetened Greek yogurt

¼ cup feta cheese, crumbled

Juice of ½ lemon

Pinch pepper

1. In a medium bowl, mix the cucumber with a pinch of salt. Spread the cucumber on the cheesecloth. Wait 2 minutes, then twist the cheesecloth to squeeze out the excess water from the cucumbers.

2. In the same bowl, mix the cucumber with the rest of the ingredients until well combined. Season with additional salt and pepper, as desired.

3. Store in an airtight container in the refrigerator for 4 to 5 days.

> **VARIATION TIP:** Use a cheese grater or food processor to grate cucumber. (If you don't like the skin, feel free to peel it before grating.) Then spread on cheesecloth and continue with step 1.

Per serving: Calories: 84; Total Fat: 5g; Saturated Fat: 3g; Cholesterol: 19mg; Sodium: 178mg; Carbohydrates: 6g; Fiber: 1g; Protein: 4g

Sweet-and-Sour Sauce

MAKES: 1¼ cups / **PREP TIME:** 5 minutes / **COOK TIME:** 10 minutes
ONE-POT, 30 MINUTES OR LESS, QUICK-PREP, VEGETARIAN, NUT-FREE, DAIRY-FREE

I don't know about you, but I love the taste of sweet-and-sour sauce, but I'm not a big fan of food dyes. This sauce is easy to make, and the food dyes are kicked to the curb. Sure, you won't get a fluorescent red color, but you will get a good-tasting recipe that you can feel good about giving to the whole family.

½ cup brown sugar

½ cup apple cider vinegar

¼ cup pineapple juice (or water)

¼ cup Ketchup (page 256)

2 tablespoons soy sauce

1 tablespoon cornstarch

Place all of the ingredients in a saucepan and bring to a boil. Reduce the heat to low and simmer, stirring frequently until thickened, about 10 minutes. Store in an airtight container in the refrigerator for up to 1 week.

INGREDIENT TIP: If you don't have time to make ketchup, use a store-bought ketchup that does not contain high-fructose corn syrup.

Per serving (¼ cup): Calories: 83: Total Fat: 0g: Saturated Fat: 0g: Cholesterol: 0mg: Sodium: 487mg: Carbohydrates: 25g: Fiber: 0g: Protein: 0g

Enchilada Sauce

MAKES: 1½ cups / **PREP TIME:** 5 minutes / **COOK TIME:** 10 minutes
30 MINUTES OR LESS, QUICK-PREP, NUT-FREE, DAIRY-FREE, GLUTEN-FREE

Enchiladas are messy to make but so delicious to eat. Most enchilada sauces you find on the shelves are loaded with ingredients from who-knows-where. This enchilada sauce is flavorful and made only of real food ingredients. Make it ahead of time so you are ready for enchiladas any day of the week.

1 to 2 tablespoons cornstarch

1 tablespoon chili powder

1 teaspoon garlic powder

½ teaspoon cumin

½ teaspoon oregano

½ teaspoon salt

¼ teaspoon pepper

2 tablespoons avocado oil

2 tablespoons tomato paste

2 cups Easy Broth (page 253)

1. In a small bowl, mix together the cornstarch, chili powder, garlic powder, cumin, oregano, salt, and pepper.

2. In a medium saucepan, heat the oil over medium heat. Add the spice mixture and whisk constantly for 1 to 2 minutes until fragrant.

3. Add the tomato paste and broth, whisking vigorously to prevent clumping.

4. Bring to a simmer and cook for 5 to 7 minutes. Remove from the heat.

5. Use immediately or store in an airtight container in the refrigerator for up to 1 week.

> **VARIATION TIP:** If consistency is too thick, add water to thin as needed but do so by a tablespoon at a time.

Per serving (½ cup): Calories: 131; Total Fat: 10g; Saturated Fat: 1g; Cholesterol: 0mg; Sodium: 593mg; Carbohydrates: 9g; Fiber: 3g; Protein: 2g

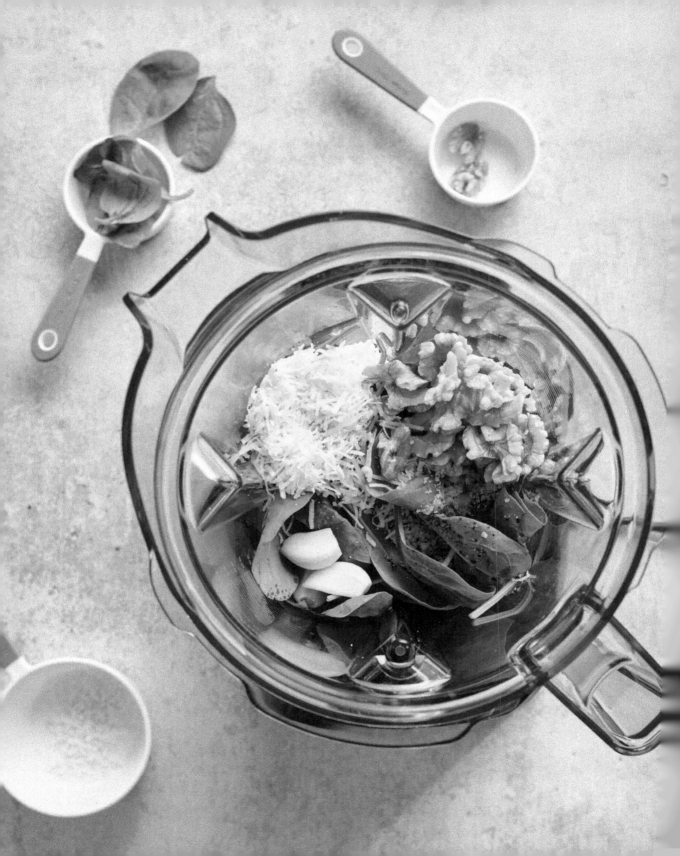

Spinach-Walnut Pesto

MAKES: 1 cup / **PREP TIME:** 5 minutes
ONE-POT, 5 INGREDIENTS OR LESS, 30 MINUTES OR LESS, QUICK-PREP, VEGETARIAN, GLUTEN-FREE

Pesto is one of those items I recommend always having on hand. It makes any meat or protein delicious and helps tie almost any dish together. The nice thing about this pesto is that you can easily find all of the ingredients in your grocery store year-round. Plus, it takes less than 5 minutes to make! If I have any pesto left over, I freeze it in 2-tablespoon portions in an ice cube tray.

2 cups spinach,
  lightly packed
⅓ cup walnuts
⅓ cup shredded
  Parmesan
½ cup extra-virgin olive oil
3 garlic cloves
½ teaspoon salt
¼ teaspoon pepper

Place all of the ingredients in a blender or food processor, and pulse until blended and smooth. Store in an airtight container in the refrigerator for up to 1 week.

> **SUBSTITUTION TIP:** To make a more traditional pesto, use basil instead of spinach—or you could use basil and spinach—and toasted pine nuts instead of walnuts.

Per serving (¼ cup): Calories: 326; Total Fat: 34g; Saturated Fat: 5g; Cholesterol: 4mg; Sodium: 409mg; Carbohydrates: 3g; Fiber: 1g; Protein: 4g

Homemade Marinara Sauce

MAKES: 8 cups / **PREP TIME:** 10 minutes / **COOK TIME:** 40 minutes
ONE-POT, QUICK-PREP, VEGETARIAN, NUT-FREE, DAIRY-FREE, GLUTEN-FREE

I grew up on marinara sauce, or as we called it in my house "gravy." There wasn't a week that went by in our house that we didn't smell fresh gravy cooking on the stovetop. We used it on pasta and pizza and sometimes we would just dip fresh bread into it. I love making this ahead of time and then having it in the refrigerator to use as needed. Sometimes I keep it chunky, and other times I blend it so it's smooth; it just depends on my mood.

1 tablespoon olive oil

1 yellow onion, chopped

5 garlic cloves, minced

1 green bell
  pepper, chopped

2 (28-ounce) cans crushed
  tomatoes

1 (6-ounce) can
  tomato paste

2 teaspoons oregano

¼ cup fresh
  parsley, chopped

¼ cup fresh
  basil, chopped

½ cup water, as needed
  for thinning

Salt

Pepper

Red pepper flakes
  (optional)

1. In a large pot, heat the oil over medium heat. Add the onion and cook for 2 to 3 minutes, then add the garlic and cook for 1 to 2 minutes more.

2. Add the bell pepper and cook for an additional 2 minutes.

3. Stir in the tomatoes, tomato paste, oregano, parsley, and basil.

4. Add about ¼ cup water to each can of tomatoes, swirl, and pour into the pot.

5. Bring the sauce to a boil, then reduce the heat to low and simmer for 30 minutes uncovered, stirring often.

6. Season with salt, pepper, and red pepper flakes, if using.

7. Thin with additional water, if needed.

8. You can leave the sauce chunky if you like or use an immersion blender to make a smooth sauce.

9. Store in an airtight container in the refrigerator for up to 1 week or freeze for up to 3 months.

INGREDIENT TIP: If you don't have fresh herbs, use 1 tablespoon of each of dried herbs instead.

Per serving (½ cup): Calories: 40; Total Fat: 1g; Saturated Fat: <1g; Cholesterol: 0mg; Sodium: 154mg; Carbohydrates: 7g; Fiber: 2g; Protein: 2g

Cauliflower Pizza Crust

MAKES: 1 crust / **PREP TIME:** 5 minutes / **COOK TIME:** 40 minutes
QUICK-PREP, VEGETARIAN, NUT-FREE, GLUTEN-FREE

Cauliflower is all the rage mostly because it is incredibly versatile. The nice thing about cauliflower is that it has a mild flavor that pairs well with all kinds of dishes. I love using it as a pizza crust because you get an extra serving of vegetables while still feeling like you are indulging.

1 head cauliflower, stems removed and chopped

½ cup grated Parmesan cheese

½ cup shredded mozzarella

2 eggs, beaten

1 teaspoon oregano

1 teaspoon garlic powder

Pinch salt

Pinch pepper

1. Preheat the oven to 400°F. Line a baking sheet with parchment paper.

2. Rice the cauliflower in a food processor.

3. In a large skillet, sauté the cauliflower over medium heat for 10 minutes (or microwave for 5 minutes).

4. When the cauliflower has cooled for about 5 minutes, lay out a cheesecloth, place cauliflower in the cloth, grab the edges, twist the cloth, and squeeze out any excess liquid from the cauliflower.

5. In a large bowl, mix together the cauliflower, Parmesan cheese, mozzarella cheese, eggs, oregano, garlic powder, salt, and pepper.

6. Using your hands or a spatula, spread the cauliflower crust out on the baking sheet.

7. Bake for 20 minutes.

8. Use the cooked crust in recipes as directed.

> **VARIATION TIP:** You can make this without removing the excess water; however, the crust will be a bit soggier. It just depends how much effort you want to put in!

Per serving: Calories: 618; Total Fat: 31g; Saturated Fat: 18g; Cholesterol: 255mg; Sodium: 1710mg; Carbohydrates: 39g; Fiber: 15g; Protein: 53g

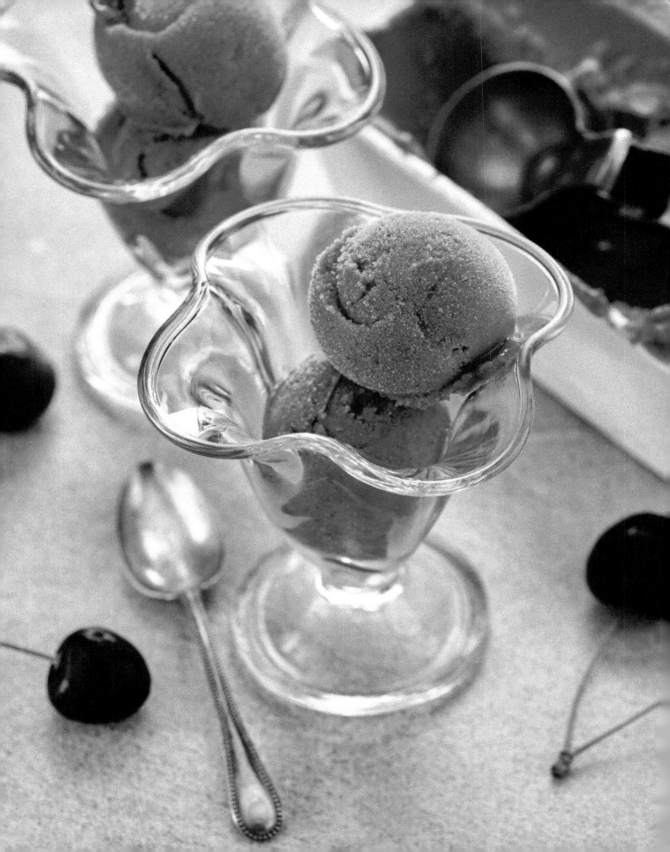

CHAPTER TWELVE

Desserts

270 Strawberry Lemonade Slushie

271 Tropical Pineapple Fruit Leather

272 Apple Nachos

273 Chili-Spiced Fruit Cups

274 Black Cherry Sorbet

275 Strawberry Shortcake Mug Cake

276 Raspberry-Lemon Bars

277 Peach Crumble

278 Easy Vanilla Ice Cream

279 Almond Butter Cookies

280 Dark Chocolate–Sea Salt Popcorn

281 S'mores Campfire Trail Mix

282 Chocolate-Covered Orange Slices

283 Fruit-and-Nut Chocolate Bark

284 Salted Chocolate–Coconut Macaroons

285 Mocha-Ricotta Mousse

287 Chocolate–Peanut Butter Freezer Fudge

289 Mocha-Cheesecake Brownies

Strawberry Lemonade Slushie

SERVES: 4 / PREP TIME: 5 minutes
5 INGREDIENTS OR LESS, 30 MINUTES OR LESS, QUICK-PREP, VEGETARIAN, NUT-FREE, DAIRY-FREE, GLUTEN-FREE

Sometimes you just want something more than water. This is something that I make when I need hydration and want something a little sweet. I loved strawberry lemonade growing up, but now I find it to be way too sweet. This slushie is a great compromise. Add some alcohol and now you've got a nice adult strawberry lemonade.

1 pound frozen
  strawberries
1 cup water
2 cups ice
Juice of 3 lemons
1 tablespoon honey

1. Put all of the ingredients in a blender and blend on high until smooth.

2. Pour into four glasses and top with fresh strawberry and lemon slices.

> **VARIATION TIP:** Add 4 ounces of vodka or rum to make this an alcoholic beverage.

Per serving: Calories: 64; Total Fat: 0g; Saturated Fat: 0g; Cholesterol: 0mg; Sodium: 2mg; Carbohydrates: 18g; Fiber: 2g; Protein: 1g

Tropical Pineapple Fruit Leather

SERVES: 6 / **PREP TIME:** 10 minutes / **COOK TIME:** 4 to 5 hours
5 INGREDIENTS OR LESS, QUICK-PREP, VEGETARIAN, NUT-FREE, DAIRY-FREE, GLUTEN-FREE

Fruit leather reminds me of lunch as a child. I suggest making this fruit leather when you have plenty to do around the house as this takes a good amount of time to cook but no real supervision is needed. If you have a dehydrator, you could use it to make this fruit leather as well.

1 pineapple, cored and chopped

1 mango, peeled and chopped

1 tablespoon honey

Juice and zest of 1 lemon

1. Preheat the oven to 200°F. Line a large baking sheet with a silicone baking mat or parchment paper.

2. Put all of the ingredients into a blender and blend on high until smooth.

3. Pour the mixture onto the baking sheet and spread it out in an even layer. Bake for 4 to 5 hours or until the center is no longer tacky.

4. Remove and let cool completely, then cut into strips and roll up in parchment paper.

5. Keep in an airtight container for up to a week.

> **TIP:** Use multiple baking sheets to make a thinner fruit leather and to speed up cooking time.

Per serving: Calories: 74; Total Fat: 0g; Saturated Fat: 0g; Cholesterol: 0mg; Sodium: 2mg; Carbohydrates: 19g; Fiber: 2g; Protein: 0g

Apple Nachos

SERVES: 6 / **PREP TIME:** 5 minutes

30 MINUTES OR LESS, QUICK-PREP, VEGETARIAN, DAIRY-FREE, GLUTEN-FREE

Move over savory nachos, apples are in the house! I have a plethora of apples as I live in upstate New York, so I'm always looking at new ways to use them. These apple nachos are a great snack or party appetizer. The apples give a nice crispness to this sweet dessert. Feel free to adjust the toppings for this dish based on what you have on hand.

½ cup dark chocolate

1 teaspoon coconut oil

2 apples, cored

¼ cup Almond Butter (page 252), melted

2 tablespoons unsweetened coconut flakes

2 tablespoons sliced almonds

2 tablespoons raisins

Cocoa nibs, dried fruit, or fresh fruit, for topping (optional)

1. In a microwave-safe bowl, melt the chocolate and coconut oil in 30-second intervals. Stir between intervals and continue until the chocolate has melted.

2. Slice the apples into wedges and arrange on a large plate.

3. Drizzle with the melted chocolate and almond butter.

4. Top with the coconut flakes, almonds, raisins, and other toppings, as desired.

> **TECHNIQUE TIP:** To melt the almond butter for easy drizzling, put it in a small saucepan on the stove over medium heat for about 5 minutes, or microwave for 30 seconds to 1 minute.

Per serving: Calories: 196; Total Fat: 13g; Saturated Fat: 5g; Cholesterol: 2mg; Sodium: 7mg; Carbohydrates: 22g; Fiber: 4g; Protein: 3g

Chili-Spiced Fruit Cups

SERVES: 8 / **PREP TIME:** 10 minutes

ONE-POT, 30 MINUTES OR LESS, QUICK-PREP, VEGETARIAN, NUT-FREE, DAIRY-FREE, GLUTEN-FREE

Fruit is a great snack and appeals to people of all ages. I decided to change up a typical fruit cup by putting a savory spin on it with lime juice, chili powder, and salt. This combination of sweet, savory, and salty is irresistible and will make you rethink how you are enjoying your fruit. Prepare it for the week or serve it at a party, or maybe both.

1 pineapple

2 mangos

1 small seedless
   watermelon

1 cucumber

Juice of 1 lime

1 teaspoon chili powder

½ teaspoon salt

1. Chop the pineapple, mangos, watermelon, and cucumber to equal-size cubes.

2. Put the fruit and cucumber cubes into a large bowl and toss with the lime juice, chili powder, and salt.

> **VARIATION TIP:** Change the fruit depending on what you have on hand or what's in season. Try adding papaya, cantaloupe, or honeydew.

Per serving: Calories: 117; Total Fat: 0g; Saturated Fat: 0g; Cholesterol: 0mg; Sodium: 152mg; Carbohydrates: 29g; Fiber: 3g; Protein: 2g

Black Cherry Sorbet

SERVES: 4 / PREP TIME: 5 minutes

ONE-POT, 5 INGREDIENTS OR LESS, 30 MINUTES OR LESS, QUICK-PREP, VEGETARIAN, NUT-FREE, DAIRY-FREE, GLUTEN-FREE

Sorbet is one of my favorite summertime treats. Of course, you can eat sorbet year-round but there is something so refreshing about it when it's hot out. Cherries are one of my favorite fruits, because they are both tart and sweet. I also love how easy this recipe is, and you can vary it by using frozen berries or other fruit.

2 pounds frozen cherries, pitted

1 cup water

½ cup maple syrup

Juice of 1 lime

1. Place all of the ingredients in a blender and blend on high until smooth.

2. Enjoy immediately or store in the freezer in an airtight container for up 1 month. When removing from freezer, let the sorbet sit on the counter for a few minutes before serving.

INGREDIENT TIP: If you only have fresh cherries, pit them, and freeze them for at least an hour or overnight before making this dessert.

Per serving: Calories: 184; Total Fat: 0g; Saturated Fat: 0g; Cholesterol: 0mg; Sodium: 4mg; Carbohydrates: 46g; Fiber: 3g; Protein: 2g

Strawberry Shortcake Mug Cake

SERVES: 1 / COOK TIME: 5 minutes
ONE-POT, 30 MINUTES OR LESS, QUICK-PREP, VEGETARIAN, GLUTEN-FREE

I've always seen this done and thought there was no way in the world it actually worked. Then, I also figured that it could be possible, but it probably didn't taste all that great. I was wrong on both counts. This mug cake does work and is delicious. It's a bit dangerous because it's so easy to make but also wonderful because it only makes one serving.

1 tablespoon butter or
  Ghee (page 251)

2 tablespoons milk
  of choice

½ teaspoon pure
  vanilla extract

¼ cup oat flour (or flour
  of choice)

½ teaspoon
  baking powder

1 tablespoon maple syrup

1 large egg

Pinch salt

2 chopped strawberries,
  plus 1 strawberry, sliced,
  for topping

1. Put the butter in a mug and microwave it for 30 seconds to 1 minute, checking every 20 seconds.

2. Whisk in the milk and the vanilla.

3. Add the flour, baking powder, syrup, egg, salt, and chopped strawberries. Whisk to combine.

4. Microwave for 90 seconds to 2 minutes or until firm.

5. Top with the remaining strawberry and enjoy immediately!

> **INGREDIENT TIP:** Make oat flour simply by placing oats in a food processor or blender and pulsing until it is ground into a fine flour.

Per serving: Calories: 371; Total Fat: 18g; Saturated Fat: 9g; Cholesterol: 221mg; Sodium: 245mg; Carbohydrates: 43g; Fiber: 5g; Protein: 12g

Raspberry-Lemon Bars

MAKES: 12 bars / **PREP TIME:** 10 minutes / **COOK TIME:** 40 minutes
ONE-POT, QUICK-PREP, VEGETARIAN, DAIRY-FREE

If you've never had a lemon bar before, now is your chance to find out what all the buzz is about. Lemon bars are tangy and sweet and satisfy the sweet tooth for all of us. I added raspberries in there to give it some extra flavor and color but feel free to add any type of berry to make it your own.

FOR THE ALMOND CRUST

Cooking oil spray

1 cup almond flour

2 tablespoons Ghee (page 251) or butter, melted

2 tablespoons honey

1 large egg

½ teaspoon pure vanilla extract

Pinch salt

FOR THE LEMON FILLING

4 large eggs

⅓ cup honey

Zest and juice of 4 lemons (½ cup lemon juice)

¼ cup tapioca flour

1 cup raspberries

TO MAKE THE ALMOND CRUST

1. Preheat the oven to 350°F. Lightly coat the inside of an 8-by-8-inch baking dish with cooking oil spray.

2. In a medium bowl, combine all of the ingredients for the almond crust. Mix well. Transfer the dough into the baking dish. Using a spatula, press the dough into the bottom of the baking dish. The dough should cover the bottom of the dish in an even layer. Bake for 15 to 20 minutes.

TO MAKE THE LEMON FILLING

1. Whisk together the eggs, honey, lemon zest, lemon juice, and tapioca flour.

2. When the almond crust has finished cooking, remove it from the oven and arrange the raspberries on top of crust in an even layer. Pour the lemon filling over the raspberries.

3. Bake for an additional 20 minutes or until cooked through.

SUBSTITUTION TIP: Make these without raspberries if you don't have any on hand or try it with blueberries, strawberries, or cherries.

Per serving (1 bar): Calories: 161; Total Fat: 9g; Saturated Fat: 2g; Cholesterol: 82mg; Sodium: 45mg; Carbohydrates: 17g; Fiber: 2g; Protein: 5g

Peach Crumble

SERVES: 8 / **PREP TIME:** 10 minutes / **COOK TIME:** 25 minutes
QUICK-PREP, VEGETARIAN, NUT-FREE, DAIRY-FREE

Crumbles are great desserts when you want something that tastes good but doesn't take a lot of effort to make. I love a good pie, but a crumble does not require nearly the amount of attention to detail. The peaches in this dish make it a home run. Feel free to use other fruit as desired and serve with a scoop of Easy Vanilla Ice Cream (page 278) on top.

FOR THE PEACH FILLING

Cooking oil spray

6 peaches, sliced

1 tablespoon honey

Juice of ½ lemon

1 tablespoon cornstarch

Pinch salt

FOR THE OAT CRUMBLE

½ cup flour

½ cup Ghee (page 251) or
    butter, melted

½ cup brown sugar

½ cup oats

½ teaspoon cinnamon

¼ teaspoon ginger

Pinch salt

TO MAKE THE PEACH FILLING

1. Preheat the oven to 350°F. Lightly coat the inside of a 10-inch pie dish with cooking oil spray.

2. In the pie dish, add all of the ingredients for the peach filling. Mix well and spread out in an even layer on the bottom of the pie dish.

TO MAKE THE OAT CRUMBLE

1. In a large bowl, mix together all of the ingredients for the oat crumble until it comes together and has a coarse or pebbly texture.

2. Sprinkle the crumble on top of the peach filling in an even layer and bake for 25 minutes. Turn the oven to broil and broil for 1 minute.

> **SUBSTITUTION TIP:** Make this recipe gluten-free by using gluten-free flour or oat flour instead of wheat flour in the crumble.

Per serving: Calories: 257; Total Fat: 16g; Saturated Fat: 9g; Cholesterol: 30mg; Sodium: 42mg; Carbohydrates: 33g; Fiber: 2g; Protein: 2g

Easy Vanilla Ice Cream

SERVES: 6 to 8 / **PREP TIME:** 30 minutes

5 INGREDIENTS OR LESS, VEGETARIAN, NUT-FREE, GLUTEN-FREE

I don't know about you, but I'm a big ice cream fan. I love a good mint chocolate chip, chocolate chip cookie dough, or s'mores ice cream. This vanilla ice cream is a simple base recipe that you can doctor up as you see fit. Once the ice cream has been churning for a few minutes, add in your favorite extra goodies, if you wish.

1½ cups whole milk

1½ cups heavy cream

¾ cups sugar

1½ teaspoons pure vanilla extract

Pinch salt

1. In a medium bowl, whisk together all of the ingredients. Whisk until the sugar is dissolved, then pour the mixture into an ice cream maker and process according to the manufacturer's instructions.

2. Enjoy immediately or store in the freezer in an airtight container for up 1 month. When removing from the freezer, let the ice cream sit on the counter for a few minutes before serving.

> **STORAGE TIP:** Store in airtight freezer-safe containers. Before covering, place a sheet of plastic wrap on the top layer of the ice cream to prevent ice crystals from forming, then cover and store in freezer.

Per serving: Calories: 341; Total Fat: 24g; Saturated Fat: 15g; Cholesterol: 89mg; Sodium: 78mg; Carbohydrates: 30g; Fiber: 0g; Protein: 3g

Almond Butter Cookies

MAKES: 18 to 20 cookies / **PREP TIME:** 15 minutes / **COOK TIME:** 15 minutes
DAIRY-FREE, 5 INGREDIENTS OR LESS, 30 MINUTES OR LESS, VEGETARIAN, GLUTEN-FREE

I'm a big fan of simple recipes. This dessert is the definition of simple. You don't have to be a baker to wow your family, friends, or coworkers with these cookies. The only warning I'll issue is these are so good you won't be able to eat just one.

1 cup Almond Butter (page 252)

1 cup coconut sugar

1 large egg

½ teaspoon pure vanilla extract

Pinch salt

1. Preheat the oven to 325°F. Line a baking sheet with parchment paper.

2. In a large bowl, mix together all of the ingredients, then refrigerate for 10 minutes.

3. Form the dough into 1-inch balls.

4. Press down with the back of a fork to flatten and sprinkle with salt.

5. Bake for 15 minutes, or until golden brown.

> **SUBSTITUTION TIP:** To make this recipe nut-free, use sunflower or pumpkin seed butter.

Per serving: Calories: 129; Total Fat: 8g; Saturated Fat: 1g; Cholesterol: 10mg; Sodium: 14mg; Carbohydrates: 14g; Fiber: 1g; Protein: 2g

Dark Chocolate–Sea Salt Popcorn

SERVES: 4 / **PREP TIME:** 5 minutes / **COOK TIME:** 10 minutes

5 INGREDIENTS OR LESS, 30 MINUTES OR LESS, QUICK-PREP, VEGETARIAN, NUT-FREE, DAIRY-FREE, GLUTEN-FREE

Popcorn is an easy-to-make dessert and enjoyable to boot. I love the combination of salty and sweet in this recipe. Be warned, the chocolate may make things messy, but if you aren't getting messy, are you really enjoying your food? I used a spoon to help drizzle the chocolate onto the popcorn, but if you aren't picky with presentation, put the popcorn in a bowl with the chocolate and toss to combine.

3 tablespoons, plus
   2 teaspoons coconut oil
½ cup popcorn kernels
⅔ cup dark chocolate
Sea salt

1. Line a baking sheet with parchment paper.

2. In a large pot, heat 3 tablespoons of oil over high heat.

3. Test out heat by adding 2 to 3 kernels until one pops. Add the remaining popcorn kernels, cover, and cook, shaking the pot occasionally to prevent burning, until the popping stops.

4. Pour the popcorn onto the baking sheet and let cool for 5 minutes.

5. Meanwhile, in a microwave-safe bowl, melt the chocolate and the remaining 2 teaspoons of coconut oil in the microwave in 30-second intervals. Stir between intervals and continue until the chocolate has melted.

6. Drizzle the chocolate over the popcorn, then sprinkle with salt, and toss.

> **INGREDIENT TIP:** Depending on the time of year and temperature of your house, you may want to refrigerate or freeze the popcorn after tossing with chocolate to help the chocolate solidify and remain solidified.

Per serving: Calories: 313; Total Fat: 22g; Saturated Fat: 17g; Cholesterol: 3mg; Sodium: 10mg; Carbohydrates: 34g; Fiber: 7g; Protein: 4g

S'mores Campfire Trail Mix

SERVES: 8 / **PREP TIME:** 5 minutes / **COOK TIME:** 15 minutes

30 MINUTES OR LESS, QUICK-PREP, VEGETARIAN, GLUTEN-FREE, DAIRY-FREE

Is there anything that screams summer more than s'mores? This campfire trail mix is easy to make and can make it feel like summer year-round. I love the addition of marshmallows, but they are not necessary for this trail mix to be delicious.

1 cup raw
  unsalted almonds

1 cup unsalted
  roasted peanuts

1½ tablespoons honey

3 tablespoons
  cocoa powder

½ teaspoon salt

2 cups pretzels

½ cup dried cranberries

1 cup dark
  chocolate morsels

1 cup small marshmallows
  (optional) (see
  Ingredient Tip)

1. Preheat the oven to 350°F. Line a baking sheet with parchment paper.

2. Spread the almonds and peanuts on baking sheet in an even layer and bake for 6 minutes.

3. Transfer the nuts to a medium bowl and toss with the honey, cocoa powder, and salt. Return the nut mixture to the baking sheet and cook for an additional 6 minutes.

4. Meanwhile, in a large bowl, combine the pretzels, cranberries, dark chocolate, and marshmallows, if using.

5. When the nuts have cooled, toss them into the pretzel mixture, and store in airtight containers until ready to eat or up to 1 week.

INGREDIENT TIP: Look for marshmallows that have no high-fructose corn syrup added to them. You may find fancier marshmallows that are square-shaped, just chop them up and toss them in!

Per serving: Calories: 355; Total Fat: 24g; Saturated Fat: 6g; Cholesterol: 0mg; Sodium: 199mg; Carbohydrates: 35g; Fiber: 6g; Protein: 8g

Chocolate-Covered Orange Slices

SERVES: 8 / PREP TIME: 25 minutes
5 INGREDIENTS OR LESS, 30 MINUTES OR LESS, VEGETARIAN, NUT-FREE, DAIRY-FREE, GLUTEN-FREE

There is something so refreshing about an orange slice. They remind me of sports growing up as we always had them for halftime and after games. This is a grown-up dessert version of orange slices that the whole family can enjoy.

3 to 4 Mandarin oranges

¾ cup dark chocolate

Flaked salt (optional)

1. Peel the oranges and separate them into sections. Place them on a paper towel–lined dish to absorb excess liquid.

2. Line a baking sheet with parchment.

3. In a microwave-safe bowl, melt the chocolate in the microwave in 30-second intervals. Stir between intervals and continue until the chocolate has melted.

4. Dip half of each orange section in the chocolate, then place on the baking sheet. Repeat until all of the orange slices are dipped halfway in chocolate.

5. Sprinkle with salt if desired and refrigerate for 15 minutes or until the chocolate has set.

> **INGREDIENT TIP:** Store these in the refrigerator until they are consumed so that the chocolate does not melt.

Per serving: Calories: 95; Total Fat: 6g; Saturated Fat: 4g; Cholesterol: 0mg; Sodium: 0mg; Carbohydrates: 13g; Fiber: 2g; Protein: 0g

Fruit-and-Nut Chocolate Bark

SERVES: 12 / **PREP TIME:** 30 minutes

5 INGREDIENTS OR LESS, 30 MINUTES OR LESS, VEGETARIAN, DAIRY-FREE, GLUTEN-FREE

Chocolate bark is great for the holidays but can be enjoyed year-round. I prefer to make this for the holidays as it makes a great gift and tends to last out of the freezer longer due to the weather. I love adding as many toppings as possible to cover the chocolate, but if you are more of a chocolate lover, feel free to cut the toppings in half and let the chocolate steal the show.

16 ounces dark chocolate

1 teaspoon coconut oil

1 cup walnuts, chopped

½ cup dried cranberries

¼ teaspoon flaked salt

1. Line a baking sheet with parchment.

2. In a microwave-safe bowl, melt the chocolate and the coconut oil in the microwave in 30-second intervals. Stir between intervals and continue until the chocolate has melted.

3. When the chocolate has melted, pour it onto baking sheet in an even layer.

4. Sprinkle the walnuts, cranberries, and salt evenly over the chocolate.

5. Freeze for 20 minutes or until you can break into pieces.

6. Break into bars and store in the refrigerator for up to 1 week or in the freezer for up to 1 month.

> **VARIATION TIP:** Vary the toppings based on what you have on hand or what you prefer. Make this nut-free by omitting the walnuts altogether.

Per serving: Calories: 259; Total Fat: 18g; Saturated Fat: 8g; Cholesterol: 5mg; Sodium: 63mg; Carbohydrates: 29g; Fiber: 4g; Protein: 3g

Salted Chocolate–Coconut Macaroons

MAKES: 24 macaroons / **PREP TIME:** 10 minutes / **COOK TIME:** 20 minutes

30 MINUTES OR LESS, QUICK-PREP, VEGETARIAN, NUT-FREE, GLUTEN-FREE, DAIRY-FREE

I have a number of friends that have dietary restrictions, including dairy-free, nut-free, and gluten-free. Most meals are easy to accommodate but dessert can be tough. This recipe fits the bill for many and is easy to whip up right before a party. Make sure you use unsweetened coconut flakes; otherwise the sweetness of the coconut will overwhelm the cookies.

½ cup maple syrup

1 teaspoon pure vanilla extract

2 large eggs

2 cups unsweetened coconut flakes

½ cup dark chocolate

1 teaspoon coconut oil

Pinch salt

1. Preheat the oven to 350°F. Line a large baking sheet with parchment paper.

2. In a large bowl, whisk together the maple syrup, vanilla, and eggs.

3. Add the coconut and mix until well combined.

4. Form the coconut mixture into 24 even-size balls. Space out the macaroons evenly on the baking sheet and bake for 20 minutes.

5. Remove from the oven and allow to cool for about 5 minutes.

6. Meanwhile, in a microwave-safe bowl, melt the chocolate and the coconut oil in the microwave in 30-second intervals. Stir between intervals and continue until the chocolate has melted.

7. Drizzle the chocolate over macaroons and sprinkle with salt.

TECHNIQUE TIP: If the mixture is not easy to roll into balls, put it in refrigerator for 5 minutes. If it still does not roll into balls, add more coconut flakes.

Per serving: Calories: 91; Total Fat: 6g; Saturated Fat: 5g; Cholesterol: 16mg; Sodium: 17mg; Carbohydrates: 8g; Fiber: 1g; Protein: 1g

Mocha-Ricotta Mousse

SERVES: 8 / **PREP TIME:** 5 minutes

ONE-POT, 5 INGREDIENTS OR LESS, 30 MINUTES OR LESS, QUICK-PREP, VEGETARIAN, NUT-FREE, GLUTEN-FREE

I love ricotta, but it's traditionally used in savory dishes. I decided one day to try it as a dessert, and the results were amazing. Not only did I love it, but it started to be something that friends would ask for at parties. The best part? It's so easy to make that I will gladly bring it to any and all parties. Pro tip: Make this directly in the ricotta container for less cleanup. You're welcome.

¼ cup chocolate chips, melted, plus 2 tablespoons for topping

2 tablespoons strongly brewed coffee or cold brew

1 (16-ounce) container ricotta

Berries, melon, pineapple, or other fruit, for dipping or for topping

1. In a medium bowl, mix the melted chocolate and coffee into the ricotta until combined.

2. Top with chocolate chips and serve with fruit for dipping.

INGREDIENT TIP: Take the ricotta out of the refrigerator a few minutes before you mix the chocolate in so that the chocolate does not harden as you are mixing it into the ricotta.

Per serving: Calories: 160; Total Fat: 11g; Saturated Fat: 7g; Cholesterol: 35mg; Sodium: 59mg; Carbohydrates: 9g; Fiber: 0g; Protein: 8g

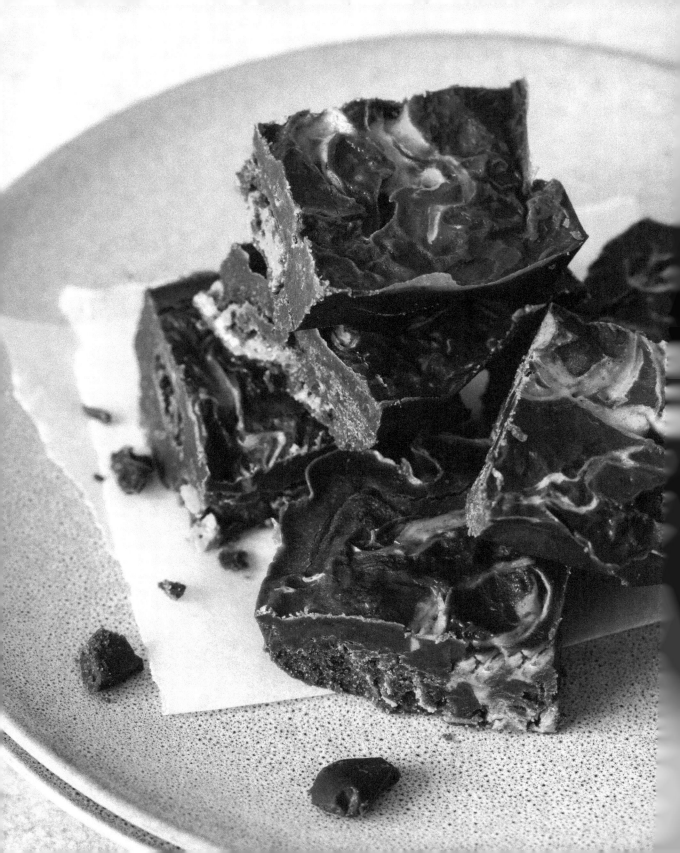

Chocolate–Peanut Butter Freezer Fudge

SERVES: 10 / **PREP TIME:** 10 minutes, plus 1 hour for freezing
5 INGREDIENTS OR LESS, VEGETARIAN, GLUTEN-FREE, DAIRY-FREE

I don't know about you, but I can't turn down anything with chocolate and peanut butter together. This recipe is no different. It's great for when you have a sweet tooth, but it's not overly sweet. I use this as a nice little treat at the end of a long day, but there is no reason you have to wait until the end of the day to enjoy it. And in case you don't want to eat a whole batch, it freezes well, too.

FOR THE CHOCOLATE

2 ounces 70 percent dark chocolate

¼ cup creamy unsweetened peanut butter

FOR THE PEANUT BUTTER LAYER

1 cup creamy unsweetened peanut butter

3 tablespoons coconut oil

3 tablespoons maple syrup

½ teaspoon pure vanilla extract

TO MAKE THE CHOCOLATE

In a microwave-safe bowl, melt the chocolate and the peanut butter in the microwave in 30-second intervals. Stir between intervals and continue until the chocolate has melted. Set aside.

TO MAKE THE PEANUT BUTTER LAYER

In a microwave-safe bowl, combine the peanut butter, coconut oil, maple syrup, and vanilla. Microwave on high in 30-second intervals. Stir between intervals and continue until the coconut oil has melted. Mix well.

CONTINUED

TO MAKE THE FUDGE

1. Line an 8-by-8-inch baking dish with parchment paper (so parchment paper hangs over side).

2. Pour in the peanut butter layer.

3. Scoop dollops of chocolate on the top of the peanut butter layer. Using a knife, swirl the chocolate dollops.

4. Place the fudge in the freezer for 45 to 60 minutes.

5. Take the fudge out of the pan by lifting up on the parchment paper. Using a serrated knife, cut into squares.

6. Enjoy immediately or place in a freezer-safe bag and keep in the freezer for up to 1 month.

> **SUBSTITUTION TIP:** Try Almond Butter (page 252) in place of peanut butter if you don't happen to have peanut butter on hand.

Per serving: Calories: 280; Total Fat: 23g; Saturated Fat: 9g; Cholesterol: 0mg; Sodium: 150mg; Carbohydrates: 13g; Fiber: 2g; Protein: 9g

Mocha-Cheesecake Brownies

MAKES: 12 brownies / **PREP TIME:** 10 minutes / **COOK TIME:** 30 minutes
QUICK-PREP, VEGETARIAN, NUT-FREE, GLUTEN-FREE

Do brownies need an introduction? I'm going to guess not, but why not gush about them with you? Brownies are always a winner, and this recipe is no different. I love using the base of this brownie recipe by itself, but I also love adding other ingredients or layers, like the cheesecake layer in this recipe. If you think you don't have time for making the cheesecake, you might want to think again and make time; it's worth it.

FOR THE BROWNIES

½ cup butter, softened, plus more for greasing

1 cup coconut sugar

⅔ cup unsweetened cocoa powder

2 large eggs

1 teaspoon pure vanilla extract

2 tablespoons brewed coffee (at room temperature) or cold brew

½ cup chocolate chips

FOR THE CHEESECAKE

8 ounces cream cheese

1 large egg

2 tablespoons maple syrup

TO MAKE THE BROWNIES

1. Preheat the oven 350°F. Grease the inside of an 8-by-8-inch baking dish with butter.

2. In a large bowl, mix together the butter, sugar, cocoa, eggs, vanilla, and coffee, then fold in the chocolate chips.

3. Pour the brownie batter into the prepared baking dish.

TO MAKE THE CHEESECAKE

1. In a separate large bowl, use a whisk (or an electric mixer) to mix the cream cheese, egg, and maple syrup.

2. Scoop dollops of cheesecake on the top of the brownie batter. Using a knife, swirl the cheesecake dollops.

3. Bake the brownies for 30 minutes or until a toothpick inserted in the center comes out clean.

> **VARIATION TIP:** You can leave out the cheesecake layer and make these as regular brownies.

Per serving: Calories: 278; Total Fat: 19g; Saturated Fat: 11g; Cholesterol: 91mg; Sodium: 136mg; Carbohydrates: 28g; Fiber: 2g; Protein: 5g

Cooking Temperatures

When you are cooking from home, it can be intimidating to know when the food is actually done, especially meat and seafood. I'd recommend starting with the USDA recommendations, listed in the chart that follows, and use a meat thermometer until you feel comfortable going by look, feel, and taste.

MEAT	MINIMUM INTERNAL TEMPERATURE
Beef, Pork, Veal, and Lamb steaks, chops, roasts	145°F and allow to rest for at least 3 minutes
Ground meats	160°F
Ham, fresh or smoked (uncooked)	145°F and allow to rest for at least 3 minutes
Poultry	165°F
Fish and Shellfish	145°F

Measurement Conversions

VOLUME EQUIVALENTS (LIQUID)

Standard	US Standard (ounces)	Metric (approximate)
2 tablespoons	1 fl. oz.	30 mL
¼ cup	2 fl. oz.	60 mL
½ cup	4 fl. oz.	120 mL
1 cup	8 fl. oz.	240 mL
1½ cups	12 fl. oz.	355 mL
2 cups or 1 pint	16 fl. oz.	475 mL
4 cups or 1 quart	32 fl. oz.	1 L
1 gallon	128 fl. oz.	4 L

OVEN TEMPERATURES

Fahrenheit (F)	Celsius (C) (approximate)
250°	120°
300°	150°
325°	165°
350°	180°
375°	190°
400°	200°
425°	220°
450°	230°

VOLUME EQUIVALENTS (DRY)

Standard	Metric (approximate)
⅛ teaspoon	0.5 mL
¼ teaspoon	1 mL
½ teaspoon	2 mL
¾ teaspoon	4 mL
1 teaspoon	5 mL
1 tablespoon	15 mL
¼ cup	59 mL
⅓ cup	79 mL
½ cup	118 mL
⅔ cup	156 mL
¾ cup	177 mL
1 cup	235 mL
2 cups or 1 pint	475 mL
3 cups	700 mL
4 cups or 1 quart	1 L

WEIGHT EQUIVALENTS

Standard	Metric (approximate)
½ ounce	15 g
1 ounce	30 g
2 ounces	60 g
4 ounces	115 g
8 ounces	225 g
12 ounces	340 g
16 ounces or 1 pound	455 g

| Resources |

Websites

Best Food Facts (http://www.bestfoodfacts.org/) provides objective information on the latest food fads and myths, as well as important nutrition information.

Eating Well (http://www.eatingwell.com/) is an online resource for clean eating, recipes, and information.

The Kitchn (https://www.thekitchn.com) is an online resource that explains how to cook almost anything you can imagine. It is a great resource for cooking techniques, recipes, and more.

Books

Salt, Fat, Acid, Heat: Mastering the Elements of Good Cooking by Samin Nosrat: A resource for those looking to understand how and why you should be cooking with certain ingredients and using specific techniques.

The Flavor Bible: The Essential Guide to Culinary Creativity, Based on the Wisdom of America's Most Imaginative Chefs by Karen Page and Andrew Dornenburg: A great resource for learning how different flavors and ingredients pair with one another.

In Defense of Food: An Eater's Manifesto by Michael Pollan: Read this book to remind you why you should eat real food and stop feeding into the diet culture.

Feel free to check out my website, *The Sassy Dietitian* (thesassydietitian.com), which is dedicated to helping people optimize their diet and lifestyles through real food nutrition. I share similar recipes to those featured in this cookbook as well as blog posts related to diet myths, sports nutrition, and general health and wellness topics.

| Index |

A

Acute inflammation, 5–6
Air-Fryer Sweet Potato Tots, 94
  in Burger Bowls, 223
Almond Butter, 252
  in Almond Butter Cookies, 279
  in Almond Butter
    Energy Bites, 86
  in Apple Nachos, 272
  in Chickpea Buddha
    Bowls, 133
  in Chocolate Chip Cookie
    Dough Overnight Oats, 57
  in Cookie Dough Dip, 85
Almond milk
  Bacon, Egg, and Cheese
    Sheet Pan Sandwiches, 63
  French Toast Overnight
    Oats, 55
Almonds
  Almond Butter, 252
  Apple-Cranberry Slaw, 116
  Apple Nachos, 272
  S'mores Campfire
    Trail Mix, 281
  Sweet 'n' Spicy Nuts
    and Seeds, 80
Apples
  Apple, Brie, and Caramelized
    Onion Burger, 227
  Apple Breakfast Sausage
    Patties, 61
  Apple-Cranberry Slaw, 116
  Apple Nachos, 272
  Cinnamon Apple Chips, 74
  Easy Apple-Tuna Salad, 169
  Pork Chops with Apples
    and Onions, 213
Artichoke hearts

Spinach Artichoke
  Roll-Ups, 176
Arugula
  Buffalo Chicken
    Cauliflower Pizza, 187
  Chickpea Buddha Bowls, 133
  Orange-Beet-Arugula
    Salad, 113
  Pesto, Prosciutto, and
    Roasted Red Pepper
    Cauliflower Pizza, 217
Asian Lettuce Wraps with
  Hoisin Sauce, 196
Asparagus
  Garlic-Dijon Asparagus, 87
  Vegetable Risotto, 139
Avocados
  Avocado-Cucumber-
    Feta Salad, 111
  Burger Bowls, 223
  Chickpea Buddha
    Bowls, 133
  Deconstructed Sushi
    Bowl, 163
  Easy Guacamole, 83
  Green Chicken
    Enchiladas, 184
  Green Power Smoothie
    Bowl, 54
  Green Shakshuka, 67
  Lemony Smoked Salmon
    Roll-Ups with Avocado, 162
  Loaded Avocado Toast, 65
  Mexican Street Corn
    Salad, 115
  Portobello Tacos, 122
  Power Quinoa Bowl, 135
  Southwest Eggs Benedict on
    Sweet Potato Toast, 69
  Spring Shrimp Rolls, 148–149

Tropical White Fish
  Ceviche, 157

B

Bacon
  Bacon, Egg, and Cheese
    Sheet Pan Sandwiches, 63
  Bacon-Wrapped Meatloaf
    Muffins, 221
  Crispy Baked Bacon, 198
  Dairy-Free Bacon Mac
    & "Cheese," 200
  Green Eggs and Ham
    Frittata, 64
  Lamb Gyros, 239
  Loaded Baked Potatoes, 199
  Loaded Baked Potato
    Soup, 104
  Pork and White Bean
    Stew, 216
Baked Crab Cakes with
  Tartar Sauce, 156
Baked Fish and Chips, 160
Barbacoa Beef Bowls, 224
Basil
  Chicken Bruschetta Pasta, 190
  Chopped Caprese Salad, 114
  Homemade Marinara
    Sauce, 266
  Roasted Red Pepper Soup
    and Ricotta
    Cheeseballs, 105
  Spaghetti Squash
    Primavera, 140
  Spring Shrimp Rolls, 148–149
BBQ Grilled Chicken, 181
BBQ Pulled Pork, 206
  in Piggy Nachos, 207
BBQ Ribs, 208

Beans, 11
    Barbacoa Beef Bowls, 224
    Beet Burger, 129
    Chicken Tortilla Soup, 109
    Classic Minestrone, 106
    One-Pot Taco Pasta, 235
    Pork and White Bean Stew, 216
    Taco Cauliflower Pizza, 222
    Tex-Mex Veggie Burger, 130
    Vegetarian Black Bean
        Enchiladas, 131
Beef
    Apple, Brie, and Caramelized
        Onion Burger, 227
    Bacon-Wrapped Meatloaf
        Muffins, 221
    Barbacoa Beef Bowls, 224
    Beef Tacos in Lettuce, 220
    Burger Bowls, 223
    Chili-Stuffed Peppers, 232
    Easy Broth, 253
    Mongolian Beef and
        Broccoli, 229
    One-Pot Taco Pasta, 235
    One-Skillet Pepper Steak, 230
    Pressure Cooker French Dip
        Sandwiches, 225–226
    Skillet Garlic-Herb Steak, 231
    Spaghetti Squash Bolognese, 234
    Spinach Meatballs and
        Zucchini Noodles, 233
    Steak and Pepper Roll-Ups, 228
    Sweet Potato and Butternut
        Squash Shepherd's
        Pie, 236–237
    Taco Cauliflower Pizza, 222
Beets
    Beet Burger, 129
    Orange-Beet-Arugula Salad, 113
Bell peppers
    Baked Crab Cakes with
        Tartar Sauce, 156
    Beef Tacos in Lettuce, 220
    Chicken Tortilla Soup, 109
    Chili-Stuffed Peppers, 232

    Chorizo Stuffed Sweet
        Potatoes, 202
    Freezer V-Egg-ie Burritos, 70–71
    Greek Lamb Bowls with
        Turmeric Cauliflower Rice and
        Cucumber Salsa, 243–244
    Green Chicken Enchiladas, 184
    Green Eggs and Ham Frittata, 64
    Green Shakshuka, 67
    Grilled Sausage, Peppers,
        and Onions, 201
    Hawaiian Pork Kebabs, 197
    High Protein Pressure Cooker
        Mac & Cheese, 142
    Homemade Marinara Sauce, 266
    Lemon Greek Chicken
        Skewers, 173
    Mexican Street Corn Salad, 115
    One-Pot Taco Pasta, 235
    One-Skillet Pepper Steak, 230
    Pesto, Prosciutto, and
        Roasted Red Pepper
        Cauliflower Pizza, 217
    Pork Bibimbap, 210
    Pork Ramen Noodle Bowls, 211
    Portobello Tacos, 122
    Power Quinoa Bowl, 135
    Quinoa Tabbouleh, 119
    Roasted Red Pepper Soup and
        Ricotta Cheeseballs, 105
    Roasted Veggie Hummus
        Panini, 128
    Sheet Pan Chicken Fajitas, 183
    Sheet Pan Sweet and Sour
        Chicken Rice Bowls, 179
    Spaghetti Squash Bolognese, 234
    Spaghetti Squash Primavera, 140
    Spring Shrimp Rolls, 148–149
    Steak and Pepper Roll-Ups, 228
    Sweet Potato and Butternut
        Squash Shepherd's
        Pie, 236–237
    Sweet Potato Crust Quiche, 68
    Taco Cauliflower Pizza, 222
    Tropical White Fish Ceviche, 157

    Vegetable Risotto, 139
    Vegetarian Black Bean
        Enchiladas, 131
    Watermelon Gazpacho, 98
Berries
    Apple-Cranberry Slaw, 116
    Berry Berry Smoothie Bowl, 53
    Blueberry-Oat Pancakes, 58
    Fruit-and-Nut Chocolate
        Bark, 283
    Harvest Kale Salad with
        Goat Cheese and Dried
        Cranberries, 118
    PB and J Protein Smoothie, 50
    Raspberry-Lemon Bars, 276
    S'mores Campfire Trail
        Mix, 281
    Strawberry–Goat
        Cheese Salad, 110
    Strawberry-Jalapeño Salsa, 82
    Strawberry Lemonade
        Slushie, 270
    Strawberry Shortcake
        Mug Cake, 275
    Strawberry Shortcake
        Overnight Oats, 56
Berry Berry Smoothie Bowl, 53
Beverages. See also Smoothies
    Quick Vanilla Latte, 52
    Strawberry Lemonade
        Slushie, 270
Black Cherry Sorbet, 274
Blueberry-Oat Pancakes, 58
Blue cheese
    Buffalo Cauliflower Bites, 90
    Buffalo Chicken Cauliflower
        Pizza, 187
Body, listening to, 10
Bowls
    Barbacoa Beef Bowls, 224
    Berry Berry Smoothie Bowl, 53
    Burger Bowls, 223
    Chickpea Buddha Bowls, 133
    Deconstructed Sushi Bowl, 163
    Egg Roll in a Bowl, 178

Greek Lamb Bowls with Turmeric
Cauliflower Rice and
Cucumber Salsa, 243–244
Green Power Smoothie Bowl, 54
Pork Ramen Noodle Bowls, 211
Power Quinoa Bowl, 135
Sesame Tofu and Brussels
Sprouts Bowl, 136–137
Sheet Pan Sweet and Sour
Chicken
Rice Bowls, 179
Brie cheese
Apple, Brie, and Caramelized
Onion Burger, 227
Broccoli
Broccoli-Walnut Salad with
Dried Cherries, 117
Easy Stovetop Phở, 100
Garlic-Parmesan Roasted
Broccoli, 88
Mongolian Beef and
Broccoli, 229
Sweet-and-Sour Eggplant, 123
Brussels sprouts
Orange-Balsamic Brussels
Sprouts, 89
Sesame Tofu and Brussels
Sprouts Bowl,
136–137
Buffalo Cauliflower Bites, 90
Buffalo Chicken Cauliflower
Pizza, 187
Burger Bowls, 223
Burgers
Apple, Brie, and Caramelized
Onion Burger, 227
Beet Burger, 129
Caprese Chicken Burgers, 177
Feta Lamb Burgers, 240
Tex-Mex Veggie Burger, 130
Butternut Squash, Mushroom, and
Goat Cheese
Cauliflower Pizza, 144
Butternut Squash Mac
& Cheese, 143

C

Cabbage
Apple-Cranberry Slaw, 116
Egg Roll in a Bowl, 178
Caprese Chicken Burgers, 177
Caramelized Onion and
Carrot Hummus, 84
in Power Quinoa Bowl, 135
Carbohydrates, 3, 5
Carnitas, 204–205
Carrots
Apple-Cranberry Slaw, 116
Asian Lettuce Wraps with
Hoisin Sauce, 196
Caramelized Onion and
Carrot Hummus, 84
Classic Minestrone, 106
Deconstructed Sushi Bowl, 163
Egg Roll in a Bowl, 178
Pork Bibimbap, 210
Pork Fried Cauliflower Rice, 209
Roasted Red Pepper Soup and
Ricotta Cheeseballs, 105
Spaghetti Squash Primavera, 140
Spring Shrimp Rolls, 148–149
Sweet Potato and Butternut
Squash Shepherd's
Pie, 236–237
Tex-Mex Veggie Burger, 130
Cauliflower
Barbacoa Beef Bowls, 224
Buffalo Cauliflower Bites, 90
Cauliflower Curry, 126
Cauliflower Pizza Crust, 267
Cilantro-Lime Cauliflower
Rice, 92
Creamy Garlic Cauliflower
Soup, 101
Dairy-Free Bacon Mac
& "Cheese," 200
Greek Lamb Bowls with
Turmeric Cauliflower Rice and
Cucumber Salsa, 243–244
Mashed Parmesan Cauliflower, 91

Pesto-Baked Cauliflower
Steaks, 125
Pork Fried Cauliflower Rice, 209
Cauliflower Pizza Crust, 267
in Buffalo Chicken
Cauliflower Pizza, 187
in Butternut Squash,
Mushroom, and Goat Cheese
Cauliflower Pizza, 144
in Pesto, Prosciutto, and
Roasted Red Pepper
Cauliflower Pizza, 217
in Taco Cauliflower Pizza, 222
Cheddar cheese
Bacon, Egg, and Cheese Sheet
Pan Sandwiches, 63
Burger Bowls, 223
Chili-Stuffed Peppers, 232
Creamy Garlic Cauliflower
Soup, 101
Freezer V-Egg-ie Burritos, 70–71
Green Chicken Enchiladas, 184
High-Protein Egg Muffins, 62
High Protein Pressure Cooker
Mac & Cheese, 142
Loaded Baked Potatoes, 199
Loaded Baked Potato
Soup, 104
One-Pot Taco Pasta, 235
Piggy Nachos, 207
Spinach Artichoke Roll-Ups, 176
Taco Cauliflower Pizza, 222
Vegetarian Black Bean
Enchiladas, 131
Cherries
Black Cherry Sorbet, 274
Broccoli-Walnut Salad with
Dried Cherries, 117
Chicken
BBQ Grilled Chicken, 181
Buffalo Chicken Cauliflower
Pizza, 187
Caprese Chicken Burgers, 177
Chicken Bruschetta Pasta, 190
Chicken Marsala, 186

Chicken *(continued)*
  Chicken Parmesan over
    Zoodles, 192
  Chicken Tortilla Soup, 109
  Crispy Baked Wings, 172
  Easy Broth, 253
  Egg Roll in a Bowl, 178
  Green Chicken Enchiladas, 184
  Grown-Up Chicken Tenders, 174
  Lemon Greek Chicken
    Skewers, 173
  Paprika-Baked Chicken
    Thighs, 180
  Pesto Chicken Alfredo with
    Spaghetti Squash, 191
  Pressure Cooker Butter
    Chicken, 182
  Pressure Cooker Chicken
    Tikka Masala, 189
  Sheet Pan Chicken Fajitas, 183
  Sheet Pan Sweet and Sour
    Chicken Rice Bowls, 179
  Skillet Peachy Chicken
    Picante, 185
  Spinach Artichoke Roll-Ups, 176
  Waldorf Chicken Salad, 175
Chickpeas
  Caramelized Onion and
    Carrot Hummus, 84
  Chickpea Buddha Bowls, 133
  Chickpea Tofu Marsala, 132
  Crunchy Chickpeas, 79
  Easy Homemade Falafel, 145
Chiles, green
  Green Shakshuka, 67
Chili-Lime Popcorn, 76
Chili-Spiced Fruit Cups, 273
Chili-Stuffed Peppers, 232
Chipotle peppers
  Barbacoa Beef Bowls, 224
  Chicken Tortilla Soup, 109
Chocolate
  Almond Butter Energy
    Bites, 86
  Apple Nachos, 272

Chocolate Chip Cookie Dough
    Overnight Oats, 57
Chocolate-Covered
    Orange Slices, 282
Chocolate–Peanut Butter
    Freezer Fudge, 287–288
Cookie Dough Dip, 85
Dark Chocolate–Sea
    Salt Popcorn, 280
Fruit-and-Nut Chocolate
    Bark, 283
Mocha-Cheesecake
    Brownies, 289
Mocha-Ricotta Mousse, 285
Salted Chocolate–Coconut
    Macaroons, 284
S'mores Campfire Trail Mix, 281
Chopped Caprese Salad, 114
Chorizo Stuffed Sweet
    Potatoes, 202
Chronic inflammation, 5–6
Cilantro
  Chorizo Stuffed Sweet
    Potatoes, 202
  Cilantro-Lime Cauliflower Rice, 92
  Honey-Lime Salmon with
    Watermelon Salsa, 164
  Lamb Lollipops with
    Chimichurri Sauce, 245
  Mexican Street Corn Salad, 115
  One-Pot Taco Pasta, 235
  Strawberry-Jalapeño Salsa, 82
  Tropical White Fish Ceviche, 157
Cilantro-Lime Cauliflower Rice, 92
  in Vegetarian Black Bean
    Enchiladas, 131
Cinnamon Apple Chips, 74
Cinnamon Toast Waffles, 59
Clams
  Grilled Clams with Lemon-
    Pepper Ghee, 152
  Linguine with Clams, 153
Classic Minestrone, 106
Clean eating
  vs. cleanses, 7

core principles, 3–4
defined, 1
foods to moderate, 9
lifestyle, 44–46
nutritional guidelines, 4
reasons for, 2
recommended foods, 8–9
and wellness concerns, 5–6
Clean Eating 101 Plan, 20–29
Cleanses, 7
Coconut
  Apple Nachos, 272
  Salted Chocolate–Coconut
    Macaroons, 284
Coconut milk
  Cauliflower Curry, 126
  Crab Bisque, 108
  Pressure Cooker Butter
    Chicken, 182
  Pressure Cooker Chicken
    Tikka Masala, 189
  Thai Peanut Ramen, 127
Coconut oil, 15
Coffee
  Mocha-Cheesecake
    Brownies, 289
  Mocha-Ricotta Mousse, 285
  Quick Vanilla Latte, 52
Complex carbohydrates, 3, 5
Condiments
  Homemade Mayo, 254
  Honey Mustard, 255
  Ketchup, 256
Cookie Dough Dip, 85
Corn
  Chicken Tortilla Soup, 109
  Mexican Street Corn
    Salad, 115
  Vegetarian Black Bean
    Enchiladas, 131
Cotija cheese
  Carnitas, 204–205
  Chorizo Stuffed Sweet
    Potatoes, 202
  Mexican Street Corn Salad, 115

Portobello Tacos, 122
Salmon Tostada Salad, 167
Cottage cheese
High Protein Pressure Cooker
Mac & Cheese, 142
Strawberry Shortcake
Overnight Oats, 56
Crab
Baked Crab Cakes with
Tartar Sauce, 156
Crab Bisque, 108
Crab Bisque, 108
Cream cheese
Mocha-Cheesecake
Brownies, 289
Spinach Artichoke Roll-Ups, 176
Creamy Garlic Cauliflower
Soup, 101
Crispy Baked Bacon, 198
in Broccoli-Walnut Salad
with Dried Cherries, 117
Crispy Baked Fish Sticks, 159
Crispy Baked Wings, 172
Crispy Garlic-Rosemary
Potato Wedges, 77
Crunchy Chickpeas, 79
in Butternut Squash,
Mushroom, and Goat Cheese
Cauliflower Pizza, 144
in Power Quinoa Bowl, 135
Cucumbers
Avocado-Cucumber-
Feta Salad, 111
Chili-Spiced Fruit Cups, 273
Deconstructed Sushi Bowl, 163
Greek Lamb Bowls with
Turmeric Cauliflower Rice and
Cucumber Salsa, 243–244
Lamb Gyros, 239
Lemony Smoked Salmon
Roll-Ups with Avocado, 162
Pork Bibimbap, 210
Quick Pickles, 259
Quinoa Tabbouleh, 119
Spring Shrimp Rolls, 148–149

Strawberry–Goat
Cheese Salad, 110
Tropical White Fish Ceviche, 157
Tzatziki, 261
Watermelon Gazpacho, 98

D

Dairy-free
Air-Fryer Sweet Potato Tots, 94
Almond Butter, 252
Almond Butter Cookies, 279
Almond Butter Energy Bites, 86
Apple Breakfast Sausage
Patties, 61
Apple Nachos, 272
Asian Lettuce Wraps with
Hoisin Sauce, 196
Baked Crab Cakes with
Tartar Sauce, 156
BBQ Grilled Chicken, 181
BBQ Pulled Pork, 206
BBQ Ribs, 208
Beef Tacos in Lettuce, 220
Beet Burger, 129
Black Cherry Sorbet, 274
Broccoli-Walnut Salad with
Dried Cherries, 117
Caramelized Onion and
Carrot Hummus, 84
Cauliflower Curry, 126
Chicken Bruschetta Pasta, 190
Chicken Marsala, 186
Chicken Tortilla Soup, 109
Chickpea Buddha Bowls, 133
Chili-Lime Popcorn, 76
Chili-Spiced Fruit Cups, 273
Chocolate-Covered
Orange Slices, 282
Chocolate–Peanut Butter
Freezer Fudge, 287–288
Cilantro-Lime Cauliflower
Rice, 92
Cinnamon Apple Chips, 74
Crab Bisque, 108

Crispy Baked Bacon, 198
Crispy Baked Wings, 172
Crispy Garlic-Rosemary
Potato Wedges, 77
Crunchy Chickpeas, 79
Dairy-Free Bacon Mac
& "Cheese," 200
Dark Chocolate–Sea
Salt Popcorn, 280
Deconstructed Sushi Bowl, 163
Easy Apple-Tuna Salad, 169
Easy Blackened Fish, 158
Easy Broth, 253
Easy Guacamole, 83
Easy Homemade Falafel, 145
Easy Stovetop Phở, 100
Egg Roll in a Bowl, 178
Enchilada Sauce, 263
Everything Bagel–Seasoned
Hard-Boiled Eggs, 81
French Toast Overnight
Oats, 55
Fruit-and-Nut Chocolate
Bark, 283
Garlic-Dijon Asparagus, 87
Gochujang, 258
Grape Leaf Pilaf, 138
Grilled Clams with Lemon-
Pepper Ghee, 152
Grilled Sausage, Peppers,
and Onions, 201
Hawaiian Pork Kebabs, 197
Homemade Marinara Sauce, 266
Homemade Mayo, 254
Honey-Lime Salmon with
Watermelon Salsa, 164
Honey Mustard, 255
Honey Mustard Pork Chops, 212
Ketchup, 256
Lamb Lollipops with
Chimichurri Sauce, 245
Lemon Lentil Soup, 107
Lemony Smoked Salmon
Roll-Ups with Avocado, 162
Loaded Avocado Toast, 65

Dairy-free *(continued)*
   Maple-Glazed Cedar
      Plank Salmon, 168
   Maple Vinaigrette, 260
   Mongolian Beef and Broccoli, 229
   One-Skillet Pepper Steak, 230
   Orange-Balsamic Brussels
      Sprouts, 89
   Paprika-Baked Chicken
      Thighs, 180
   Peach Crumble, 277
   Pesto-Baked Cauliflower
      Steaks, 125
   Poached Eggs, 248
   Pork and White Bean Stew, 216
   Pork Bibimbap, 210
   Pork Chops with Apples
      and Onions, 213
   Pork Fried Cauliflower Rice, 209
   Pork Ramen Noodle Bowls, 211
   Pressure Cooker Chicken
      Tikka Masala, 189
   Quick Pickles, 259
   Raspberry-Lemon Bars, 276
   Salted Chocolate–Coconut
      Macaroons, 284
   Sassy BBQ Sauce, 257
   Sesame Tofu and Brussels
      Sprouts Bowl, 136–137
   Sheet Pan Chicken Fajitas, 183
   Sheet Pan Sweet and Sour
      Chicken Rice Bowls, 179
   Skillet Garlic-Herb Steak, 231
   Skillet Peachy Chicken
      Picante, 185
   S'mores Campfire Trail Mix, 281
   Southwest Eggs Benedict on
      Sweet Potato Toast, 69
   Spaghetti Squash, 249
   Spicy Shrimp Tacos, 150
   Spring Shrimp Rolls, 148–149
   Steak and Pepper Roll-Ups, 228
   Strawberry-Jalapeño Salsa, 82
   Strawberry Lemonade
      Slushie, 270

   Sweet-and-Sour Eggplant, 123
   Sweet-and-Sour Sauce, 262
   Sweet Potato Salmon
      Cakes, 165
   Taco Seasoning, 250
   Tex-Mex Veggie Burger, 130
   Thai Peanut Ramen, 127
   Tropical Pineapple Fruit
      Leather, 271
   Tropical White Fish
      Ceviche, 157
   Turmeric Rice, 93
   Vegetarian Black Bean
      Enchiladas, 131
   Watermelon Gazpacho, 98
Dairy-Free Bacon Mac &
   "Cheese," 200
Dairy products, 9, 14
Dark Chocolate–Sea Salt
   Popcorn, 280
Deconstructed Sushi Bowl, 163
Desserts, 44
Diet, 2
Digestion, 6
Dips and spreads
   Caramelized Onion and
      Carrot Hummus, 84
   Cookie Dough Dip, 85
   Easy Guacamole, 83
   Strawberry-Jalapeño Salsa, 82
Dressings
   Maple Vinaigrette, 260

E

Easy Apple-Tuna Salad, 169
Easy Blackened Fish, 158
Easy Broth, 253
   in Barbacoa Beef Bowls, 224
   in Enchilada Sauce, 263
   in Mashed Parmesan
      Cauliflower, 91
   in Pork and White Bean Stew, 216
   in Pressure Cooker Lamb
      Meatballs, 241

   in Sweet Potato and
      Butternut Squash
      Shepherd's Pie, 236–237
   in Turmeric Rice, 93
Easy Guacamole, 83
   in Salmon Tostada Salad, 167
Easy Stovetop Phở, 100
Easy Vanilla Ice Cream, 278
Eggplants
   Roasted Veggie Hummus
      Panini, 128
   Sheet Pan Eggplant
      Parmesan, 124
   Sweet-and-Sour Eggplant, 123
Egg Roll in a Bowl, 178
Eggs
   Bacon, Egg, and Cheese Sheet
      Pan Sandwiches, 63
   Cauliflower Pizza Crust, 267
   Easy Homemade Falafel, 145
   Egg Roll in a Bowl, 178
   Everything Bagel–Seasoned
      Hard-Boiled Eggs, 81
   Freezer V-Egg-ie Burritos, 70–71
   Green Eggs and Ham
      Frittata, 64
   Green Shakshuka, 67
   High-Protein Egg Muffins, 62
   Homemade Mayo, 254
   Poached Eggs, 248
   Pork Bibimbap, 210
   Pork Fried Cauliflower Rice, 209
   Power Quinoa Bowl, 135
   Raspberry-Lemon Bars, 276
   Salted Chocolate–Coconut
      Macaroons, 284
   Sweet Potato Crust Quiche, 68
Enchilada Sauce, 263
   in Vegetarian Black Bean
      Enchiladas, 131
Energy, 6
Equipment, 14–15
Everything Bagel–Seasoned
   Hard-Boiled Eggs, 81
Exercise, 45

F

Fatigue, 6
Fats, 3, 5, 9, 11
Feta cheese
Avocado-Cucumber-
Feta Salad, 111
Feta Lamb Burgers, 240
Greek Lamb Bowls with Turmeric
Cauliflower Rice and
Cucumber Salsa, 243–244
Green Shakshuka, 67
Lamb Kofta Kebabs, 238
Mediterranean Fish in
Parchment, 161
Orange-Beet-Arugula Salad, 113
Power Quinoa Bowl, 135
Pressure Cooker Lamb
Meatballs, 241
Quinoa Tabbouleh, 119
Salmon Tostada Salad, 167
Tzatziki, 261
Fish
Baked Fish and Chips, 160
Crispy Baked Fish Sticks, 159
Deconstructed Sushi Bowl, 163
Easy Apple-Tuna Salad, 169
Easy Blackened Fish, 158
Honey-Lime Salmon with
Watermelon Salsa, 164
Lemony Smoked Salmon
Roll-Ups with Avocado, 162
Maple-Glazed Cedar
Plank Salmon, 168
Mediterranean Fish in
Parchment, 161
Salmon Tostada Salad, 167
Sweet Potato Salmon
Cakes, 165
Tropical White Fish Ceviche, 157
5 ingredients or less
Air-Fryer Sweet Potato Tots, 94
Almond Butter, 252
Almond Butter Cookies, 279
Almond Butter Energy Bites, 86

Avocado-Cucumber-
Feta Salad, 111
BBQ Grilled Chicken, 181
BBQ Pulled Pork, 206
Berry Berry Smoothie Bowl, 53
Black Cherry Sorbet, 274
Buffalo Cauliflower Bites, 90
Caprese Chicken Burgers, 177
Caramelized Onion and
Carrot Hummus, 84
Chili-Lime Popcorn, 76
Chocolate-Covered
Orange Slices, 282
Chocolate–Peanut Butter
Freezer Fudge, 287–288
Cilantro-Lime Cauliflower Rice, 92
Cinnamon Apple Chips, 74
Cookie Dough Dip, 85
Crispy Baked Bacon, 198
Crispy Garlic-Rosemary
Potato Wedges, 77
Crunchy Chickpeas, 79
Dark Chocolate–Sea
Salt Popcorn, 280
Easy Broth, 253
Easy Guacamole, 83
Easy Vanilla Ice Cream, 278
Five-Ingredient Veggie
Lasagna, 141
Fruit-and-Nut Chocolate
Bark, 283
Garlic-Dijon Asparagus, 87
Garlic-Parmesan Roasted
Broccoli, 88
Ghee, 251
Gochujang, 258
Grilled Clams with Lemon-
Pepper Ghee, 152
Grilled Sausage, Peppers,
and Onions, 201
Honey Mustard Pork Chops, 212
Lemon Meringue Smoothie, 51
Lemony Smoked Salmon
Roll-Ups with Avocado, 162
Loaded Avocado Toast, 65

Maple Vinaigrette, 260
Mashed Parmesan Cauliflower, 91
Mocha-Ricotta Mousse, 285
Mussels Marinara, 154
Orange-Balsamic Brussels
Sprouts, 89
Parmesan Crisps, 75
PB and J Protein Smoothie, 50
Pesto-Baked Cauliflower
Steaks, 125
Poached Eggs, 248
Quick Vanilla Latte, 52
Sheet Pan Chicken Fajitas, 183
Skillet Garlic-Herb Steak, 231
Spaghetti Squash, 249
Spinach-Walnut Pesto, 265
Spring Shrimp Rolls, 148–149
Strawberry-Jalapeño Salsa, 82
Strawberry Lemonade
Slushie, 270
Tropical Pineapple Fruit
Leather, 271
Turmeric Rice, 93
Tzatziki, 261
Five-Ingredient Veggie
Lasagna, 141
Freezer staples, 13–14
Freezer V-Egg-ie Burritos, 70–71
French Toast Overnight Oats, 55
Fruit-and-Nut Chocolate Bark, 283
Fruits, 8, 13. See also specific

G

Garlic-Dijon Asparagus, 87
Garlic-Parmesan Roasted
Broccoli, 88
Ghee, 251
in Buffalo Chicken
Cauliflower Pizza, 187
in Chickpea Tofu Marsala, 132
in Grilled Clams with Lemon-
Pepper Ghee, 152
in Linguine with Clams, 153
in Loaded Baked Potatoes, 199

Ghee *(continued)*
in Loaded Baked Potato
Soup, 104
in Mashed Parmesan
Cauliflower, 91
in Paprika-Baked Chicken
Thighs, 180
in Peach Crumble, 277
in Pesto Chicken Alfredo with
Spaghetti Squash, 191
in Raspberry-Lemon Bars, 276
in Simple French Onion Soup, 99
in Skillet Garlic-Herb Steak, 231
in Skillet Peachy Chicken
Picante, 185
in Southwest Eggs Benedict on
Sweet Potato
Toast, 69
in Strawberry Shortcake
Mug Cake, 275
in Sweet 'n' Spicy Nuts
and Seeds, 80
Ginger
Asian Lettuce Wraps with
Hoisin Sauce, 196
Deconstructed Sushi Bowl, 163
Easy Stovetop Phở, 100
Egg Roll in a Bowl, 178
Mongolian Beef and Broccoli, 229
One-Skillet Pepper Steak, 230
Pressure Cooker Butter
Chicken, 182
Pressure Cooker Chicken
Tikka Masala, 189
Steak and Pepper Roll-Ups, 228
Sweet-and-Sour Eggplant, 123
Thai Peanut Ramen, 127
Gluten-free
Air-Fryer Sweet Potato Tots, 94
Almond Butter, 252
Almond Butter Cookies, 279
Almond Butter Energy Bites, 86
Apple, Brie, and Caramelized
Onion Burger, 227

Apple Breakfast Sausage
Patties, 61
Apple-Cranberry Slaw, 116
Apple Nachos, 272
Avocado-Cucumber-
Feta Salad, 111
Bacon-Wrapped Meatloaf
Muffins, 221
Baked Crab Cakes with
Tartar Sauce, 156
Barbacoa Beef Bowls, 224
BBQ Grilled Chicken, 181
Beef Tacos in Lettuce, 220
Berry Berry Smoothie Bowl, 53
Black Cherry Sorbet, 274
Blueberry-Oat Pancakes, 58
Broccoli-Walnut Salad with
Dried Cherries, 117
Buffalo Chicken Cauliflower
Pizza, 187
Burger Bowls, 223
Butternut Squash, Mushroom,
and Goat Cheese
Cauliflower Pizza, 144
Caprese Chicken Burgers, 177
Caramelized Onion and
Carrot Hummus, 84
Carnitas, 204–205
Cauliflower Curry, 126
Cauliflower Pizza Crust, 267
Chicken Marsala, 186
Chicken Tortilla Soup, 109
Chickpea Buddha Bowls, 133
Chickpea Tofu Marsala, 132
Chili-Lime Popcorn, 76
Chili-Spiced Fruit Cups, 273
Chili-Stuffed Peppers, 232
Chocolate Chip Cookie Dough
Overnight Oats, 57
Chocolate-Covered
Orange Slices, 282
Chocolate–Peanut Butter
Freezer Fudge, 287–288
Chopped Caprese Salad, 114

Chorizo Stuffed Sweet
Potatoes, 202
Cilantro-Lime Cauliflower Rice, 92
Cinnamon Apple Chips, 74
Cookie Dough Dip, 85
Crab Bisque, 108
Creamy Garlic Cauliflower
Soup, 101
Crispy Baked Bacon, 198
Crispy Baked Fish Sticks, 159
Crispy Baked Wings, 172
Crunchy Chickpeas, 79
Dairy-Free Bacon Mac
& "Cheese," 200
Dark Chocolate–Sea
Salt Popcorn, 280
Easy Apple-Tuna Salad, 169
Easy Blackened Fish, 158
Easy Broth, 253
Easy Guacamole, 83
Easy Vanilla Ice Cream, 278
Enchilada Sauce, 263
Everything Bagel–Seasoned
Hard-Boiled Eggs, 81
Feta Lamb Burgers, 240
Five-Ingredient Veggie
Lasagna, 141
French Toast Overnight Oats, 55
Fruit-and-Nut Chocolate
Bark, 283
Garlic-Dijon Asparagus, 87
Garlic-Parmesan Roasted
Broccoli, 88
Ghee, 251
Grape Leaf Pilaf, 138
Greek Lamb Bowls with
Turmeric Cauliflower Rice and
Cucumber Salsa, 243–244
Green Chicken Enchiladas, 184
Green Eggs and Ham Frittata, 64
Green Power Smoothie Bowl, 54
Green Shakshuka, 67
Grilled Sausage, Peppers,
and Onions, 201

Grown-Up Chicken Tenders, 174
Harvest Kale Salad with
    Goat Cheese and Dried
    Cranberries, 118
High-Protein Egg Muffins, 62
High Protein Pressure Cooker
    Mac & Cheese, 142
Homemade Cream of
    Mushroom Soup, 102–103
Homemade Marinara
    Sauce, 266
Homemade Mayo, 254
Honey-Lime Salmon with
    Watermelon Salsa, 164
Honey Mustard, 255
Honey Mustard Pork Chops, 212
Ketchup, 256
Lamb Gyros, 239
Lamb Kofta Kebabs, 238
Lamb Lollipops with
    Chimichurri Sauce, 245
Lemon Greek Chicken
    Skewers, 173
Lemon Lentil Soup, 107
Lemon Meringue Smoothie, 51
Lemony Smoked Salmon
    Roll-Ups with Avocado, 162
Loaded Baked Potatoes, 199
Loaded Baked Potato Soup, 104
Maple Vinaigrette, 260
Mashed Parmesan Cauliflower, 91
Mediterranean Fish in
    Parchment, 161
Mexican Street Corn Salad, 115
Mocha-Cheesecake
    Brownies, 289
Mocha-Ricotta Mousse, 285
Orange-Balsamic Brussels
    Sprouts, 89
Orange-Beet-Arugula Salad, 113
Paprika-Baked Chicken
    Thighs, 180
Parmesan Crisps, 75
PB and J Protein Smoothie, 50

Pesto, Prosciutto, and
    Roasted Red Pepper
    Cauliflower Pizza, 217
Pesto-Baked Cauliflower
    Steaks, 125
Pesto Chicken Alfredo with
    Spaghetti Squash, 191
Piggy Nachos, 207
Poached Eggs, 248
Pork and White Bean Stew, 216
Pork Chops with Apples
    and Onions, 213
Portobello Tacos, 122
Power Quinoa Bowl, 135
Pressure Cooker Butter
    Chicken, 182
Pressure Cooker Chicken
    Tikka Masala, 189
Pumpkin Spice Baked
    Oatmeal Bars, 60
Quick Pickles, 259
Quick Vanilla Latte, 52
Quinoa Tabbouleh, 119
Salmon Tostada Salad, 167
Salted Chocolate–Coconut
    Macaroons, 284
Scallop Risotto, 155
Sheet Pan Chicken Fajitas, 183
Sheet Pan Eggplant
    Parmesan, 124
Skillet Garlic-Herb Steak, 231
Skillet Peachy Chicken
    Picante, 185
S'mores Campfire Trail Mix, 281
Southwest Eggs Benedict on
    Sweet Potato Toast, 69
Spaghetti Squash, 249
Spaghetti Squash Bolognese, 234
Spaghetti Squash Primavera, 140
Spicy Shrimp Tacos, 150
Spinach Artichoke Roll-Ups, 176
Spinach Meatballs and
    Zucchini Noodles, 233
Spinach-Walnut Pesto, 265

Strawberry–Goat
    Cheese Salad, 110
Strawberry-Jalapeño Salsa, 82
Strawberry Lemonade
    Slushie, 270
Strawberry Shortcake
    Mug Cake, 275
Strawberry Shortcake
    Overnight Oats, 56
Stuffed Pork Tenderloin, 215
Sweet 'n' Spicy Nuts
    and Seeds, 80
Sweet Potato and Butternut
    Squash Shepherd's
    Pie, 236–237
Sweet Potato Crust Quiche, 68
Sweet Potato Salmon
    Cakes, 165
Taco Cauliflower Pizza, 222
Taco Seasoning, 250
Tropical Pineapple Fruit
    Leather, 271
Tropical White Fish Ceviche, 157
Turmeric Rice, 93
Tzatziki, 261
Vegetable Risotto, 139
Vegetarian Black Bean
    Enchiladas, 131
Waldorf Chicken Salad, 175
Watermelon Gazpacho, 98
Goat cheese
    Butternut Squash, Mushroom,
        and Goat Cheese
        Cauliflower Pizza, 144
    Butternut Squash Mac
        & Cheese, 143
    Harvest Kale Salad with
        Goat Cheese and Dried
        Cranberries, 118
    Roasted Veggie Hummus
        Panini, 128
    Strawberry–Goat
        Cheese Salad, 110
    Stuffed Pork Tenderloin, 215

Gochujang, 258
   in Deconstructed Sushi Bowl, 163
   in Easy Stovetop Phở, 100
   in Pork Bibimbap, 210
   in Sesame Tofu and Brussels
     Sprouts Bowl, 136–137
Grape Leaf Pilaf, 138
Greek Lamb Bowls with Turmeric
   Cauliflower Rice and
   Cucumber Salsa, 243–244
Green Chicken Enchiladas, 184
Green Eggs and Ham Frittata, 64
Green Power Smoothie Bowl, 54
Green Shakshuka, 67
Grilled Clams with Lemon-
   Pepper Ghee, 152
Grilled Sausage, Peppers,
   and Onions, 201
Grown-Up Chicken Tenders, 174
Gut health, 6

H

Harvest Kale Salad with
   Goat Cheese and Dried
   Cranberries, 118
Hawaiian Pork Kebabs, 197
Healthy fats, 3, 5, 9, 11
Healthy Lifestyle Plan, 37–43
Herbs, 8, 12. *See also specific*
High-Protein Egg Muffins, 62
High Protein Pressure Cooker
   Mac & Cheese, 142
Homemade Cream of Mushroom
   Soup, 102–103
Homemade Marinara Sauce, 266
   in Chicken Parmesan
     over Zoodles, 192
   in Five-Ingredient Veggie
     Lasagna, 141
   in Mussels Marinara, 154
   in Sheet Pan Eggplant
     Parmesan, 124
   in Spinach Meatballs and
     Zucchini Noodles, 233

Homemade Mayo, 254
   in Baked Crab Cakes with
     Tartar Sauce, 156
   in Carnitas, 204–205
   in Easy Apple-Tuna Salad, 169
   in Honey Mustard, 255
   in Southwest Eggs Benedict
     on Sweet Potato Toast, 69
   in Waldorf Chicken Salad, 175
Honey-Lime Salmon with
   Watermelon Salsa, 164
Honey Mustard, 255
   in Grown-Up Chicken
     Tenders, 174
   in Honey Mustard Pork
     Chops, 212
Honey Mustard Pork Chops, 212
Hummus
   Caramelized Onion and
     Carrot Hummus, 84
   Greek Lamb Bowls with
     Turmeric Cauliflower Rice and
     Cucumber Salsa, 243–244
   Roasted Veggie Hummus
     Panini, 128
Hydration, 3–4

I

Ice Cream, Easy Vanilla, 278
Inflammation, 5–6
Ingredient staples, 11–14

J

Jalapeño peppers
   Cauliflower Curry, 126
   Chicken Tortilla Soup, 109
   Easy Guacamole, 83
   Green Chicken Enchiladas, 184
   Green Shakshuka, 67
   Honey-Lime Salmon with
     Watermelon Salsa, 164
   One-Pot Taco Pasta, 235
   Piggy Nachos, 207

Skillet Peachy Chicken
   Picante, 185
Strawberry-Jalapeño Salsa, 82
Tropical White Fish Ceviche, 157

K

Kale
   Green Eggs and Ham
     Frittata, 64
   Green Shakshuka, 67
   Harvest Kale Salad with
     Goat Cheese and Dried
     Cranberries, 118
   Pork and White Bean Stew, 216
   Sweet Potato Crust Quiche, 68
   Vegetable Risotto, 139
Ketchup, 256
   in Burger Bowls, 223
   in Grown-Up Chicken
     Tenders, 174
   in Sweet-and-Sour Sauce, 262

L

Lamb
   Feta Lamb Burgers, 240
   Greek Lamb Bowls with Turmeric
     Cauliflower Rice and
     Cucumber Salsa, 243–244
   Lamb Gyros, 239
   Lamb Kofta Kebabs, 238
   Lamb Lollipops with
     Chimichurri Sauce, 245
   Pressure Cooker Lamb
     Meatballs, 241
Legumes, 9, 11
Lemons
   Avocado-Cucumber-
     Feta Salad, 111
   Caramelized Onion and
     Carrot Hummus, 84
   Chickpea Buddha Bowls, 133
   Garlic-Dijon Asparagus, 87
   Grape Leaf Pilaf, 138

Greek Lamb Bowls with Turmeric Cauliflower Rice and Cucumber Salsa, 243–244
Grilled Clams with Lemon-Pepper Ghee, 152
Homemade Mayo, 254
Lamb Kofta Kebabs, 238
Lamb Lollipops with Chimichurri Sauce, 245
Lemon Greek Chicken Skewers, 173
Lemon Lentil Soup, 107
Lemon Meringue Smoothie, 51
Lemony Smoked Salmon Roll-Ups with Avocado, 162
Maple-Glazed Cedar Plank Salmon, 168
Maple Vinaigrette, 260
Mediterranean Fish in Parchment, 161
Peach Crumble, 277
Pressure Cooker Lamb Meatballs, 241
Quinoa Tabbouleh, 119
Raspberry-Lemon Bars, 276
Scallop Risotto, 155
Shrimp Pesto Pasta, 151
Strawberry Lemonade Slushie, 270
Sweet Potato Salmon Cakes, 165
Tropical Pineapple Fruit Leather, 271
Tzatziki, 261
Vegetable Risotto, 139
Lentil Soup, Lemon, 107
Lettuce
    Asian Lettuce Wraps with Hoisin Sauce, 196
    Beef Tacos in Lettuce, 220
    Burger Bowls, 223
    Easy Apple-Tuna Salad, 169
    Portobello Tacos, 122
    Salmon Tostada Salad, 167
    Spring Shrimp Rolls, 148–149

Limes
    Barbacoa Beef Bowls, 224
    Black Cherry Sorbet, 274
    Carnitas, 204–205
    Chili-Lime Popcorn, 76
    Chili-Spiced Fruit Cups, 273
    Chili-Stuffed Peppers, 232
    Cilantro-Lime Cauliflower Rice, 92
    Easy Guacamole, 83
    Honey-Lime Salmon with Watermelon Salsa, 164
    Lamb Gyros, 239
    Mexican Street Corn Salad, 115
    One-Pot Taco Pasta, 235
    Portobello Tacos, 122
    Spicy Shrimp Tacos, 150
    Spring Shrimp Rolls, 148–149
    Strawberry-Jalapeño Salsa, 82
    Thai Peanut Ramen, 127
    Tropical White Fish Ceviche, 157
Linguine with Clams, 153
Loaded Avocado Toast, 65
Loaded Baked Potatoes, 199
Loaded Baked Potato Soup, 104

M

Macronutrients, 3, 5
Mangos
    Chili-Spiced Fruit Cups, 273
    Tropical Pineapple Fruit Leather, 271
    Tropical White Fish Ceviche, 157
Maple-Glazed Cedar Plank Salmon, 168
Maple Vinaigrette, 260
    in Harvest Kale Salad with Goat Cheese and Dried Cranberries, 118
    in Strawberry–Goat Cheese Salad, 110
Mashed Parmesan Cauliflower, 91
Meal plans
    about, 16, 19–20
    Clean Eating 101, 20–29

Healthy Lifestyle, 37–43
    shortcuts, 45–46
    Wellness, 29–36
Meal prepping, 25, 45–46
Meats, 14. See also specific
Mediterranean Fish in Parchment, 161
Melons
    Chili-Spiced Fruit Cups, 273
    Honey-Lime Salmon with Watermelon Salsa, 164
    Watermelon Gazpacho, 98
Mexican Street Corn Salad, 115
Mint
    Grape Leaf Pilaf, 138
    Lamb Kofta Kebabs, 238
    Lamb Lollipops with Chimichurri Sauce, 245
Mocha-Cheesecake Brownies, 289
Mocha-Ricotta Mousse, 285
Mongolian Beef and Broccoli, 229
Mozzarella cheese
    Buffalo Chicken Cauliflower Pizza, 187
    Caprese Chicken Burgers, 177
    Cauliflower Pizza Crust, 267
    Chicken Parmesan over Zoodles, 192
    Chopped Caprese Salad, 114
    Five-Ingredient Veggie Lasagna, 141
    Pesto, Prosciutto, and Roasted Red Pepper Cauliflower Pizza, 217
    Sheet Pan Eggplant Parmesan, 124
    Spinach-Sausage-Pumpkin Pasta Bake, 203
    Sweet Potato Crust Quiche, 68
Mushrooms
    Burger Bowls, 223
    Butternut Squash, Mushroom, and Goat Cheese Cauliflower Pizza, 144
    Chicken Marsala, 186

Mushrooms *(continued)*
   Chickpea Tofu Marsala, 132
   Easy Stovetop Phở, 100
   Homemade Cream of
      Mushroom Soup, 102–103
   Pork Bibimbap, 210
   Pork Ramen Noodle Bowls, 211
   Portobello Tacos, 122
   Power Quinoa Bowl, 135
   Sweet Potato and Butternut
      Squash Shepherd's
      Pie, 236–237
   Tex-Mex Veggie Burger, 130
   Thai Peanut Ramen, 127
   Vegetarian Black Bean
      Enchiladas, 131
Mussels Marinara, 154

N

Noodles
   Easy Stovetop Phở, 100
   Pork Ramen Noodle Bowls, 211
   Thai Peanut Ramen, 127
Nut-free
   Air-Fryer Sweet Potato Tots, 94
   Apple, Brie, and Caramelized
      Onion Burger, 227
   Apple Breakfast Sausage
      Patties, 61
   Avocado-Cucumber-
      Feta Salad, 111
   Bacon-Wrapped Meatloaf
      Muffins, 221
   Baked Crab Cakes with
      Tartar Sauce, 156
   Baked Fish and Chips, 160
   Barbacoa Beef Bowls, 224
   BBQ Grilled Chicken, 181
   BBQ Pulled Pork, 206
   BBQ Ribs, 208
   Beef Tacos in Lettuce, 220
   Beet Burger, 129
   Black Cherry Sorbet, 274
   Buffalo Cauliflower Bites, 90

Buffalo Chicken Cauliflower
   Pizza, 187
Burger Bowls, 223
Butternut Squash, Mushroom,
   and Goat Cheese
   Cauliflower Pizza, 144
Butternut Squash Mac
   & Cheese, 143
Caramelized Onion and
   Carrot Hummus, 84
Cauliflower Curry, 126
Cauliflower Pizza Crust, 267
Chicken Bruschetta Pasta, 190
Chicken Marsala, 186
Chicken Parmesan over
   Zoodles, 192
Chicken Tortilla Soup, 109
Chickpea Tofu Marsala, 132
Chili-Lime Popcorn, 76
Chili-Spiced Fruit Cups, 273
Chili-Stuffed Peppers, 232
Chocolate-Covered
   Orange Slices, 282
Chopped Caprese Salad, 114
Chorizo Stuffed Sweet
   Potatoes, 202
Cilantro-Lime Cauliflower Rice, 92
Cinnamon Apple Chips, 74
Cinnamon Toast Waffles, 59
Classic Minestrone, 106
Crab Bisque, 108
Creamy Garlic Cauliflower
   Soup, 101
Crispy Baked Bacon, 198
Crispy Baked Wings, 172
Crispy Garlic-Rosemary
   Potato Wedges, 77
Crunchy Chickpeas, 79
Dairy-Free Bacon Mac
   & "Cheese," 200
Dark Chocolate–Sea
   Salt Popcorn, 280
Easy Apple-Tuna Salad, 169
Easy Blackened Fish, 158
Easy Broth, 253

Easy Guacamole, 83
Easy Homemade Falafel, 145
Easy Stovetop Phở, 100
Easy Vanilla Ice Cream, 278
Enchilada Sauce, 263
Everything Bagel–Seasoned
   Hard-Boiled Eggs, 81
Feta Lamb Burgers, 240
Five-Ingredient Veggie
   Lasagna, 141
Freezer V-Egg-ie Burritos, 70–71
Garlic-Dijon Asparagus, 87
Garlic-Parmesan Roasted
   Broccoli, 88
Ghee, 251
Grape Leaf Pilaf, 138
Greek Lamb Bowls with
   Turmeric Cauliflower Rice and
   Cucumber Salsa, 243–244
Green Chicken Enchiladas, 184
Green Eggs and Ham Frittata, 64
Green Shakshuka, 67
Grilled Clams with Lemon-
   Pepper Ghee, 152
Grilled Sausage, Peppers,
   and Onions, 201
Grown-Up Chicken Tenders, 174
Hawaiian Pork Kebabs, 197
High-Protein Egg Muffins, 62
High Protein Pressure Cooker
   Mac & Cheese, 142
Homemade Cream of
   Mushroom Soup, 102–103
Homemade Marinara Sauce, 266
Homemade Mayo, 254
Honey-Lime Salmon with
   Watermelon Salsa, 164
Honey Mustard, 255
Honey Mustard Pork
   Chops, 212
Ketchup, 256
Lamb Gyros, 239
Lamb Kofta Kebabs, 238
Lamb Lollipops with
   Chimichurri Sauce, 245

Lemon Greek Chicken Skewers, 173
Lemon Lentil Soup, 107
Lemon Meringue Smoothie, 51
Lemony Smoked Salmon Roll-Ups with Avocado, 162
Linguine with Clams, 153
Loaded Avocado Toast, 65
Loaded Baked Potatoes, 199
Loaded Baked Potato Soup, 104
Maple-Glazed Cedar Plank Salmon, 168
Maple Vinaigrette, 260
Mashed Parmesan Cauliflower, 91
Mediterranean Fish in Parchment, 161
Mexican Street Corn Salad, 115
Mocha-Cheesecake Brownies, 289
Mocha-Ricotta Mousse, 285
Mongolian Beef and Broccoli, 229
Mussels Marinara, 154
One-Pot Taco Pasta, 235
One-Skillet Pepper Steak, 230
Orange-Balsamic Brussels Sprouts, 89
Paprika-Baked Chicken Thighs, 180
Parmesan Crisps, 75
Peach Crumble, 277
Piggy Nachos, 207
Poached Eggs, 248
Pork and White Bean Stew, 216
Pork Bibimbap, 210
Pork Chops with Apples and Onions, 213
Pork Ramen Noodle Bowls, 211
Portobello Tacos, 122
Power Quinoa Bowl, 135
Pressure Cooker Butter Chicken, 182
Pressure Cooker Chicken Tikka Masala, 189
Pressure Cooker French Dip Sandwiches, 225–226

Pressure Cooker Lamb Meatballs, 241
Quick Pickles, 259
Quick Vanilla Latte, 52
Quinoa Tabbouleh, 119
Roasted Red Pepper Soup and Ricotta Cheeseballs, 105
Roasted Veggie Hummus Panini, 128
Salmon Tostada Salad, 167
Salted Chocolate–Coconut Macaroons, 284
Sassy BBQ Sauce, 257
Scallop Risotto, 155
Sesame Tofu and Brussels Sprouts Bowl, 136–137
Sheet Pan Chicken Fajitas, 183
Sheet Pan Eggplant Parmesan, 124
Sheet Pan Sweet and Sour Chicken Rice Bowls, 179
Simple French Onion Soup, 99
Skillet Garlic-Herb Steak, 231
Skillet Peachy Chicken Picante, 185
Southwest Eggs Benedict on Sweet Potato Toast, 69
Spaghetti Squash, 249
Spaghetti Squash Bolognese, 234
Spaghetti Squash Primavera, 140
Spicy Shrimp Tacos, 150
Spinach Artichoke Roll-Ups, 176
Spinach Meatballs and Zucchini Noodles, 233
Spinach-Sausage-Pumpkin Pasta Bake, 203
Steak and Pepper Roll-Ups, 228
Strawberry-Jalapeño Salsa, 82
Strawberry Lemonade Slushie, 270
Strawberry Shortcake Overnight Oats, 56
Stuffed Pork Tenderloin, 215
Sweet-and-Sour Eggplant, 123
Sweet-and-Sour Sauce, 262

Sweet Potato and Butternut Squash Shepherd's Pie, 236–237
Sweet Potato Crust Quiche, 68
Sweet Potato Salmon Cakes, 165
Taco Cauliflower Pizza, 222
Taco Seasoning, 250
Tropical Pineapple Fruit Leather, 271
Tropical White Fish Ceviche, 157
Turmeric Rice, 93
Tzatziki, 261
Vegetable Risotto, 139
Vegetarian Black Bean Enchiladas, 131
Watermelon Gazpacho, 98
Nutritional guidelines, 4

O

Oats
Almond Butter Energy Bites, 86
Baked Fish and Chips, 160
Beet Burger, 129
Blueberry-Oat Pancakes, 58
Chocolate Chip Cookie Dough Overnight Oats, 57
Easy Homemade Falafel, 145
French Toast Overnight Oats, 55
Pumpkin Spice Baked Oatmeal Bars, 60
Strawberry Shortcake Overnight Oats, 56
One-pot
Almond Butter, 252
Almond Butter Energy Bites, 86
Apple-Cranberry Slaw, 116
Asian Lettuce Wraps with Hoisin Sauce, 196
Avocado-Cucumber-Feta Salad, 111
Barbacoa Beef Bowls, 224
BBQ Pulled Pork, 206
BBQ Ribs, 208
Beef Tacos in Lettuce, 220

One-pot (continued)
  Black Cherry Sorbet, 274
  Burger Bowls, 223
  Carnitas, 204–205
  Cauliflower Curry, 126
  Chicken Tortilla Soup, 109
  Chili-Spiced Fruit Cups, 273
  Classic Minestrone, 106
  Cookie Dough Dip, 85
  Crab Bisque, 108
  Creamy Garlic Cauliflower
    Soup, 101
  Crispy Baked Bacon, 198
  Easy Apple-Tuna Salad, 169
  Easy Broth, 253
  Easy Guacamole, 83
  Easy Stovetop Phở, 100
  Egg Roll in a Bowl, 178
  Garlic-Parmesan Roasted
    Broccoli, 88
  Ghee, 251
  Gochujang, 258
  Grape Leaf Pilaf, 138
  Green Shakshuka, 67
  High Protein Pressure Cooker
    Mac & Cheese, 142
  Homemade Cream of
    Mushroom Soup, 102–103
  Homemade Marinara Sauce, 266
  Homemade Mayo, 254
  Honey Mustard, 255
  Ketchup, 256
  Lemon Lentil Soup, 107
  Linguine with Clams, 153
  Loaded Baked Potatoes, 199
  Loaded Baked Potato Soup, 104
  Maple Vinaigrette, 260
  Mashed Parmesan Cauliflower, 91
  Mediterranean Fish in
    Parchment, 161
  Mocha-Ricotta Mousse, 285
  Mongolian Beef and Broccoli, 229
  Mussels Marinara, 154
  One-Pot Taco Pasta, 235
  One-Skillet Pepper Steak, 230

  Parmesan Crisps, 75
  Pesto-Baked Cauliflower
    Steaks, 125
  Piggy Nachos, 207
  Poached Eggs, 248
  Pork and White Bean Stew, 216
  Pork Bibimbap, 210
  Pork Chops with Apples
    and Onions, 213
  Pork Fried Cauliflower Rice, 209
  Pressure Cooker Butter
    Chicken, 182
  Pressure Cooker Chicken
    Tikka Masala, 189
  Quick Pickles, 259
  Raspberry-Lemon Bars, 276
  Roasted Veggie Hummus
    Panini, 128
  Sassy BBQ Sauce, 257
  Skillet Garlic-Herb Steak, 231
  Skillet Peachy Chicken
    Picante, 185
  Spaghetti Squash, 249
  Spinach-Walnut Pesto, 265
  Spring Shrimp Rolls, 148–149
  Strawberry–Goat Cheese
    Salad, 110
  Strawberry-Jalapeño Salsa, 82
  Strawberry Shortcake
    Mug Cake, 275
  Sweet-and-Sour Eggplant, 123
  Sweet-and-Sour Sauce, 262
  Thai Peanut Ramen, 127
  Turmeric Rice, 93
  Tzatziki, 261
  Vegetable Risotto, 139
One-Pot Taco Pasta, 235
One-Skillet Pepper Steak, 230
Onions
  Apple, Brie, and Caramelized
    Onion Burger, 227
  Caramelized Onion and
    Carrot Hummus, 84
  Carnitas, 204–205
  Easy Homemade Falafel, 145

  Grilled Sausage, Peppers,
    and Onions, 201
  Pork Chops with Apples
    and Onions, 213
  Simple French Onion Soup, 99
Oranges
  Carnitas, 204–205
  Chocolate-Covered
    Orange Slices, 282
  Mongolian Beef and Broccoli, 229
  Orange-Balsamic Brussels
    Sprouts, 89
  Orange-Beet-Arugula Salad, 113
  Tropical White Fish Ceviche, 157

P

Pancakes, Blueberry-Oat, 58
Pantry staples, 11–12
Paprika-Baked Chicken Thighs, 180
Parmesan cheese
  Bacon-Wrapped Meatloaf
    Muffins, 221
  Cauliflower Pizza Crust, 267
  Chicken Parmesan over
    Zoodles, 192
  Classic Minestrone, 106
  Crispy Baked Fish Sticks, 159
  Garlic-Parmesan Roasted
    Broccoli, 88
  Green Eggs and Ham Frittata, 64
  Grown-Up Chicken Tenders, 174
  Linguine with Clams, 153
  Mashed Parmesan Cauliflower, 91
  Mussels Marinara, 154
  Parmesan Crisps, 75
  Pesto Chicken Alfredo with
    Spaghetti Squash, 191
  Roasted Red Pepper Soup and
    Ricotta Cheeseballs, 105
  Scallop Risotto, 155
  Sheet Pan Eggplant
    Parmesan, 124
  Shrimp Pesto Pasta, 151
  Spaghetti Squash Bolognese, 234

Spaghetti Squash Primavera, 140
Spinach Artichoke Roll-Ups, 176
Spinach Meatballs and
    Zucchini Noodles, 233
Spinach-Sausage-Pumpkin
    Pasta Bake, 203
Spinach-Walnut Pesto, 265
Sweet Potato and Butternut
    Squash Shepherd's
    Pie, 236–237
Vegetable Risotto, 139
Pasta
    Butternut Squash Mac
        & Cheese, 143
    Chicken Bruschetta Pasta, 190
    Classic Minestrone, 106
    Dairy-Free Bacon Mac
        & "Cheese," 200
    High Protein Pressure Cooker
        Mac & Cheese, 142
    Linguine with Clams, 153
    One-Pot Taco Pasta, 235
    Shrimp Pesto Pasta, 151
    Spinach-Sausage-Pumpkin
        Pasta Bake, 203
PB and J Protein Smoothie, 50
Peaches
    Peach Crumble, 277
    Skillet Peachy Chicken
        Picante, 185
Peanut butter
    Asian Lettuce Wraps with
        Hoisin Sauce, 196
    Berry Berry Smoothie Bowl, 53
    Chocolate–Peanut Butter
        Freezer Fudge, 287–288
    PB and J Protein Smoothie, 50
    Spring Shrimp Rolls, 148–149
    Thai Peanut Ramen, 127
Peanuts
    Asian Lettuce Wraps with
        Hoisin Sauce, 196
    S'mores Campfire Trail Mix, 281
Pears
    Waldorf Chicken Salad, 175

Peas
    Pork Fried Cauliflower Rice, 209
Pecans
    Strawberry–Goat Cheese
        Salad, 110
Pepitas
    Sweet 'n' Spicy Nuts
        and Seeds, 80
Pesto, Prosciutto, and Roasted Red
        Pepper Cauliflower Pizza, 217
Pesto-Baked Cauliflower
        Steaks, 125
Pesto Chicken Alfredo with
        Spaghetti Squash, 191
Physical activity, 4
Piggy Nachos, 207
Pineapple
    Chili-Spiced Fruit Cups, 273
    Green Power Smoothie Bowl, 54
    Hawaiian Pork Kebabs, 197
    Sheet Pan Sweet and Sour
        Chicken Rice Bowls, 179
    Tropical Pineapple Fruit
        Leather, 271
Pizzas
    Buffalo Chicken Cauliflower
        Pizza, 187
    Butternut Squash, Mushroom,
        and Goat Cheese
        Cauliflower Pizza, 144
    Pesto, Prosciutto, and
        Roasted Red Pepper
        Cauliflower Pizza, 217
    Taco Cauliflower Pizza, 222
Poached Eggs, 248
    in Loaded Avocado Toast, 65
    in Southwest Eggs Benedict
        on Sweet Potato Toast, 69
Popcorn
    Chili-Lime Popcorn, 76
    Dark Chocolate–Sea
        Salt Popcorn, 280
Pork. See also Bacon; Sausage
    Apple Breakfast Sausage
        Patties, 61

Asian Lettuce Wraps with
    Hoisin Sauce, 196
BBQ Pulled Pork, 206
BBQ Ribs, 208
Carnitas, 204–205
Easy Broth, 253
Hawaiian Pork Kebabs, 197
Honey Mustard Pork
    Chops, 212
Pork and White Bean Stew, 216
Pork Bibimbap, 210
Pork Chops with Apples
    and Onions, 213
Pork Fried Cauliflower Rice, 209
Pork Ramen Noodle Bowls, 211
Stuffed Pork Tenderloin, 215
Portion size, 3
Portobello Tacos, 122
Potatoes. See also Sweet potatoes
    Crispy Garlic-Rosemary
        Potato Wedges, 77
    Loaded Baked Potatoes, 199
    Loaded Baked Potato Soup, 104
Power Quinoa Bowl, 135
Pressure Cooker Butter
    Chicken, 182
Pressure Cooker Chicken
    Tikka Masala, 189
Pressure Cooker French Dip
    Sandwiches, 225–226
Pressure Cooker Lamb
    Meatballs, 241
Processed foods, 2
Prosciutto
    Pesto, Prosciutto, and
        Roasted Red Pepper
        Cauliflower Pizza, 217
Proteins, 3, 5, 9, 14. See also
        specific
Pumpkin purée
    Green Power Smoothie Bowl, 54
    Pumpkin Spice Baked
        Oatmeal Bars, 60
    Spinach-Sausage-Pumpkin
        Pasta Bake, 203

Q

Quick Pickles, 259
  in Burger Bowls, 223
Quick-prep
  Air-Fryer Sweet Potato Tots, 94
  Almond Butter, 252
  Almond Butter Energy Bites, 86
  Apple, Brie, and Caramelized
    Onion Burger, 227
  Apple Breakfast Sausage
    Patties, 61
  Apple Nachos, 272
  Asian Lettuce Wraps with
    Hoisin Sauce, 196
  Avocado-Cucumber-
    Feta Salad, 111
  Bacon, Egg, and Cheese Sheet
    Pan Sandwiches, 63
  Baked Crab Cakes with
    Tartar Sauce, 156
  Baked Fish and Chips, 160
  Barbacoa Beef Bowls, 224
  BBQ Pulled Pork, 206
  BBQ Ribs, 208
  Beef Tacos in Lettuce, 220
  Beet Burger, 129
  Berry Berry Smoothie Bowl, 53
  Black Cherry Sorbet, 274
  Blueberry-Oat Pancakes, 58
  Broccoli-Walnut Salad with
    Dried Cherries, 117
  Buffalo Cauliflower Bites, 90
  Buffalo Chicken Cauliflower
    Pizza, 187
  Burger Bowls, 223
  Butternut Squash, Mushroom,
    and Goat Cheese
    Cauliflower Pizza, 144
  Caprese Chicken Burgers, 177
  Caramelized Onion and
    Carrot Hummus, 84
  Carnitas, 204–205
  Cauliflower Curry, 126
  Cauliflower Pizza Crust, 267

Chicken Bruschetta Pasta, 190
Chicken Marsala, 186
Chicken Tortilla Soup, 109
Chickpea Buddha Bowls, 133
Chili-Lime Popcorn, 76
Chili-Spiced Fruit Cups, 273
Chili-Stuffed Peppers, 232
Chocolate Chip Cookie Dough
  Overnight Oats, 57
Chopped Caprese Salad, 114
Chorizo Stuffed Sweet
  Potatoes, 202
Cilantro-Lime Cauliflower Rice, 92
Cinnamon Apple Chips, 74
Cinnamon Toast Waffles, 59
Classic Minestrone, 106
Cookie Dough Dip, 85
Crab Bisque, 108
Creamy Garlic Cauliflower
  Soup, 101
Crispy Baked Bacon, 198
Crispy Baked Fish Sticks, 159
Crispy Baked Wings, 172
Crispy Garlic-Rosemary
  Potato Wedges, 77
Crunchy Chickpeas, 79
Dairy-Free Bacon Mac
  & "Cheese," 200
Dark Chocolate–Sea
  Salt Popcorn, 280
Deconstructed Sushi Bowl, 163
Easy Apple-Tuna Salad, 169
Easy Blackened Fish, 158
Easy Broth, 253
Easy Guacamole, 83
Easy Stovetop Phở, 100
Egg Roll in a Bowl, 178
Enchilada Sauce, 263
Everything Bagel–Seasoned
  Hard-Boiled Eggs, 81
Feta Lamb Burgers, 240
Freezer V-Egg-ie Burritos,
  70–71
French Toast Overnight Oats, 55
Garlic-Dijon Asparagus, 87

Garlic-Parmesan Roasted
  Broccoli, 88
Ghee, 251
Gochujang, 258
Grape Leaf Pilaf, 138
Greek Lamb Bowls with
  Turmeric Cauliflower Rice and
  Cucumber Salsa, 243–244
Green Eggs and Ham Frittata, 64
Green Power Smoothie Bowl, 54
Green Shakshuka, 67
Grilled Clams with Lemon-
  Pepper Ghee, 152
Grilled Sausage, Peppers,
  and Onions, 201
Harvest Kale Salad with
  Goat Cheese and Dried
  Cranberries, 118
High-Protein Egg Muffins, 62
High Protein Pressure Cooker
  Mac & Cheese, 142
Homemade Cream of
  Mushroom Soup, 102–103
Homemade Marinara Sauce, 266
Honey-Lime Salmon with
  Watermelon Salsa, 164
Honey Mustard, 255
Ketchup, 256
Lamb Gyros, 239
Lemon Lentil Soup, 107
Lemon Meringue Smoothie, 51
Lemony Smoked Salmon
  Roll-Ups with Avocado, 162
Linguine with Clams, 153
Loaded Avocado Toast, 65
Loaded Baked Potatoes, 199
Loaded Baked Potato Soup, 104
Maple Vinaigrette, 260
Mashed Parmesan Cauliflower, 91
Mediterranean Fish in
  Parchment, 161
Mexican Street Corn Salad, 115
Mocha-Cheesecake
  Brownies, 289
Mocha-Ricotta Mousse, 285

Mongolian Beef and Broccoli, 229

Mussels Marinara, 154

One-Pot Taco Pasta, 235

Orange-Balsamic Brussels Sprouts, 89

Paprika-Baked Chicken Thighs, 180

Parmesan Crisps, 75

PB and J Protein Smoothie, 50

Peach Crumble, 277

Pesto, Prosciutto, and Roasted Red Pepper Cauliflower Pizza, 217

Pesto-Baked Cauliflower Steaks, 125

Piggy Nachos, 207

Poached Eggs, 248

Pork and White Bean Stew, 216

Pork Bibimbap, 210

Pork Chops with Apples and Onions, 213

Pork Fried Cauliflower Rice, 209

Pork Ramen Noodle Bowls, 211

Portobello Tacos, 122

Power Quinoa Bowl, 135

Pressure Cooker Butter Chicken, 182

Pressure Cooker Chicken Tikka Masala, 189

Pressure Cooker French Dip Sandwiches, 225–226

Pressure Cooker Lamb Meatballs, 241

Pumpkin Spice Baked Oatmeal Bars, 60

Quick Pickles, 259

Quick Vanilla Latte, 52

Quinoa Tabbouleh, 119

Raspberry-Lemon Bars, 276

Roasted Red Pepper Soup and Ricotta Cheeseballs, 105

Roasted Veggie Hummus Panini, 128

Salmon Tostada Salad, 167

Salted Chocolate–Coconut Macaroons, 284

Sassy BBQ Sauce, 257

Scallop Risotto, 155

Sheet Pan Chicken Fajitas, 183

Sheet Pan Eggplant Parmesan, 124

Sheet Pan Sweet and Sour Chicken Rice Bowls, 179

Shrimp Pesto Pasta, 151

Simple French Onion Soup, 99

Skillet Garlic-Herb Steak, 231

Skillet Peachy Chicken Picante, 185

S'mores Campfire Trail Mix, 281

Southwest Eggs Benedict on Sweet Potato Toast, 69

Spaghetti Squash, 249

Spaghetti Squash Bolognese, 234

Spaghetti Squash Primavera, 140

Spicy Shrimp Tacos, 150

Spinach Artichoke Roll-Ups, 176

Spinach Meatballs and Zucchini Noodles, 233

Spinach-Sausage-Pumpkin Pasta Bake, 203

Spinach-Walnut Pesto, 265

Strawberry–Goat Cheese Salad, 110

Strawberry-Jalapeño Salsa, 82

Strawberry Lemonade Slushie, 270

Strawberry Shortcake Mug Cake, 275

Strawberry Shortcake Overnight Oats, 56

Sweet-and-Sour Eggplant, 123

Sweet-and-Sour Sauce, 262

Sweet 'n' Spicy Nuts and Seeds, 80

Sweet Potato and Butternut Squash Shepherd's Pie, 236–237

Sweet Potato Salmon Cakes, 165

Taco Cauliflower Pizza, 222

Taco Seasoning, 250

Tex-Mex Veggie Burger, 130

Thai Peanut Ramen, 127

Tropical Pineapple Fruit Leather, 271

Turmeric Rice, 93

Vegetable Risotto, 139

Waldorf Chicken Salad, 175

Watermelon Gazpacho, 98

Quick Vanilla Latte, 52

Quinoa
  Chickpea Buddha Bowls, 133
  Power Quinoa Bowl, 135
  Quinoa Tabbouleh, 119

R

Raspberry-Lemon Bars, 276

Recipes, about, 16–17

Refrigerator staples, 13–14

Rice
  Deconstructed Sushi Bowl, 163
  Grape Leaf Pilaf, 138
  Mongolian Beef and Broccoli, 229
  One-Skillet Pepper Steak, 230
  Pork Bibimbap, 210
  Scallop Risotto, 155
  Sesame Tofu and Brussels Sprouts Bowl, 136–137
  Sheet Pan Sweet and Sour Chicken Rice Bowls, 179
  Turmeric Rice, 93
  Vegetable Risotto, 139

Ricotta cheese
  Five-Ingredient Veggie Lasagna, 141
  Mocha-Ricotta Mousse, 285
  Roasted Red Pepper Soup and Ricotta Cheeseballs, 105

Roasted Red Pepper Soup and Ricotta Cheeseballs, 105

Roasted Veggie Hummus Panini, 128

Rosemary
  Crispy Garlic-Rosemary
    Potato Wedges, 77
  Homemade Cream of
    Mushroom Soup, 102–103

S

Salads
  Apple-Cranberry Slaw, 116
  Avocado-Cucumber-
    Feta Salad, 111
  Broccoli-Walnut Salad with
    Dried Cherries, 117
  Chopped Caprese Salad, 114
  Easy Apple-Tuna Salad, 169
  Harvest Kale Salad with
    Goat Cheese and Dried
    Cranberries, 118
  Mexican Street Corn Salad, 115
  Orange-Beet-Arugula Salad, 113
  Quinoa Tabbouleh, 119
  Salmon Tostada Salad, 167
  Strawberry–Goat
    Cheese Salad, 110
  Waldorf Chicken Salad, 175
Salmon
  Deconstructed Sushi Bowl, 163
  Honey-Lime Salmon with
    Watermelon Salsa, 164
  Lemony Smoked Salmon
    Roll-Ups with Avocado, 162
  Maple-Glazed Cedar
    Plank Salmon, 168
  Salmon Tostada Salad, 167
  Sweet Potato Salmon Cakes, 165
Salted Chocolate–Coconut
  Macaroons, 284
Sandwiches and wraps. See
  also Burgers; Tacos
  Asian Lettuce Wraps with
    Hoisin Sauce, 196
  Bacon, Egg, and Cheese Sheet
    Pan Sandwiches, 63
  Carnitas, 204–205

Freezer V-Egg-ie Burritos, 70–71
Lamb Gyros, 239
Lemony Smoked Salmon
  Roll-Ups with Avocado, 162
Pressure Cooker French Dip
  Sandwiches, 225–226
Roasted Veggie Hummus
  Panini, 128
Sheet Pan Chicken Fajitas, 183
Spring Shrimp Rolls, 148–149
Sassy BBQ Sauce, 257
  in BBQ Grilled Chicken, 181
  in BBQ Pulled Pork, 206
  in BBQ Ribs, 208
  in Crispy Baked Wings, 172
  in Piggy Nachos, 207
Sauces. See also Condiments;
  Dressings
  Enchilada Sauce, 263
  Gochujang, 258
  Homemade Marinara Sauce, 266
  Sassy BBQ Sauce, 257
  Spinach-Walnut Pesto, 265
  Strawberry-Jalapeño Salsa, 82
  Sweet-and-Sour Sauce, 262
  Tzatziki, 261
Sausage
  Apple Breakfast Sausage
    Patties, 61
  Chorizo Stuffed Sweet
    Potatoes, 202
  Grilled Sausage, Peppers,
    and Onions, 201
  Spinach-Sausage-Pumpkin
    Pasta Bake, 203
Scallop Risotto, 155
Sesame Tofu and Brussels
  Sprouts Bowl, 136–137
Sheet Pan Chicken Fajitas, 183
Sheet Pan Eggplant Parmesan, 124
Sheet Pan Sweet and Sour
  Chicken Rice Bowls, 179
Shrimp
  Shrimp Pesto Pasta, 151
  Spicy Shrimp Tacos, 150

Spring Shrimp Rolls, 148–149
Simple French Onion Soup, 99
Skillet Garlic-Herb Steak, 231
Skillet Peachy Chicken Picante, 185
Smoothies
  Berry Berry Smoothie Bowl, 53
  Green Power Smoothie Bowl, 54
  Lemon Meringue Smoothie, 51
  PB and J Protein Smoothie, 50
S'mores Campfire Trail Mix, 281
Snacks, 36. See also Dips
  and spreads
  Almond Butter Energy Bites, 86
  Cinnamon Apple Chips, 74
  Crunchy Chickpeas, 79
  Everything Bagel–Seasoned
    Hard-Boiled Eggs, 81
  Parmesan Crisps, 75
  Sweet 'n' Spicy Nuts
    and Seeds, 80
Soups
  Chicken Tortilla Soup, 109
  Classic Minestrone, 106
  Crab Bisque, 108
  Creamy Garlic Cauliflower
    Soup, 101
  Easy Broth, 253
  Easy Stovetop Phở, 100
  Homemade Cream of
    Mushroom Soup, 102–103
  Lemon Lentil Soup, 107
  Loaded Baked Potato Soup, 104
  Pork and White Bean Stew, 216
  Roasted Red Pepper Soup and
    Ricotta Cheeseballs, 105
  Simple French Onion Soup, 99
  Thai Peanut Ramen, 127
  Watermelon Gazpacho, 98
Southwest Eggs Benedict on
  Sweet Potato Toast, 69
Spaghetti Squash, 249
  in Pesto Chicken Alfredo with
    Spaghetti Squash, 191
  in Spaghetti Squash
    Bolognese, 234

in Spaghetti Squash
Primavera, 140
Spices, 8, 12
Spicy Shrimp Tacos, 150
Spinach
Butternut Squash, Mushroom,
and Goat Cheese
Cauliflower Pizza, 144
Classic Minestrone, 106
Green Eggs and Ham Frittata, 64
Green Power Smoothie Bowl, 54
Pork Ramen Noodle Bowls, 211
Power Quinoa Bowl, 135
Spinach Artichoke Roll-Ups, 176
Spinach Meatballs and
Zucchini Noodles, 233
Spinach-Sausage-Pumpkin
Pasta Bake, 203
Spinach-Walnut Pesto, 265
Strawberry—Goat
Cheese Salad, 110
Stuffed Pork Tenderloin, 215
Thai Peanut Ramen, 127
Spinach-Walnut Pesto, 265
in Caprese Chicken Burgers, 177
in Pesto, Prosciutto, and
Roasted Red Pepper
Cauliflower Pizza, 217
in Pesto-Baked Cauliflower
Steaks, 125
in Pesto Chicken Alfredo with
Spaghetti Squash, 191
in Shrimp Pesto Pasta, 151
Spring Shrimp Rolls, 148–149
Squash
Butternut Squash, Mushroom,
and Goat Cheese
Cauliflower Pizza, 144
Butternut Squash Mac
& Cheese, 143
Harvest Kale Salad with
Goat Cheese and Dried
Cranberries, 118
Roasted Veggie Hummus
Panini, 128

Spaghetti Squash, 249
Spaghetti Squash Bolognese, 234
Spaghetti Squash Primavera, 140
Sweet Potato and Butternut
Squash Shepherd's
Pie, 236–237
Steak and Pepper Roll-Ups, 228
Strawberry—Goat Cheese
Salad, 110
Strawberry-Jalapeño Salsa, 82
in Salmon Tostada Salad, 167
Strawberry Lemonade
Slushie, 270
Strawberry Shortcake
Mug Cake, 275
Strawberry Shortcake
Overnight Oats, 56
Stuffed Pork Tenderloin, 215
Sugars, 3, 9
Sweet-and-Sour Eggplant, 123
Sweet-and-Sour Sauce, 262
in Sheet Pan Sweet and Sour
Chicken Rice Bowls, 179
in Sweet-and-Sour Eggplant, 123
Sweeteners, 9, 12
Sweet 'n' Spicy Nuts and
Seeds, 80
in Harvest Kale Salad with
Goat Cheese and Dried
Cranberries, 118
Sweet potatoes
Air-Fryer Sweet Potato Tots, 94
Baked Fish and Chips, 160
Chickpea Buddha Bowls, 133
Chorizo Stuffed Sweet
Potatoes, 202
Dairy-Free Bacon Mac
& "Cheese," 200
Freezer V-Egg-ie Burritos, 70–71
Harvest Kale Salad with
Goat Cheese and Dried
Cranberries, 118
Power Quinoa Bowl, 135
Southwest Eggs Benedict on
Sweet Potato Toast, 69

Sweet Potato and Butternut
Squash Shepherd's
Pie, 236–237
Sweet Potato Crust Quiche, 68
Sweet Potato Salmon Cakes, 165
Swiss cheese
Pressure Cooker French Dip
Sandwiches, 225–226
Simple French Onion Soup, 99

T

Taco Cauliflower Pizza, 222
Tacos
Beef Tacos in Lettuce, 220
Portobello Tacos, 122
Spicy Shrimp Tacos, 150
Taco Seasoning, 250
in Beef Tacos in Lettuce, 220
in Chicken Tortilla Soup, 109
in One-Pot Taco Pasta, 235
in Portobello Tacos, 122
in Sheet Pan Chicken Fajitas, 183
in Spicy Shrimp Tacos, 150
in Taco Cauliflower Pizza, 222
in Vegetarian Black Bean
Enchiladas, 131
Tex-Mex Veggie Burger, 130
Thai Peanut Ramen, 127
30 minutes or less, 164
Air-Fryer Sweet Potato Tots, 94
Almond Butter, 252
Almond Butter Cookies, 279
Almond Butter Energy Bites, 86
Apple Breakfast Sausage
Patties, 61
Apple Nachos, 272
Asian Lettuce Wraps with
Hoisin Sauce, 196
Avocado-Cucumber-
Feta Salad, 111
Bacon, Egg, and Cheese Sheet
Pan Sandwiches, 63
Baked Crab Cakes with
Tartar Sauce, 156

30 minutes or less *(continued)*
  Beef Tacos in Lettuce, 220
  Berry Berry Smoothie Bowl, 53
  Black Cherry Sorbet, 274
  Blueberry-Oat Pancakes, 58
  Broccoli-Walnut Salad with
    Dried Cherries, 117
  Buffalo Chicken Cauliflower
    Pizza, 187
  Burger Bowls, 223
  Caprese Chicken Burgers, 177
  Caramelized Onion and
    Carrot Hummus, 84
  Cauliflower Curry, 126
  Chicken Bruschetta Pasta, 190
  Chickpea Buddha Bowls, 133
  Chili-Lime Popcorn, 76
  Chili-Spiced Fruit Cups, 273
  Chocolate-Covered
    Orange Slices, 282
  Chopped Caprese Salad, 114
  Cilantro-Lime Cauliflower Rice, 92
  Cinnamon Toast Waffles, 59
  Cookie Dough Dip, 85
  Creamy Garlic Cauliflower
    Soup, 101
  Crispy Baked Bacon, 198
  Crispy Baked Fish Sticks, 159
  Dark Chocolate–Sea
    Salt Popcorn, 280
  Deconstructed Sushi Bowl, 163
  Easy Apple-Tuna Salad, 169
  Easy Blackened Fish, 158
  Easy Guacamole, 83
  Easy Homemade Falafel, 145
  Egg Roll in a Bowl, 178
  Enchilada Sauce, 263
  Everything Bagel–Seasoned
    Hard-Boiled Eggs, 81
  Feta Lamb Burgers, 240
  Freezer V-Egg-ie Burritos,
    70–71
  Fruit-and-Nut Chocolate
    Bark, 283
  Gochujang, 258

Greek Lamb Bowls with
  Turmeric Cauliflower Rice and
  Cucumber Salsa, 243–244
Green Power Smoothie Bowl, 54
Green Shakshuka, 67
Grilled Clams with Lemon-
  Pepper Ghee, 152
Grilled Sausage, Peppers,
  and Onions, 201
Harvest Kale Salad with
  Goat Cheese and Dried
  Cranberries, 118
High-Protein Egg Muffins, 62
High Protein Pressure Cooker
  Mac & Cheese, 142
Homemade Mayo, 254
Honey Mustard, 255
Ketchup, 256
Lamb Lollipops with
  Chimichurri Sauce, 245
Lemon Meringue Smoothie, 51
Lemony Smoked Salmon
  Roll-Ups with Avocado, 162
Linguine with Clams, 153
Loaded Avocado Toast, 65
Maple-Glazed Cedar
  Plank Salmon, 168
Maple Vinaigrette, 260
Mashed Parmesan Cauliflower, 91
Mediterranean Fish in
  Parchment, 161
Mexican Street Corn Salad, 115
Mocha-Ricotta Mousse, 285
Mongolian Beef and Broccoli, 229
Mussels Marinara, 154
One-Pot Taco Pasta, 235
Parmesan Crisps, 75
PB and J Protein Smoothie, 50
Pesto, Prosciutto, and
  Roasted Red Pepper
  Cauliflower Pizza, 217
Piggy Nachos, 207
Poached Eggs, 248
Pork Bibimbap, 210
Pork Fried Cauliflower Rice, 209

Pork Ramen Noodle Bowls, 211
Portobello Tacos, 122
Pressure Cooker Chicken
  Tikka Masala, 189
Pressure Cooker Lamb
  Meatballs, 241
Quick Pickles, 259
Quick Vanilla Latte, 52
Roasted Veggie Hummus
  Panini, 128
Salmon Tostada Salad, 167
Salted Chocolate–Coconut
  Macaroons, 284
Sassy BBQ Sauce, 257
Sheet Pan Sweet and Sour
  Chicken Rice Bowls, 179
Shrimp Pesto Pasta, 151
Skillet Garlic-Herb Steak, 231
S'mores Campfire Trail Mix, 281
Southwest Eggs Benedict on
  Sweet Potato Toast, 69
Spicy Shrimp Tacos, 150
Spinach-Walnut Pesto, 265
Spring Shrimp Rolls, 148–149
Strawberry–Goat
  Cheese Salad, 110
Strawberry-Jalapeño Salsa, 82
Strawberry Lemonade
  Slushie, 270
Strawberry Shortcake
  Mug Cake, 275
Sweet-and-Sour Eggplant, 123
Sweet-and-Sour Sauce, 262
Sweet 'n' Spicy Nuts
  and Seeds, 80
Sweet Potato Salmon
  Cakes, 165
Taco Cauliflower Pizza, 222
Taco Seasoning, 250
Thai Peanut Ramen, 127
Tzatziki, 261
Waldorf Chicken Salad, 175
Watermelon Gazpacho, 98
Tofu
  Chickpea Tofu Marsala, 132

Sesame Tofu and Brussels
Sprouts Bowl, 136–137
Tomatoes
Burger Bowls, 223
Caprese Chicken Burgers, 177
Cauliflower Curry, 126
Chicken Bruschetta Pasta, 190
Chicken Tortilla Soup, 109
Chili-Stuffed Peppers, 232
Chopped Caprese Salad, 114
Classic Minestrone, 106
Feta Lamb Burgers, 240
Green Chicken Enchiladas, 184
Homemade Marinara Sauce, 266
Lamb Gyros, 239
Loaded Avocado Toast, 65
Mediterranean Fish in
Parchment, 161
Mexican Street Corn Salad, 115
One-Pot Taco Pasta, 235
Piggy Nachos, 207
Pressure Cooker Chicken
Tikka Masala, 189
Quinoa Tabbouleh, 119
Roasted Red Pepper Soup and
Ricotta Cheeseballs, 105
Sassy BBQ Sauce, 257
Shrimp Pesto Pasta, 151
Skillet Peachy Chicken
Picante, 185
Southwest Eggs Benedict on
Sweet Potato Toast, 69
Spaghetti Squash Bolognese, 234
Spaghetti Squash Primavera, 140
Stuffed Pork Tenderloin, 215
Sweet Potato and Butternut
Squash Shepherd's
Pie, 236–237
Taco Cauliflower Pizza, 222
Watermelon Gazpacho, 98
Tools, 14–15
Tropical Pineapple Fruit
Leather, 271
Tropical White Fish Ceviche, 157
Tuna

Easy Apple-Tuna Salad, 169
Turmeric Rice, 93
Tzatziki, 261
in Greek Lamb Bowls with
Turmeric Cauliflower Rice and
Cucumber Salsa, 243–244
in Lamb Gyros, 239

V

Vegetable Risotto, 139
Vegetables, 8, 13. *See also specific*
Easy Broth, 253
High-Protein Egg Muffins, 62
Vegetarian
Air-Fryer Sweet Potato Tots, 94
Almond Butter, 252
Almond Butter Cookies, 279
Almond Butter Energy Bites, 86
Apple-Cranberry Slaw, 116
Apple Nachos, 272
Avocado-Cucumber-
Feta Salad, 111
Beet Burger, 129
Berry Berry Smoothie Bowl, 53
Black Cherry Sorbet, 274
Blueberry-Oat Pancakes, 58
Buffalo Cauliflower Bites, 90
Butternut Squash, Mushroom,
and Goat Cheese
Cauliflower Pizza, 144
Butternut Squash Mac
& Cheese, 143
Caramelized Onion and
Carrot Hummus, 84
Cauliflower Curry, 126
Cauliflower Pizza Crust, 267
Chickpea Buddha Bowls, 133
Chickpea Tofu Marsala, 132
Chili-Lime Popcorn, 76
Chili-Spiced Fruit Cups, 273
Chocolate Chip Cookie Dough
Overnight Oats, 57
Chocolate-Covered
Orange Slices, 282

Chocolate–Peanut Butter
Freezer Fudge, 287–288
Chopped Caprese Salad, 114
Cilantro-Lime Cauliflower Rice, 92
Cinnamon Apple Chips, 74
Cinnamon Toast Waffles, 59
Classic Minestrone, 106
Cookie Dough Dip, 85
Creamy Garlic Cauliflower
Soup, 101
Crispy Garlic-Rosemary
Potato Wedges, 77
Crunchy Chickpeas, 79
Dark Chocolate–Sea
Salt Popcorn, 280
Easy Guacamole, 83
Easy Homemade Falafel, 145
Easy Vanilla Ice Cream, 278
Everything Bagel–Seasoned
Hard-Boiled Eggs, 81
Five-Ingredient Veggie
Lasagna, 141
Freezer V-Egg-ie Burritos, 70–71
French Toast Overnight Oats, 55
Fruit-and-Nut Chocolate
Bark, 283
Garlic-Dijon Asparagus, 87
Garlic-Parmesan Roasted
Broccoli, 88
Ghee, 251
Gochujang, 258
Grape Leaf Pilaf, 138
Green Power Smoothie Bowl, 54
Green Shakshuka, 67
Harvest Kale Salad with Goat
Cheese and Dried
Cranberries, 118
High-Protein Egg Muffins, 62
High Protein Pressure Cooker
Mac & Cheese, 142
Homemade Cream of
Mushroom Soup, 102–103
Homemade Marinara Sauce, 266
Homemade Mayo, 254
Honey Mustard, 255

Vegetarian (continued)
Ketchup, 256
Lemon Lentil Soup, 107
Lemon Meringue Smoothie, 51
Loaded Avocado Toast, 65
Maple Vinaigrette, 260
Mashed Parmesan Cauliflower, 91
Mexican Street Corn Salad, 115
Mocha-Cheesecake
Brownies, 289
Mocha-Ricotta Mousse, 285
Orange-Balsamic Brussels
Sprouts, 89
Orange-Beet-Arugula
Salad, 113
Parmesan Crisps, 75
PB and J Protein Smoothie, 50
Peach Crumble, 277
Pesto-Baked Cauliflower
Steaks, 125
Poached Eggs, 248
Portobello Tacos, 122
Power Quinoa Bowl, 135
Pumpkin Spice Baked
Oatmeal Bars, 60
Quick Pickles, 259
Quick Vanilla Latte, 52
Quinoa Tabbouleh, 119
Raspberry-Lemon Bars, 276
Roasted Red Pepper Soup and
Ricotta Cheeseballs, 105
Roasted Veggie Hummus
Panini, 128
Salted Chocolate–Coconut
Macaroons, 284
Sassy BBQ Sauce, 257
Sesame Tofu and Brussels
Sprouts Bowl, 136–137
Sheet Pan Eggplant
Parmesan, 124
Simple French Onion Soup, 99
S'mores Campfire Trail Mix, 281
Southwest Eggs Benedict on
Sweet Potato Toast, 69
Spaghetti Squash, 249

Spaghetti Squash Primavera, 140
Spinach-Walnut Pesto, 265
Strawberry–Goat Cheese
Salad, 110
Strawberry-Jalapeño Salsa, 82
Strawberry Lemonade
Slushie, 270
Strawberry Shortcake
Mug Cake, 275
Strawberry Shortcake
Overnight Oats, 56
Sweet-and-Sour Eggplant, 123
Sweet-and-Sour Sauce, 262
Sweet 'n' Spicy Nuts
and Seeds, 80
Sweet Potato Crust Quiche, 68
Taco Seasoning, 250
Tex-Mex Veggie Burger, 130
Thai Peanut Ramen, 127
Tropical Pineapple Fruit
Leather, 271
Turmeric Rice, 93
Tzatziki, 261
Vegetable Risotto, 139
Vegetarian Black Bean
Enchiladas, 131
Watermelon Gazpacho, 98
Vegetarian Black Bean
Enchiladas, 131

W

Waffles, Cinnamon Toast, 59
Waldorf Chicken Salad, 175
Walnuts
Broccoli-Walnut Salad with
Dried Cherries, 117
Fruit-and-Nut Chocolate
Bark, 283
Orange-Beet-Arugula Salad, 113
Pumpkin Spice Baked
Oatmeal Bars, 60
Spinach-Walnut Pesto, 265
Sweet 'n' Spicy Nuts
and Seeds, 80

Tex-Mex Veggie Burger, 130
Waldorf Chicken Salad, 175
Water, 3–4, 45
Watermelon Gazpacho, 98
Wellness Plan, 29–36
Whole foods, 3
Whole grains, 9, 11

Y

Yogurt, Greek
Apple-Cranberry Slaw, 116
Berry Berry Smoothie
Bowl, 53
Blueberry-Oat Pancakes, 58
Chili-Stuffed Peppers, 232
Chocolate Chip Cookie Dough
Overnight Oats, 57
Cookie Dough Dip, 85
High-Protein Egg Muffins, 62
Lamb Kofta Kebabs, 238
Lemon Greek Chicken
Skewers, 173
Lemon Meringue Smoothie, 51
Loaded Baked Potatoes, 199
Mexican Street Corn Salad, 115
Pressure Cooker Butter
Chicken, 182
Tzatziki, 261
Waldorf Chicken Salad, 175

Z

Zucchini
Chicken Parmesan over
Zoodles, 192
Five-Ingredient Veggie
Lasagna, 141
Lemon Greek Chicken
Skewers, 173
Sheet Pan Sweet and Sour
Chicken Rice Bowls, 179
Shrimp Pesto Pasta, 151
Spinach Meatballs and
Zucchini Noodles, 233
Steak and Pepper Roll-Ups, 228

| About the Author |

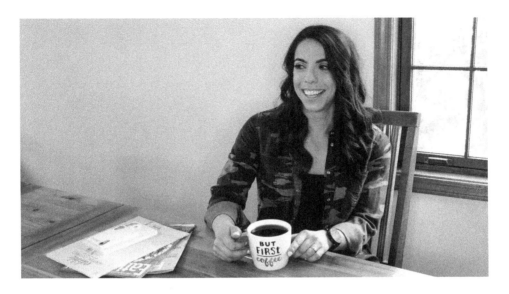

Laura Ligos, MBA, RDN, CSSD, is a sports dietitian and online real food blogger, educator, and nutrition expert. She received her bachelor of science degree in Nutrition Sciences from Cornell University. She went on to complete her dietetic internship and master of business administration at Dominican University. As a lifelong athlete, she knew her passion was in sports nutrition as well as teaching people how to cook and build a real food lifestyle. She educates people in her hometown as well as through her blog at thesassydietitian.com and on her Instagram account (@thesassydietitian). Laura is also a CrossFit Level 2 trainer at her local CrossFit gym where she loves coaching her athletes and helping them live an active life through movement and nutrition. She currently resides in Albany, NY, with her husband and her wheaten terrier pup, Bode, who you can see running through sprinklers daily on her Instagram account.

CPSIA information can be obtained
at www.ICGtesting.com
Printed in the USA
LVHW070456190122
708830LV00007B/254

9 781641 526068